Case Studies in Blood Disorders

Case Studies in Blood Disorders

Editor: Harper Lawrence

AMERICAN
MEDICAL PUBLISHERS
www.americanmedicalpublishers.com

AMERICAN
MEDICAL PUBLISHERS
www.americanmedicalpublishers.com

Cataloging-in-Publication Data

Case studies in blood disorders / edited by Harper Lawrence.
p. cm.
Includes bibliographical references and index.
ISBN 979-8-88740-592-6
1. Blood--Diseases. 2. Blood--Diseases--Genetic aspects. 3. Blood--Diseases--Pathophysiology.
4. Blood--Diseases--Treatment. 5. Hematology. I. Lawrence, Harper.
RC636 .D57 2023
616.15--dc23

American Medical Publishers,
41 Flatbush Avenue,
1st Floor, New York,
NY 11217, USA

ISBN 979-8-88740-592-6 (Hardback)

Contents

Preface

Blood disorders, also known as hematologic disorders, refer to a wide range of medical conditions that affect the components of blood or its ability to function properly. These disorders can involve abnormalities in white blood cells, red blood cells, platelets, or the plasma that carries them. A few of the common blood disorders are anemia, hemophilia, and various types of leukemia. Other examples include thrombocytopenia, which is a condition marked by low platelet counts, and sickle cell disease, a genetic disorder causing abnormal red blood cells. Prominent symptoms of these disorders are dizziness, rapid heartbeat and fatigue. Some of the treatments which are used for managing blood disorders are blood and platelet transfusions, corticosteroids, and anticoagulants. This book contains some path-breaking studies on blood disorders. It will serve as a valuable source of reference for graduate and postgraduate students.

The researches compiled throughout the book are authentic and of high quality, combining several disciplines and from very diverse regions from around the world. Drawing on the contributions of many researchers from diverse countries, the book's objective is to provide the readers with the latest achievements in the area of research. This book will surely be a source of knowledge to all interested and researching the field.

In the end, I would like to express my deep sense of gratitude to all the authors for meeting the set deadlines in completing and submitting their research chapters. I would also like to thank the publisher for the support offered to us throughout the course of the book. Finally, I extend my sincere thanks to my family for being a constant source of inspiration and encouragement.

Editor

1

Immune Thrombocytopenia following COVID-19 Vaccine

Sonal Prasad,[1] Roopam Jariwal,[2] Moujidin Adebayo,[2] Sara Jaka,[2] Greti Petersen,[2] and Everardo Cobos[2]

[1]*Ross University School of Medicine, Bridgetown, Barbados*
[2]*Department of Internal Medicine, UCLA at Kern Medical Center, Bakersfield, CA 93306, USA*

Correspondence should be addressed to Roopam Jariwal; roopamj27@gmail.com

Academic Editor: Pier Paolo Piccaluga

Several vaccines have been developed and are being administered against severe acute respiratory syndrome coronavirus 2 (SARS-CoV-2). Common side effects include fever, chills, headache, myalgia, and soreness at the injection site. However, some rare adverse effects have also been reported. We present a case of induced thrombocytopenia presenting with petechiae and mucosal bleeding which developed as an adverse response after first-dose administration of the Moderna COVID-19 vaccine.

1. Introduction

Immune thrombocytopenic purpura (ITP) is an acquired thrombocytopenia characterized by a platelet count less than 100×10^9/L caused by autoantibodies against platelet antigens leading to increased platelet destruction and decreased platelet production [1]. Many vaccines such as influenza, varicella, measles, mumps, and rubella are known to induce ITP [2]. More recently, cases of thrombocytopenia following COVID-19 vaccination have been reported since the initiation of mass vaccinations. Two different types of immune thrombocytopenia are being reported which include vaccine-induced immune thrombocytopenia (VIT) and vaccine-induced immune thrombotic thrombocytopenia (VITT). The messenger RNA (mRNA) vaccines against SARS-CoV-2 are the first of their kind with different mechanisms of action. Understanding of the clinical manifestations in response to vaccination, their pathogenesis, and subsequent treatment of related thrombocytopenia is still evolving.

2. Case

A 58-year-old Hispanic male with hypertension and diabetes presented to our hospital for acute onset of mucosal bleeding, petechiae, and easy bruising. He denied any previous history of spontaneous bleeding or easy bruising. Physical examination was notable for diffuse petechiae along the arms, legs, and abdomen along with numerous oral lesions and gingival bleeding (Figure 1). He was noted to have a platelet count of 3×10^9/L with all other cell lines within normal limits. In addition, the following labs were also within normal limits: prothrombin time, partial thromboplastin time, fibrinogen, d-dimer, bilirubin, lactate dehydrogenase, and haptoglobin. Coombs test to detect red blood cell antibodies was negative. Peripheral blood smear showed sparse platelets, no platelet clumping, and normal morphology of all other cells. Platelet antibodies were all negative. Viral studies for human immunodeficiency virus and hepatitis A, B, and C were all nonreactive. The antinuclear antibody test for autoimmune workup was negative. The platelet factor 4 antibody test was weakly positive, but the confirmatory serotonin-release assay was negative. Ultrasound of the abdomen showed hepatic steatosis and mild splenomegaly with the spleen measuring 12.6 cm in length. These tests were obtained to rule out disseminated intravascular coagulation, hemolytic uremic syndrome, thrombotic thrombocytopenic purpura, heparin-induced thrombocytopenia, and viral-induced thrombocytopenia. Further history taking elucidated that the patient had not had any recent upper respiratory infection or COVID-19 infection. COVID-19 test was negative. The patient had

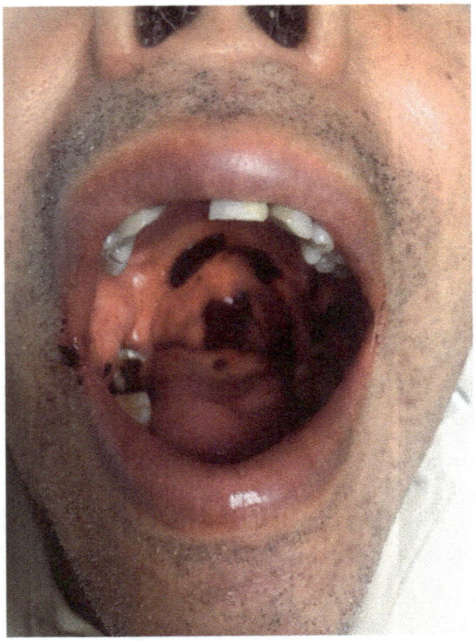

Figure 1: Significant gingival and oral mucosal bleeding.

received his first dose of the Moderna COVID-19 vaccine on April 28, 2021; three weeks prior to the development of spontaneous bleeding. After a comprehensive and exhaustive workup of all well-known precipitants of ITP returned negative, a diagnosis of idiopathic thrombocytopenic purpura was made.

We treated the patient with high-dose dexamethasone 40 mg/day for four days and transfused five units of platelets, but his platelet count continued to be refractory with counts of 7×10^9/L. He was then started on intravenous immunoglobulin (IVIG) 1 g/kg for two days. After two doses of IVIG, his platelet count improved to 39×10^9/L, with the resolution of his mucosal bleeding, and he was discharged home. Five days later, the patient re-presented to our hospital with recurrent gingival bleeding, this time with a platelet count of 7×10^9/L. He was transfused one unit of platelets, started on high-dose dexamethasone 40 mg/day for four days, and IVIG 1 g/kg for two days. Four days into admission, his platelet count improved to 41×10^9/L, and he was again discharged home. Patient was not discharged on a tapering regimen of steroid medication. Five days after his second hospital discharge, he presented for a third time once more with gingival bleeding with a platelet count $<3 \times 10^9$/L. This time, we treated the patient with three platelet transfusions, two doses of IVIG 1 g/kg, as well as romiplostim—a thrombopoietin receptor agonist (TPO-RA)—starting at 1 mcg/kg and increasing by 1 mcg weekly, and fostamatinib—an inhibitor of spleen tyrosine kinase (SYK)—100 mg twice daily. The patient received a total of two doses of romiplostim with improvement in the platelet count to 18×10^9/L and resolution of symptoms. He was then discharged home with fostamatinib 100 mg twice daily with a close follow-up in the hematology clinic. Ten days after hospital discharge, the patient's platelet count increased to 81×10^9/L with no recurrence in bleeding. His most recent platelet count is 109×10^9/L, and he is maintained on fostamatinib 100 mg twice daily. Patient refused to receive the second dose of the Moderna vaccine as well as any other vaccine type.

3. Discussion

With the widespread administration of COVID-19 vaccines to combat and curb the pandemic, adverse reactions have been reported including rare instances of thrombocytopenia and thrombosis. More specifically, there have been reported cases of both vaccine-induced immune thrombocytopenia (VIT) and vaccine-induced immune thrombotic thrombocytopenia (VITT). VITT presents within 4–30 days of vaccination with symptoms of thrombocytopenia and thrombosis including cerebral venous sinus thrombosis, splanchnic thrombosis [1], pulmonary embolism, and deep vein thrombosis. Significant laboratory findings in VITT include low fibrinogen, elevated d-dimer, and low platelets [3]. VIT has been noted to present with thrombocytopenia within 1–23 days with symptoms of bleeding, bruising, and petechiae [1]. Laboratory findings in VIT are only remarkable for severely low platelet count.

Clinical manifestations of VIT and VITT are similar to heparin-induced thrombocytopenia (HIT). In HIT, patients develop an antibody directed against endogenous platelet factor 4 (PF4) in complex with heparin, after exposure to heparin. This antibody activates platelets resulting in thrombosis. Recent reports show that patients with VIT and VITT secondary to Pfizer and Moderna COVID-19 vaccines have antibodies against PF4 on the enzyme-linked immunosorbent assay (ELISA) [4], a similar finding reported in HIT. Our patient presented with symptoms and laboratory findings concerning HIT, yet he had no prior exposure to heparin. As VIT rose amongst our differential diagnoses, we obtained an ELISA to see if there were antibodies against PF4. This test resulted as weakly positive. In HIT, a serotonin-release assay (SRA) can be used as a confirmatory test for antibodies against PF4—SRA performed on our patient's serum sample resulted negative. However, the confirmatory test does not seem to hold the same clinical significance in VIT and VITT as in HIT. Many cases report that only an ELISA test was performed, and no other confirmatory test was utilized to make the diagnosis of VIT/VITT. Although SRA is highly sensitive for HIT, one study showed evidence of patients with HIT who were SRA-negative [5]. Hence, SRA may not be needed to accurately make the diagnosis of VIT or VITT. However, as there are conflicting reports regarding the need for the confirmatory test, further investigation is required. In another article with positive cases of VITT, HIT, the ELISA was used to detect anti-PF4 antibodies and were positive; however, the rapid non-ELISA tests were negative. Hence, they recommend that it might be beneficial to repeat testing with a different ELISA method as they suggest that the antibodies present in these patients could have an epitope that is not recognized by the currently available assays [6].

There is confounding evidence whether VIT and VITT occur via the same mechanism or if they are the same reaction with a spectrum of manifestations. A review of the literature shows that VITT has been the predominantly reported thrombocytopenia in adenoviral vector-based vaccines such as AstraZeneca [1, 3, 4] and Johnson & Johnson [1], whereas VIT has mostly been reported in mRNA-based vaccines such as Pfizer and Moderna [4]. However, more research is needed to establish a correlation between the occurrence of VIT and VITT with the type of COVID-19 vaccine being administered.

Our patient received the Moderna vaccine and three weeks later presented with isolated thrombocytopenia which we ultimately diagnosed as VIT. We cannot be sure whether the patient had preexisting ITP but not by history, and there was no prior documentation. Of reported cases of VIT, most patients responded to treatment with corticosteroids and IVIG [7]. In one case report, a 22-year-old healthy male developed VIT after receiving the Pfizer vaccine and was treated with dexamethasone 40 mg/day for four days, a platelet transfusion, and IVIG 1 g/kg for two days which eventually led to resolution of the VIT [8]. Refractory cases of thrombocytopenia to both steroids and IVIG may benefit from a thrombopoietic agent. We treated our patient with multiple doses of steroids, IVIG, and platelet transfusions, yet his platelet count remained persistently low. The platelet count increased but declined soon afterwards. Due to his recurrent presentations and hospitalizations, we resorted to a combination of a TPO-RA—romiplostim—and a SYK inhibitor—fostamatinib. This drug combination was finally able to stabilize and increase our patient's platelet count. A case report published in the Journal of Blood Medicine utilized romiplostim alone as a second-line agent to success for VIT after steroids and IVIG were unsuccessful. With our review of the literature, the combination of TPO-RA and SYK inhibitors for treatment of refractory VIT has not been reported elsewhere. However, no specific algorithm has shown efficacy for treatment [6].

Our case is unique in that multiple treatment modalities were employed to increase platelet count with multiple rounds of steroids, platelet transfusions, and IVIG, despite which, our patient's platelet count remained low. Finally, treatment with TPO-RA and SYK inhibitors was able to stabilize his platelet count.

4. Conclusion

COVID-19 vaccine-induced ITP is a rare adverse effect that needs continued surveillance. Since the mechanism of COVID-19 VIT is unclear, it is worthwhile to further investigate the use of TPO-RA and SYK inhibitors as treatment options. Vaccination against SARS-CoV-2 is imperative to control the global pandemic, and clinicians need to be aware of and have a low index of suspicion on making the diagnosis of VIT or VITT. It is important to acknowledge that some patients may not respond to the standard accepted treatment with steroids and IVIG. Cases similar to ours may benefit from therapy with TPO-RA and the SYK inhibitor when first-line therapy with steroids and IVIG are unsuccessful.

Consent

Written informed consent was obtained from the patient for their anonymized information to be published in this article.

References

[1] K. J. Welsh, J. Baumblatt, W. Chege, R. Goud, and N. Nair, "Thrombocytopenia including immune thrombocytopenia after receipt of mRNA COVID-19 vaccines reported to the vaccine adverse event reporting system (VAERS)," *Vaccine*, vol. 39, no. 25, pp. 3329–3332, 2021.

[2] J. M. Helms, K. T. Ansteatt, J. C. Roberts et al., "Severe, refractory immune thrombocytopenia occurring after SARS-CoV-2 vaccine," *Journal of Blood Medicine*, vol. 12, pp. 221–224, 2021.

[3] M. Scully, D. Singh, R. Lown et al., "Pathologic antibodies to platelet factor 4 after ChAdOx1 nCoV-19 vaccination," *New England Journal of Medicine*, vol. 384, no. 23, pp. 2202–2211, 2021.

[4] D. B. Cines and J. B. Bussel, "SARS-CoV-2 vaccine-induced immune thrombotic thrombocytopenia," *New England Journal of Medicine*, vol. 384, no. 23, pp. 2254–2256, 2021.

[5] T. E. Warkentin, I. Nazy, J. I. Sheppard, J. W. Smith, J. G. Kelton, and D. M. Arnold, "Serotonin-release assay-negative heparin-induced thrombocytopenia," *American Journal of Hematology*, vol. 95, no. 1, pp. 38–47, 2020.

[6] S. Pavord, M. Scully, B. J. Hunt et al., "Clinical features of vaccine-induced immune thrombocytopenia and thrombosis," *New England Journal of Medicine*, vol. 385, no. 18, pp. 1680–1689, 2021.

[7] E. J. Lee, D. B. Cines, T. Gernsheimer et al., "Thrombocytopenia following Pfizer and Moderna SARS-CoV-2 vaccination," *American Journal of Hematology*, vol. 96, no. 5, pp. 534–537, 2021.

[8] O. Tarawneh and H. Tarawneh, "Immune thrombocytopenia in a 22-year-old post COVID-19 vaccine," *American Journal of Hematology*, vol. 96, no. 5, pp. E133–E134, 2021.

2

Long-Term Zidovudine Therapy and Whether it is a Trigger of Vitamin B12 Deficiency: A Case Study of Megaloblastic Anemia at the University of Zambia Teaching Hospital

Natasha Mupeta Kaweme, Sahar Mounir Nagib Butress, and Hamakwa Muluti Mantina

University Teaching Hospital, Private Bag RW1X Ridgeway, Nationalist Road, Lusaka 10101, Zambia

Correspondence should be addressed to Hamakwa Muluti Mantina; muluti70@gmail.com

Academic Editor: Gergely Feher

Macrocytic anemia is frequently observed in adult HIV-infected patients treated with nucleoside reverse transcriptase inhibitors and with vitamin B12 and folate deficiency. In this case report, we discuss a 52-year-old nonvegetarian male on long-term antiretroviral therapy for 5 years, presenting with severe macrocytic anemia (hemoglobin, 3.7 g/dL; mean corpuscular volume, 119.6 fL) and leukopenia ($2.71 * 10^9$/L), who was diagnosed with megaloblastic anemia caused by vitamin B12 deficiency following laboratory investigations. Parenteral vitamin B12 replacement therapy was initiated, with an early response observed. Notwithstanding, the treatment response was not sustained as the patient later presented with refractory anemia and persistence of macrocytosis. Discontinuation of zidovudine with concurrent vitamin B12 administration promptly improved the patient's clinical deficiency symptoms. At the end of 3 months, the patient had a complete hematological recovery. The deficiency of vitamin B12 disrupts DNA synthesis inhibiting effective hematopoiesis in all cell lines, particularly erythroid precursors and further promotes reversible bone marrow failure. Long-term ART therapy with zidovudine causes cytotoxicity in myeloid and erythroid precursors and induces bone marrow suppression. Whether long-term zidovudine consumption induced lower levels of vitamin B12 and subsequent megaloblastic anemia requires in-depth research and exploration.

1. Introduction

Anemia is a frequent hematological complication of human immunodeficiency virus (HIV) infection, and its incidence is adversely associated with advanced HIV disease, poor treatment outcomes, and increased risk of patient mortality [1, 2]. Although the causes of anemia in the general population are multifactorial in origin with various pathophysiological mechanisms, the most common etiology globally is iron deficiency, among other nutritional deficiencies such as folic acid and vitamin B12 [1]. In the setting of HIV infection, several factors, including chronic disease, the direct/indirect influence of HIV infection on hematopoietic stem/progenitor cells [3], altered cytokine milieu, opportunistic infections, and ART (antiretroviral therapy)-induced toxicity, result in impaired hematopoiesis and suppressed proliferation and differentiation of hematopoietic stem/progenitor cells, thus leading to cytopenias, anemia, thrombocytopenia, and neutropenia [4–6].

Although the burden of anemia among persons living with HIV in Zambia has not been fully established, a recent study by Cao et al. reported that the prevalence of anemia among adults living with HIV was higher in Southern Africa than that in East Africa. Furthermore, anemia in HIV infection was common among all groups in the population [2] and was higher in advanced HIV disease, among women, infants, and children in developing countries [7, 8]. Other factors, including socioeconomic factors, marital status, monthly income, and educational status, influence the severity of anemia among persons living with HIV [9].

Macrocytic anemia, defined as an increase in red blood cell mean corpuscular volume (MCV) of greater than 100 femtoliters (fL) in the setting of anemia, is a key observation in patients on long-term nucleoside reverse transcriptase inhibitors (NRTIs) [10, 11]. The exact mechanism by which NRTIs such as zidovudine led to macrocytosis in HIV-infected persons is yet to be explored. NRTIs interfere with mitochondrial DNA synthesis by inhibiting polymerases responsible for erythrocyte formation. Interference with mitochondrial DNA synthesis impairs the synthesis of erythroid precursors in the bone marrow (megaloblastic erythropoiesis) and consequently, macrocytosis [12–14]. Similarly, Reddy et al. hypothesized that zidovudine suppressed erythropoiesis and inhibited erythroid stem cells resulting in red cell aplasia, decreased reticulocyte counts and hemoglobin levels without hemolysis or blood loss [15], and increased MCV and erythropoietin levels [16]. A study conducted 3 decades ago highlighted that life-threatening hematological toxicity was probably attributed to transient depletion of mitochondrial DNA and sensitivity of DNA polymerase in some cell mitochondria [17].

At present, zidovudine and stavudine are less commonly used, as novel ART combinations with safer toxicity profiles have been introduced. In pediatric patients, zidovudine has been extensively used for treating HIV and preventing perinatal transmission of HIV in neonates [18]. However, the adverse mitochondrial toxicity of zidovudine favors the use of abacavir or tenofovir alafenamide. Zidovudine-induced bone marrow toxicity is common in patients with advanced disease and is related to early long-term high-dose therapy [19]. Generally, stavudine is associated with significant toxicity and increases the risk of macrocytosis, limiting its use in clinical practice [10].

According to the Zambia Consolidated HIV guidelines 2020 (currently in use), zidovudine-based regimens are the preferred second-line regimen for patients failing on tenofovir or abacavir-based regimens. A major concern for this arises from a recent study in Zambia that demonstrated high prevalence of HIV drug resistance, including thymidine analog mutations that confer resistance or reduced susceptibility to zidovudine, stavudine, and other NRTIs in adolescents and young adult patients [20].

This case study will discuss our experience with a patient who presented with macrocytic anemia associated with a history of long-term zidovudine consumption coupled with vitamin B12 deficiency and hypothesize the importance of a pragmatic approach to the diagnosis and management of macrocytic anemia in persons living with HIV to ensure the provision of quality health care in a resource-limited setting.

2. Case Presentation

A 52-year-old nonvegetarian male was referred to our hematology department with a one-month history of swelling of both lower limbs, progressive generalized body weakness, and severe anemia. He was diagnosed with HIV infection in 2010 and was on antiretroviral drugs for approximately 11 years at the time of presentation. The patient reported that his initial regimen was tenofovir/emtricitabine/efavirenz. He had no prior history of alcohol consumption and reported no HIV-related opportunistic infections during his course of treatment. His physical examination was significant for severe palmar and conjunctival pallor.

Initial laboratory results showed bicytopenia, hemoglobin 3.7 g/dL (reference range, 14.3–18.3), white cell count $2.71 * 10^9$/L (reference range, 4.00–10.00), and a normal platelet count of $301 * 10^9$/L (reference range, 150–400) with an elevated mean corpuscular volume (MCV) and mean cell hemoglobin (MCH) of 119.6 femtoliters (fL) (reference range, 79.1–98.9) and 40.2 picograms (pg) (reference range, 27.0–32.0), respectively. Peripheral blood differential counts were 55.3% neutrophils, 33.6% lymphocytes, 10.7% monocytes, 0.4% eosinophils, and no basophils. The peripheral blood smear showed anisopoikilocytosis, ovalomacrocytosis, and hypersegmented neutrophils. Serum vitamin B12 was 66.2 pg/ml (reference range, 211–946), and serum folate was 7.75 ng/ml (reference range 4.6–34).

A comprehensive metabolic panel, including kidney function tests, liver function tests, and a lipid panel, was within the normal range. Additional investigations such as stool for occult blood and echocardiogram/electrocardiogram showed no abnormalities. The patient had a complete viral suppression (target not detected) with an absolute CD4 count of 451 cells/μL (reference range, 410–1590).The laboratory test results indicating a significant deficiency of vitamin B12 (66.2 pg/ml) and peripheral blood smear findings of hypersegmented neutrophils and oval macrocytes led the team to the diagnosis of megaloblastic anemia.

The patient received 4 units of packed cells while admitted, and parenteral vitamin B12 at 1000 mcg daily was initiated. At subsequent clinic visits, recovery of blood cell counts with normalization of MCV and MCH parameters was noted. The serum intrinsic factor antibody test result was equivocal. Despite this, maintenance of vitamin B12 at weekly and then monthly dosing was continued.

Two months after initiation of vitamin B12, the patient presented to our outpatient clinic with a complaint of generalized body weakness and heart palpitations with severe conjunctival pallor and tachycardia on examination. A complete blood count showed severe anemia with hemoglobin 3.6 g/dl, white cell count $2.41 * 10^9$/l, MCV 114.1 fL, MCH 36.4 pg, and a normal platelet count. Peripheral blood smear findings were consistent with the initial report but showed significant numbers of round macrocytes, occasional oval macrocytes, and hypersegmented neutrophils. The patient's laboratory workup is summarized in Table 1.

After a detailed review of the patient's drug history, it was found that his antiretroviral medication was changed to an AZT-based regimen (zidovudine/lamivudine/efavirenz) in 2017 for unknown reasons. We decided to admit the patient for packed cell transfusion, and a consult was sent to the infectious disease unit to revise the treatment regimen. Following transfusion, the patient was discharged on vitamin B12, folic acid, and a dolutegravir-based regimen (tenofovir disoproxil fumarate/lamivudine/dolutegravir) based on the current WHO recommendations for first-line and second-line antiretroviral regimens. The patient was closely followed up in the outpatient department and experienced complete recovery of hemoglobin, red cell count, MCV, and MCH count with an improving absolute

Table 1: Laboratory results at initial diagnosis and at follow-up visits.

Laboratory parameters	Reference range	Initial laboratory results	Laboratory results over time following parenteral B12 supplementation			
			Post transfusion and B12 initiation	2 months post B12 supplementation	21 days post AZT discontinuation	3 months post AZT discontinuation
Hemoglobin (g/dL)	14.3–18.3	3.7	8.6	3.6	10.4	14.9
Red cell count (*10^{12}/L)	4.50–5.50	0.92	2.50	0.99	3.22	5.13
White cell count (*10^9/L)	4.00–10.00	2.71	2.58	2.41	2.61	3.56
Platelet count (*10^9/L)	150–400	301	320	281	188	200
Differential count (%)						
Neutrophils	40–70%	55.3%	51.9%	45.7%	36.3%	27.1%
Lymphocytes	20–40%	33.6%	36.4%	40.2%	52.5%	59.0%
Monocytes	2–10%	10.7%	9.7%	13.7%	7.7%	9.6
Eosinophils	0.04–0.4%	0.4%	1.6%	0.4%	3.1%	3.7
Basophils	0.02–0.2%	0.0%	0.4%	0.0%	0.4%	0.6%
MCV (fL)	79.1–98.9	119.6	98.8	114.1	103.4	87.3
MCH (pg)	27.0–32.0	40.2	34.4	35.4	32.3	29.0
Absolute neutrophil count (*10^9/L)	2.00–7.00	1.50	1.34	1.10	0.95	0.96
Urea (mmol/L)	2.80–7.10	4.12	—	—	—	4.83
Creatinine (μmol/L)	59.0–104.0	58.3	—	62.4	—	89.6
Total bilirubin (mmol/L)	2.0–21.0	32.3	—	—	—	6.2
ALT (U/L)	0.0–45.0	20.0	—	17.1	—	8.2
AST U/L)	0.0–35.0	24.2	—	—	—	31.4
Lactate dehydrogenase (IU/L)	135–247	176	—	—	—	—

neutrophil count within 3 months. At present, the patient reports good physical health with stable blood counts.

3. Discussion

Macrocytic anemia is broadly classified as [1] megaloblastic associated with vitamin B12 and folate deficiency and [2] the nonmegaloblastic moiety associated with chronic alcoholism, liver disease, hypothyroidism, hereditary spherocytosis, and states of increased red cell consumption such as hemolysis or high turnover in pregnancy [21]. The most common cause of megaloblastic anemia is vitamin B12 deficiency caused by malabsorption due to the absence of intrinsic factors caused by pernicious anemia or following gastric surgery, transcobalamin II deficiency, duodenal and colonic inflammatory damage from celiac disease, or infection with the tapeworm *Diphyllobothrium latum*, and insufficient dietary intake. Common drugs such as phenytoin, trimethoprim, valproic acid, hydroxyurea, methotrexate, azathioprine, zidovudine, and other antiretroviral drugs can also cause macrocytic anemia [22].

Early identification and prompt treatment of vitamin B12 deficiency, a reversible and treatable cause of ineffective hematopoiesis, can significantly improve the survival outcomes of persons living with HIV. Our patient experienced refractory anemia and mild leukopenia despite continued treatment with parenteral vitamin B12 with no concern for other nutritional factors, opportunistic infections, or progression of HIV disease. At the initial diagnosis and confirmation of vitamin B12 deficiency and megaloblastic anemia, the patient showed an early response to vitamin B12 supplements; however, this early response was not sustained. We hypothesized that the relapse of megaloblastic anemia was probably associated with significantly low vitamin B12 levels, higher MCV levels, and the persistence of mitochondrial toxicity or the presence of mitochondrial DNA mutations induced by zidovudine which might elicit more severe mitochondrial dysfunction [21].

Although the patient's folate level of 7.75 ng/ml (reference range 4.6–34) was within the normal range (lower limit of normal), concern for 'masked' folate deficiency after initiation of vitamin B12 was speculated. Vitamin B12 deficient cells are unable to utilize folate, and only upon treatment with vitamin B12, folate can be utilized. As a result, underlying folate deficiency can manifest with a significant decrease in folate levels of less than 2 ng/ml. Concurrent administration of folate with vitamin B12 will avert a suboptimal response of anemia to vitamin B12 alone. Measurement of red cell folate assay, serum methylmalonic acid, and homocysteine levels could have confirmed the likelihood of folate deficiency or combined nutritional deficiency. However, the tests were not performed due to financial constraints. In vitamin B12 deficiency, both metabolites increase proportionally to the severity of deficiency, whereas in pure folate deficiency, only homocysteine levels are elevated and methylmalonic acid is normal [23].

Desk review has not revealed any study that has explored the possibility of an association between zidovudine therapy and lower levels of vitamin B12 and folate and its impact on hematopoiesis and erythropoiesis. Notwithstanding, Puspasari et al. hypothesized that interference of mitochondrial DNA synthesis induced by zidovudine resulted in hematological interference in the form of reduced vitamin B12 and folate levels in blood which in turn, led to megaloblastic anemia and oral lesions [24, 25].

Cotrimoxazole prophylaxis is commonly used in Zambia for the prevention of pneumocystis jirovecii pneumonia, isosporiasis, toxoplasmosis, malaria, and other HIV-related and non-HIV-related diseases. It is initiated in adult patients with a CD4 count of less than 350 cells/μL or having stage II, III, or IV disease according to the WHO clinical staging and discontinued when the CD4 count is greater than or equal to 350 cells/μL for two consecutive values at least 6 months apart while on ART (Zambia Consolidated Guidelines for Treatment and Prevention of HIV Infection, 2020). Trimethoprim is considered a weak inhibitor of dihydrofolate reductase that can interfere with folic acid metabolism and promote megaloblastic changes at high doses [7]. In this case study, the patient reported no history of cotrimoxazole consumption; therefore, it was excluded as a possible cause of megaloblastic anemia.

Neutropenia is a common concomitant feature in megaloblastic anemia. Vitamin B12 and folate deficiency interferes with effective hematopoiesis and induces bone marrow suppression [26], decreased myeloid production, and adverse neutropenia which increases the risk of infection. Other etiologies, including bacterial and viral infections, immunodeficiency and underlying chronic disease, are commonly associated with leukopenia and neutropenia. In patients with infection due to neutropenia, underlying vitamin B12 deficiency may exacerbate the susceptibility to cytopenias [27].

Our patient had chronic but asymptomatic neutropenia, persisting for over three months. Notwithstanding, a gradual improvement in the total white cell count was observed with vitamin B12 treatment and zidovudine discontinuation. We hypothesized that the presence of chronic neutropenia could have been a result of prolonged or advanced vitamin deficiency in underlying HIV infection, although the patient had complete viral suppression. About 4 decades ago, Kaplan and Basford hypothesized that megaloblastic anemia of vitamin B12 and folate deficiency was associated with morphological and quantitative abnormalities in developing leucocytes, resulting in reduced leucocyte numbers with nuclei hypersegmentation [28].

Appropriate treatment of vitamin B12 deficiency provides rapid resolution of clinical deficiency symptoms and prompt hematological recovery. Our patient's biological markers reached normal values or improved within 3 months of zidovudine discontinuation and vitamin B12 supplementation. Furthermore, the patient had no clinical features consistent with deficiency. Initial response to vitamin B12 can be determined by reticulocytosis occurring within a week after starting treatment. Complete hematological recovery and normalization of MCV are estimated to be between 2 and 8 weeks [29]. The persistence of macrocytosis is not affected by the duration of zidovudine therapy. Yu et al. showed that a higher MCV took longer to normalize, with a percentage of patients having persistent macrocytosis 2 years after zidovudine cessation [21].

The treatment and follow-up of patients on antiretroviral drugs require a multidisciplinary approach, including ART specialists, hematologists, nutritionists, and pharmacologists, to ensure early identification of drug-induced macrocytosis and prompt intervention. Early nutritional intervention can ensure optimal nutrition and health status in persons receiving ART. Rezaei et al. suggested that combined administration of vitamin B12 and folate supplements had a beneficial effect on the hematological status of HIV-infected persons receiving HAART [30]. An urgent revision of first-line and second-line therapies to include novel integrase inhibitors such as dolutegravir, also currently available in resource-limited settings, can reduce the incidence of zidovudine-related macrocytic anemia. Zidovudine is avoided in patients with low hemoglobin levels due to its additive effect on anemia and myelotoxicity. Monthly monitoring of hemoglobin levels after switching and re-initiating ART drugs for three months should be mandatory.

Among the significant limitations in the management of our patient were the inability to measure serum methylmalonic acid and homocysteine levels to increase the sensitivity and precision of the diagnosis of vitamin B12, folate, or combined deficiency. These metabolites are useful markers when the clinical picture is equivocal. Second, a reticulocyte count was not possible, given the unavailability of methylene blue stain. Reticulocytopenia suggests vitamin B12 deficiency in megaloblastic anemia. The seminal limitation was the inability to assess vitamin B12 and folate serum levels following treatment to monitor response. The recent literature has revealed that monitoring vitamin B12 is not necessary for patients receiving replacement therapy.

4. Conclusion

Macrocytic anemia is frequently observed in HIV patients on long-term nucleoside reverse transcriptase inhibitors such as zidovudine. In this case study, we have discussed the history, presentation, and laboratory workup of a patient with refractory anemia and elevated mean corpuscular volume and mean corpuscular hemoglobin on long-term zidovudine therapy coupled with vitamin B12 deficiency, thus supporting a diagnosis of megaloblastic anemia. It may be possible that increased zidovudine toxicity was exacerbated by vitamin B12 deficiency, as each is associated with bone marrow suppression. Discontinuation of zidovudine and treatment with parenteral vitamin B12 resulted in a rapid resolution of the patient's clinical deficiency symptoms.

It is evident that anemia is prevalent among people living with HIV infection, and therefore, more attention is required for a tailored, safer choice of ART regimens to minimize drug-related hematological toxicities. It is highly recommended that older treatment regimens be discarded in preference for safer novel regimens that have demonstrated improved survival outcomes while minimizing adverse events. Accordingly, we propose a detailed study that will explore the link between long-term zidovudine therapy and lower levels of vitamin B12 and folate.

Abbreviations

ART: Antiretroviral therapy
DNA: Deoxyribonucleic acid
HAART: Highly active antiretroviral therapy
MCH: Mean corpuscular hemoglobin
MCV: Mean corpuscular volume
HIV: Human immunodeficiency virus
NRTIs: Nucleoside reverse transcriptase inhibitors.

Authors' Contributions

NMK performed literature research and wrote the final manuscript. SMNB devised the study and conducted a critical review of the manuscript. HMM conceived and revised the final manuscript. All authors read and approved the final manuscript.

Acknowledgments

The authors thank the entire hematology department for their continued support and Mr. Elemson Muyanga for his dedicated assistance in editing the final manuscript.

References

[1] K. W. Zerihun, G. A. Bikis, and E. A. Muhammad, "Prevalence and associated factors of anemia among adult human immune deficiency virus positive patients on anti-retroviral therapy at Debre Tabor hospital, Northwest Ethiopia," *BMC Research Notes*, vol. 12, no. 1, p. 168, 2019.

[2] G. Cao, Y. Wang, Y. Wu, W. Jing, J. Liu, and M. Liu, "Prevalence of anemia among people living with HIV: a systematic review and meta-analysis," *eClinicalMedicine*, vol. 44, Article ID 101283, 2022.

[3] T. Tsukamoto, S. Gorantla, and V. Rodrigues, "Editorial: direct and indirect interactions of HIV with host cells," *Frontiers in Cellular and Infection Microbiology*, vol. 11, Article ID 771370, 2021.

[4] T. A. Ageru, M. M. Koyra, K. D. Gidebo, and T. L. Abiso, "Anemia and its associated factors among adult people living with human immunodeficiency virus at Wolaita Sodo University teaching referral hospital," *PLoS One*, vol. 14, no. 10, Article ID e0221853, 2019.

[5] C. Durandt, J. C. Potgieter, J. Mellet et al., "HIV and haematopoiesis," *South African Medical Journal*, vol. 109, pp. 40–45, 2019.

[6] A. Marchionatti and M. M. Parisi, "Anemia and thrombocytopenia in people living with HIV/AIDS: a narrative literature review," *International Health*, vol. 13, no. 2, pp. 98–109, 2021.

[7] Y. Berhane, D. Haile, and T. Tolessa, "Anemia in HIV/aids patients on antiretroviral treatment at ayder specialized hospital, mekele, Ethiopia: a case-control study," *Journal of Blood Medicine*, vol. 11, pp. 379–387, 2020.

[8] A. I. Abioye, C. T. Andersen, C. R. Sudfeld, and W. W. Fawzi, "Anemia, iron status, and HIV: a systematic review of the evidence," *Advances in Nutrition*, vol. 11, no. 5, pp. 1334–1363, 2020.

[9] K. B. Gebremedhin and T. B. Haye, "Factors associated with anemia among people living with HIV/AIDS taking ART in Ethiopia," *Advances in Hematology*, vol. 2019, Article ID 9614205, 8 pages, 2019.

[10] D. Genn é, P. Sudre, D. Anwar, C. Saa ï, and B. Hirschel, "Causes of macrocytosis in HIV-infected patients not treated with zidovudine," *Journal of Infection*, vol. 40, no. 2, pp. 160–163, 2000.

[11] C. A. Moore and A. Adil, *Macrocytic Anemia*, StatPearlsPublishing, Treasure Island, FL, USA, 2021.

[12] D. Pertiwi, Suradi, T. I. Winarni, and A. N. Probandari, "The length of AZT consumption and homocysteine levels are protective factors of macrocytic anemia among adult HIV-infected patients: a case-control study in central java province, Indonesia," *Bangladesh Journal of Medical Science*, vol. 19, no. 4, pp. 638–645, 2020.

[13] F. Romanelli, K. Empey, and C. Pomeroy, "Macrocytosis as an indicator of medication (zidovudine) adherence in patients with HIV infection," *AIDS Patient Care and STDs*, vol. 16, no. 9, pp. 405–411, 2002.

[14] W. D. Kufel, "Nucleoside reverse transcriptase inhibitor (NRTI) associated macrocytosis," *International Journal of Virology AIDS*, vol. 3, no. 1, 2016.

[15] D. M. Y. Reddy, A. Lokesh, V. Sivaranjani, S. V. Lakshmi, and M. V. Subbaiah, "Zidovudine induced hematological disorders and hyperpigmentation," *World Journal of Pharmacy and Pharmaceutical Sciences*, vol. 6, no. 10, pp. 1284–1290, 2017.

[16] J. Prashant, S. Amit, S. Mumtaz, and S. Ashok, "Zidovudine-induced anemia in HIV/AIDS," *New Indian Journal of Pediatrics*, vol. 5, no. 1, pp. 47–49, 2016.

[17] R. Yarchoan, K. Weinhold, H. K. Lyerly et al., "Administration of 3'-AZIDO-3'-DEOXYTHYMIDINE, an inhibitor of htlv-III/lav replication, to patients with aids or aids-related complex," *The Lancet*, vol. 327, no. 8481, pp. 575–580, 1986.

[18] "Antiretroviral medication zidovudine (ZDV, retrovir) | NIH," https://clinicalinfo.hiv.gov/en/guidelines.

[19] Z. Getaneh, W. Wale, B. Chanie et al., "Magnitude and associated factors of anemia among AZT based HAART experienced adult HIV patients at University of Gondar comprehensive specialized referral hospital, Northwest, Ethiopia, 2019: a retrospective cohort study," *BMC Infectious Diseases*, vol. 21, no. 1, p. 1016, 2021.

[20] S. Miti, R. Handema, L. Mulenga et al., "Prevalence and characteristics of HIV drug resistance among antiretroviral treatment (ART) experienced adolescents and young adults living with HIV in Ndola, Zambia," *PLoS One*, vol. 15, no. 8, Article ID e0236156, 2020.

[21] I. Yu, R. N. Greenberg, T. N. Crawford, A. C. Thornton, and T. Myint, "Persistence of macrocytosis after discontinuation of zidovudine in HIV-infected patients," *Journal of the International Association of Physicians in AIDS Care*, vol. 16, no. 5, pp. 512–515, 2017.

[22] Y. H. Wu, M. J. Hwang, Y. P. Lee, and C. P. Chiang, "Atrophic glossitis in pernicious anemia patients can be treated to normal in two weeks by intramuscular injection of vitamin B12," *Journal of Dental Science*, vol. 15, no. 4, pp. 558-559, 2020.

[23] S. P. Stabler and A. C. Antony, *Megaloblastic Anemia*, Cancer Therapy Advisor, New York, NJ, USA, 2019.

[24] D. Puspasari, D. M. D. Herawati, and I. Sufiawati, "Association between serum B12 and folate levels and manifestations of oral lesions in HIV adult patients," *Malaysian Journal of Nutrition*, vol. 24, no. 4, pp. 507–513, 2018.

[25] C. H. Shiboski, H. Chen, R. Secours et al., "High accuracy of common HIV-related oral disease diagnoses by non-oral health specialists in the AIDS clinical trial group," *PLoS One*, vol. 10, no. 7, Article ID e0131001, 2015.

[26] D. Rs and K. Majmundar, "B12 deficiency as a cause of neutropenic sepsis," *Annals of Hematology and Oncology*, vol. 4, no. 11, p. 1181, 2017.

[27] H. Sarbay, "Investigation of the incidence of vitamin B12 deficiency in leukopenia and neutropenia secondary to infection," *International Journal of Contemporary Pediatrics*, vol. 7, no. 1, pp. 42–45, 2019.

[28] S. S. Kaplan and R. E. Basford, "Effect of vitamin B12 and folic acid deficiencies on neutrophil function," *Blood*, vol. 47, no. 5, pp. 801–805, 1976.

[29] R. Carmel, "How i treat cobalamin (vitamin B12) deficiency," *Blood*, vol. 112, no. 6, pp. 2214–2221, 2008.

[30] E. Rezaei, H. Sedigh Ebrahim-Saraie, H. Heidari et al., "Impact of vitamin supplements on HAART related hematological abnormalities in HIV-infected patients," *Medical Journal of the Islamic Republic of Iran*, vol. 30, p. 350, 2016.

3

Disseminated *Mycobacterium tuberculosis*: An Unusual Presentation with Associated Hemophagocytic Lymphohistiocytosis

Ahmed Arfa, Nivin Omar, Kulsum Bano, and Natasha M. Savage

Department of Pathology, Medical College of Georgia at Augusta University, Augusta, Georgia

Correspondence should be addressed to Natasha M. Savage; nsavage@augusta.edu

Academic Editor: Tomas Jose Gonzalez-Lopez

Hemophagocytic lymphohistiocytosis (HLH) is a rare, potentially fatal, and systemic hyperinflammatory syndrome with exacerbated and uncontrolled activation of histiocytes and lymphocytes against mature cells. Secondary HLH can occur in association with a myriad of underlying infections or malignancies. Our patient is a 38-year-old male prisoner with poorly controlled diabetes and no known other medical conditions. He was referred to our emergency department with three-week history of worsening malaise, weight loss, fever, bruising, and shortness of breath; imaging showed pneumomediastinum, lung nodule, and adrenal mass. Biopsy of the lung nodule revealed acid-fast bacilli. Furthermore, bone marrow biopsy showed foci of necrosis with associated acid-fast bacilli and hemophagocytosis highlighted by CD163 stain; consequently, secondary HLH was suggested. Hence, lab results were reviewed and found to satisfy five of the eight secondary HLH criteria. Moreover, ferritin was >10,000 ng/ml, which has been suggested to be highly suspicious for HLH. The patient was started on anti-MAC therapy. Unfortunately, the patient's status declined rapidly; he developed multi-organ failure and succumbed to disease. Later, his culture confirmed *Mycobacterium tuberculosis*. In conclusion, we presented a rare and challenging case of secondary HLH associated with disseminated *Mycobacterium tuberculosis*. A high index of suspicion is required for early diagnosis and treatment, and pathologists should be aware of *Mycobacterium tuberculosis*' association with secondary HLH.

1. Introduction

Hemophagocytic lymphohistiocytosis (HLH) is a systemic, hyperinflammatory syndrome with uncontrolled activation of histiocytes and lymphocytes against mature cells and their hematopoietic precursors within the reticuloendothelial system [1]. Additionally, there is cytokine overproduction, and consequently, hypercytokinemia (so called "cytokine storm") can cause end-organ failure and death. It can be misdiagnosed as sepsis, among other entities, given significant clinical and laboratory overlap [2]. HLH is classified into two forms, primary or familial, which is due to a variety of genetic defects, and secondary or acquired, which is associated with a myriad of causes including infections, malignancies, and autoimmune diseases [3]. Although HLH secondary to infection is predominantly viral in origin, especially Epstein–Barr virus (EBV), bacteria such as mycobacteria, fungi, and protozoa can trigger secondary HLH as well [4]. *Mycobacterium tuberculosis* (MTB) has diverse clinical presentations and complications; thus, it can be a great challenge for clinicians to diagnose. It is rarely complicated by HLH [1, 5]. Furthermore, spontaneous pneumomediastinum is a rare presentation of MTB [6]. Despite this, our patient presented with spontaneous pneumomediastinum and developed secondary HLH. Tuberculosis-associated HLH (TB-HLH) has high mortality rate [1, 5], and a high index of suspicion is required by pathologists and clinicians alike to start prompt treatment with anti-tuberculous therapy (ATT) [7]. We report an unusual presentation of disseminated MTB associated with secondary HLH in a patient with uncontrolled diabetes mellitus.

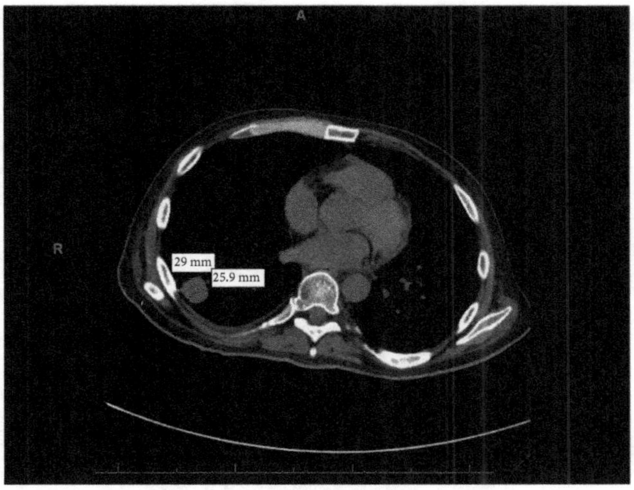

Figure 1: CT chest imaging showing increase in size of right lower lobe lung nodule.

2. Case Description

A 38-year-old incarcerated male patient with a medical history of newly diagnosed type 2 diabetes mellitus and tobacco abuse was transferred to our inpatient facility for further evaluation of spontaneous pneumomediastinum. Three weeks prior to presentation, the patient noted increasing fatigue, shortness of breath on exertion, weight loss, and rash. On day of hospital admission, he was found to have mild splenomegaly and petechial rash involving the abdominal wall and lower extremities, with no other pertinent positive findings on physical examination. He underwent computerized tomography (CT) scans of chest, abdomen, and pelvis at an outside facility, which revealed a right lower lobe lung nodule, left adrenal mass, and small pneumomediastinum.

Initial laboratory examination revealed normocytic anemia, hemoglobin of 8 g/dL, white blood cell (WBC) count of 9,300/mm^3, platelet count of 76,000/mm^3, absolute reticulocyte count of 1.7, fibrinogen of 321 mg/dL, prothrombin time /international normalized ratio (PT/INR) of 11.0 seconds/1.0, activated partial thromboplastin time (aPPT) of 26.3 seconds, lactate dehydrogenase (LDH) of 1138 U/L, haptoglobin <30 mg/dL, ferritin of 10,398 ng/mL, iron saturation of 68%, total iron binding capacity of 137 mcg/dL, total bilirubin of 0.7 mg/dL, aspartate aminotransferase (AST) of 66 U/L, alanine aminotransferase (ALT) of 57 U/L, and creatinine of 0.54 mg/dL. Bronchoscopy on hospital day 2 ruled out airway trauma as a cause for pneumomediastinum. Repeat CT imaging showed increase in size of right lower lobe lung nodule and stable size of left adrenal nodule (Figure 1).

Differential diagnosis based on initial presentation included primary lung malignancy metastatic to adrenal gland versus malignancy of unknown primary versus infectious process. Differential diagnosis for cytopenia included anemia of chronic disease secondary to presumed malignancy, marrow infiltration secondary to metastatic disease or other marrow infiltrative process, and/or HLH related to malignancy or infection. On day 7 of admission, patient underwent CT guided biopsy of the right lower lobe lung nodule, which revealed numerous acid-fast bacilli (AFB), without evidence of malignancy. A bone marrow biopsy performed on day 14 revealed prominent increase in macrophages with hemophagocytosis within aspirate smears (Figure 2(a)). The bone marrow biopsy showed small areas of necrosis (Figure 2(b)). CD163 stain further highlighted the hemophagocytosis (Figure 2(c)). Acid-fast microorganisms were noted on FITE stain (Figure 2(d)). The H Score [8] was utilized, and a score of 195 was obtained, indicating an 80–88% probability of HLH. Hence, a preliminary diagnosis of disseminated mycobacterial infection with secondary HLH was made. Initial suspicion was for *Mycobacterium avium* complex (MAC), and the patient was initiated on empiric anti-MAC therapy with amikacin, rifampin, ethambutol, and azithromycin. Unfortunately, before HLH directed therapy could be initiated, the patient had clinical deterioration with multiorgan failure (acute liver and renal failure), disseminated intravascular coagulation, and acute hypoxic respiratory failure requiring mechanical ventilation. The patient's clinical condition continued to rapidly deteriorate, and he subsequently expired on day 18. Posthumously, we received results of AFB cultures from bronchoalveolar lavage indicating MTB infection.

3. Discussion

HLH is a life threating disorder first described in 1952 as "familial hemophagocytic reticulosis." It is associated with hyperinflammatory syndrome and cytokine storm as a result of uncontrolled, exacerbated Th_1-cell and macrophage activation with diminished ability of cytotoxic T-cells and natural killer (NK) cells clearing up the target antigen. This results in ineffective inflammatory response and uncontrolled histiocytic phagocytosis of blood trilinear precursors and the mature blood elements in bone marrow. There are two forms of the disease: primary form also referred to as familial HLH and secondary or acquired HLH [1]. The primary autosomal recessive form has an incidence rate of 1 : 50,000 live births. The median survival rate is less than two months after diagnosis if left untreated [9]. It typically presents during infancy or early childhood, and it may be triggered by infections [10]. Secondary HLH can occur secondary to many underlying diseases including lymphoma (anaplastic large cell lymphoma, NK/T-cell lymphoma nasal type, Hodgkin lymphoma, and so on), infection (EBV, cytomegalovirus, herpes simplex viruses, adenovirus, and so on), autoimmune disease (lupus, systemic idiopathic juvenile arthritis, and so on), post-allogeneic stem cell transplant (immunologic reaction at engraftment), or medication-related hypersensitivity (carbamazepine, phenobarbital, sulfamethoxazole, and so on).

In secondary HLH, it is important to identify the underlying cause as the prognosis varies greatly based at least in part by different underlying conditions. Although infection-related HLH is predominantly viral in origin, especially EBV, bacteria such as mycobacteria, fungi, and protozoa can

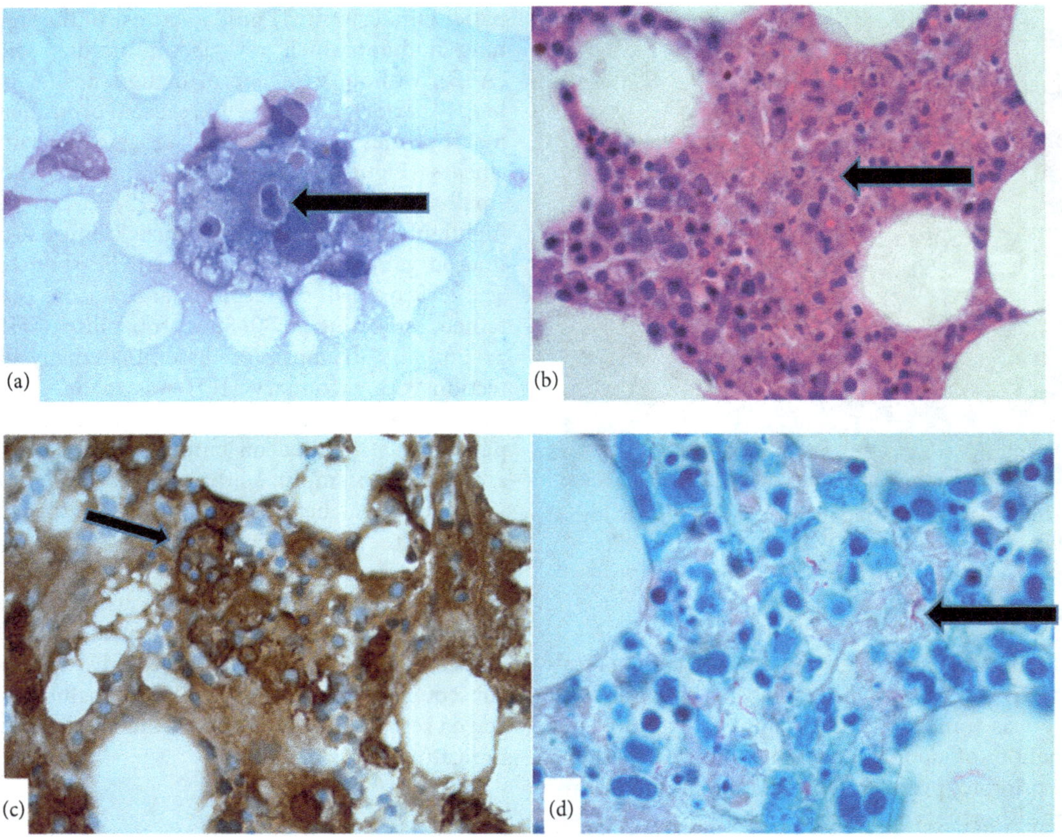

FIGURE 2: 40x magnification. (a) Bone marrow aspirate smear showing histiocyte with hemophagocytosis. (b) Bone marrow biopsy H&E stain showing foci of necrosis by normal bone marrow. (c) CD163 stain showing histiocyte engulfing other hematopoietic cell (rosette appearance). (d) FITE stain showing acid-fast bacilli.

trigger secondary HLH as well [4, 11]. TB-HLH was first reported in 1980s [8]. MTB is an obligate intracellular pathogen that induces TH1-mediated cytotoxicity with activation of NK-cells and macrophages resulting in the release of chemokines and cytokines including TNF-α, IFN-γ, IL-1, IL-6, IL-18, and GM-CSF, thus resulting in a cytokine storm [1]. In Per Tseng et. al's study 23% of all infection induced HLH was related to MTB. It was also associated with longer duration of symptoms and a higher mortality rate [5]. This was reflected in our patient's case, as our patient died as a result of TB-HLH.

Most TB-HLH patients present with a fever of unknown origin (FOU), hepatosplenomegaly, and cytopenias [12]. However, to the best of our knowledge, this is the first reported TB-HLH case to present with spontaneous pneumothorax. Our patient had multiple risk factors contributing to the development of TB including a history of type 2 diabetes and incarceration.

TB-HLH has a varied course, with an overall high mortality. Given the rarity of the condition and typical delays in diagnosis, patients with TB-associated HLH tend to have poorer outcomes, with reported mortality ranging from 50% [13] to 100% [1] without treatment. Padhi et al. reported that based on a literature review performed from January 1975 to March 2014, there was 63 cases of TB-HLH with a reported fatality rate of 49% (31 of the 63 patients studied) [1].

Bhattacharyya et al. reported that there may be a delay in diagnosis of HLH for multiple reasons including concordant liver failure and coagulopathy. In our case, our patient developed liver dysfunction and coagulopathy, which may have obscured/delayed the TB-HLH diagnosis [5]. Moreover, there is significant clinical overlap between HLH and septic shock, thus further complicating diagnosis; however, HLH can be diagnosed if there is a mutation in a known causative gene (primary/familial) or if at least five of eight HLH-2004 criteria are met (secondary) as shown in Table 1. Our patient fulfilled total five criteria out of eight as per HLH-2004 protocol including (cytopenias, fever, splenomegaly, hemophagocytosis, and hyperferritinemia). A new scoring system was introduced in 2014 called H Score which helps to avoid underdiagnosis of HLH. It consists of nine variables as shown in Table 2. There is a possible number of points assigned to each variable, and then the H Score is calculated. Our patient had a score of 195, indicating an 80–88% probability of HLH.

Regarding therapy, the goal of treatment in HLH is to curtail the widespread inflammation and multi-organ failure caused by excessive activation of the immune system [15]. This consists of a regimen of immune therapy plus chemotherapy aimed at suppressing the cytokine storm associated with HLH. When a precipitating cause is identified, therapy is aimed at treating the underlying condition such as ATT for patients with TB-HLH, which may be sufficient in cases with mild presentation. Two treatment protocols have

TABLE 1: HLH 2004 criteria [14].

Molecular diagnosis consistent with primary HLH (gene mutations)	Homozygosity or compound heterozygosity is required (*PRAF1*, *STX11*, *RAB27A*, *STXBP2*, *UNC13D*, *SH2D1A*, *BIRC4*)
Below criteria are for secondary HLH (at least 5 of 8 criteria must be present)	
Fever	≥38.5 C
Splenomegaly	Spleen palpated >3 cm below the left costal margin
Hemophagocytosis	In bone marrow, spleen, lymph nodes, or liver
NK-cell activity	Low or absent according to local laboratory references
Soluble CD25	(i.e., soluble IL-2 receptor) ≥ 2,400 U/ml
Ferritin	≥500 μg/L
Cytopenias (affecting ≥2 of 3 lineages)	Hemoglobin <9 g/dL Platelets $<100 \times 10^9$/L Neutrophils $<1 \times 10^9$/L
Hypertriglyceridemia and/or hypofibrinogenemia	Fasting triglycerides >265 mg/dL Fibrinogen <150 mg/dL

TABLE 2: H Score criteria [14].

Parameter	Status	Score
Known underlying immunosuppression	No	0
	Yes	18
Organomegaly	No	0
	Hepatomegaly or splenomegaly	+23
	Hepatomegaly and splenomegaly	+38
Number of cytopenias	1 lineage	0
	2 lineages	+24
	3 lineages	+34
Ferritin, ng/mL (or μg/L)	<2000 = 0	0
	2000–6000	+35
	>6000	+50
Triglyceride, mg/dL (mmol/L)	<132.7 (<1.5)	0
	132.7–354 (1.5–4)	+44
	>354 (>4)	+64
Fibrinogen, mg/dL (g/L)	>250 (>2.5)	0
	<250 (<2.5)	+30
AST, U/L	<30	0
	>30	+19
Temperature, °F (°C)	<101.1 (38.4)	0
	101.1–102.9 (38.4–39.4)	+33
	>102.9 (>39.4)	+49
Hemophagocytosis in bone marrow aspirate	No	0
	Yes	+35

been developed in the treatment of primary HLH, HLH-94 [7] and HLH-2004 [16], which include agents such as dexamethasone, etoposide, and cyclosporine as back bones of therapy. Patients are initially placed on an induction regimen with these agents. Those who recover are weaned off therapy, while those who do not respond proceed to hematopoietic stem cell transplant. No clear guidelines exist on timing of initiation of immunomodulatory therapy in cases of secondary HLH.

Specifically, in the case of TB-HLH, literature review reveals that patients have been treated with ATT alone or ATT in combination with HLH-specific therapy. Patients who were started on ATT with or without immunotherapy had better outcomes than those who received no treatment at all [13]. Often, treatment with agents such as etoposide and cyclosporine is not feasible due to fulminant multi-organ failure at time of diagnosis, as was seen in our case. This further highlights the need for increased awareness of HLH, with paramount importance given to a search for secondary causes such as TB, as early diagnosis and prompt initiation of treatment could be lifesaving in an otherwise fatal illness.

4. Conclusion

TB-HLH is a life-threatening condition often with delay in diagnosis and a high fatality rate. A high index of suspicion is required by pathologists and clinicians as it may present with unusual findings such as spontaneous pneumomediastinum. Prompt treatment with ATT and potentially HLH-directed therapy may dramatically result in a better outcome.

References

[1] S. Padhi, K. Ravichandran, J. Sahoo, R. B. Varghese, and A. Basheer, "Hemophagocytic lymphohistiocytosis: an unusual complication in disseminated mycobacterium tuberculosis," *Lung India*, vol. 32, no. 6, p. 593, 2015.

[2] Z. Hindi, A. A. Khaled, and A. Abushahin, "Hemophagocytic syndrome masquerading as septic shock: an approach to such dilemma," *SAGE Open Medical Case Reports*, vol. 5, Article ID 2050313X17746309, 2017.

[3] G. E. Janka, "Familial and acquired hemophagocytic lymphohistiocytosis," *Annual Review of Medicine*, vol. 63, no. 1, pp. 233–246, 2012.

[4] G. Janka and U. Zur Stadt, "Familial and acquired hemophagocytic lymphohistiocytosis," *Hematology*, vol. 2005, no. 1, pp. 82–88, 2005.

[5] P. Aggarwal, G. Kumar, N. Dev, and P. Kumari, "Haemophagocytic lymphohistiocytosis: a cause for rare but fatal outcome in tuberculosis," *BMJ Case Reports*, vol. 2012, Article ID bcr2012006982, 2012.

[6] M. Das, U. C. M. Natchu, R. Lodha, and S. K. Kabra, "Pneumomediastinum and subcutaneous emphysema in acute miliary tuberculosis," *The Indian Journal of Pediatrics*, vol. 71, no. 6, pp. 553-554, 2004.

[7] H. Trottestam, A. Horne, M. Aricò et al., "Chemoimmunotherapy for hemophagocytic lymphohistiocytosis: long-term results of the HLH-94 treatment protocol," *Blood*, vol. 118, no. 17, pp. 4577–4584, 2011.

[8] L. Fardet, L. Galicier, O. Lambotte et al., "Development and validation of the HScore, a score for the diagnosis of reactive hemophagocytic syndrome," *Arthritis & Rheumatology*, vol. 66, no. 9, pp. 2613–2620, 2014.

[9] J.-I. Henter, G. Elinder, O. Söder, and A. Öst, "Incidence in sweden and clinical features of familial hemophagocytic lymphohistiocytosis," *Acta Paediatrica*, vol. 80, no. 4, pp. 428–435, 1991.

[10] J.-I. Henter, A. Ehrnst, J. Andersson, and G. Elinder, "Familial hemophagocytic lymphohistiocytosis and viral infections," *Acta Paediatrica*, vol. 82, no. 4, pp. 369–372, 1993.

[11] E. Campo, E. Condom, M.-J. Miro, M.-C. Cid, and V. Romagosa, "Tuberculosis-associated hemophagocytic syndrome: a systemic process," *Cancer*, vol. 58, no. 12, pp. 2640–2645, 1986.

[12] Y. Zhang, G. Liang, H. Qin, Y. Li, and X. Zeng, "Tuberculosis-associated hemophagocytic lymphohistiocytosis with initial presentation of fever of unknown origin in a general hospital: an analysis of 8 clinical cases," *Medicine*, vol. 96, no. 16, Article ID e6575, 2017.

[13] P. K. Brastianos, J. W. Swanson, M. Torbenson, J. Sperati, and P. C. Karakousis, "Tuberculosis-associated haemophagocytic syndrome," *The Lancet Infectious Diseases*, vol. 6, no. 7, pp. 447–454, 2006.

[14] Y. Zhang, G. Liang, H. Qin, Y. Li, and X. Zeng, "Tuberculosis-associated hemophagocytic lymphohistiocytosis with initial presentation of fever of unknown origin in a general hospital An analysis of 8 clinical cases," *Medicine (Baltimore)*, vol. 96, no. 16, pp. 2728–2738, 2017.

[15] P. La Rosée, A. Horne, M. Hines et al., "Recommendations for the management of hemophagocytic lymphohistiocytosis in adults," *Blood*, vol. 133, no. 23, pp. 2465–2477, 2019.

[16] E. Bergsten, A. Horne, M. Aricó et al., "Confirmed efficacy of etoposide and dexamethasone in HLH treatment: long-term results of the cooperative HLH-2004 study," *Blood*, vol. 130, no. 25, pp. 2728–2738, 2017.

4

A Curious Case of Pseudothrombocytopenia due to *In Vitro* Agglutination

Le Zhong, Juskaran Chadha, and Ali Ameri

Department of Medicine, Zucker School of Medicine at Hofstra/Northwell at Lenox Hill Hospital, 100 E 77th St., New York, NY 10075, USA

Correspondence should be addressed to Le Zhong; lzhong@northwell.edu

Academic Editor: Sergio Storti

Pseudothrombocytopenia (PTCP) is a laboratory phenomenon that can occur in hospitalized patients, with approximately 0.1 to 0.2% due to ethylenediaminetetraacetic acid (ETDA). The EDTA-dependent mechanism of PTCP occurs due to a conformational change of platelet surface glycoprotein IIb/IIIa (GPIIb/IIIa) caused by EDTA, which allows natural IgM or IgG auto-antibodies to bind to GPIIb/IIIa, leading to platelet agglutination. In most cases, PTCP resolves when a repeat blood sample is drawn in collection tubes containing either citrate or heparin. Here, we report a case of a 23-year-old female presenting with symptoms of gastroenteritis. She exhibited PTCP with blood draws obtained in not only collection tubes containing ETDA, but also with collection tubes containing heparin and citrate, which is highly unusual. The lack of resolution of platelet clumping in collection tubes containing either heparin or citrate suggests that heparin or citrate may also cause conformational changes to platelet surface glycoproteins in a similar mechanism as that of EDTA that allows binding of certain auto-antibodies.

1. Introduction and Case Presentation

A 23-year-old female with history of childhood asthma and eczema presented to the hospital's emergency department (ED) with 4 hours of epigastric abdominal pain, vomiting, and diarrhea. Review of systems was negative for fevers, chills, or any signs or symptoms of bleeding. Vital signs were stable on arrival. Examination revealed no signs of bleeding, including no rashes, petechia, purpura, or ecchymoses on skin examination.

Laboratory studies were obtained in the ED, including a blood draw obtained in a collection tube containing ethylenediaminetetraacetic acid (EDTA) obtained via venipuncture and analyzed for a complete blood count (CBC) using a Sysmex XN-10 CBC analyzer (Table 1). Notably, the initial CBC revealed a platelet count of 11×10^9/L; WBC count and hemoglobin were within the reference ranges. Repeat CBC obtained in EDTA later the same day after admission to the hospital showed platelet count of 10×10^9/L. Given the initially reported thrombocytopenia to 11×10^9/L in the absence of any significant hematological history, the initial clinical concern was for idiopathic thrombocytopenic purpura (ITP) and the patient was treated with one dose of oral dexamethasone 40 mg.

Given the finding of severe thrombocytopenia without signs or symptoms of mucocutaneous bleeding, alternate etiologies of the patient's thrombocytopenia besides ITP were suspected and a peripheral blood smear was prepared from the blood draw sample obtained in EDTA. Examination of a peripheral smear of blood samples collected into tube containing EDTA on Day 1 revealed significant platelet clumping (Figure 1). On the peripheral smear, platelet clumping can be found by examining the smear under 40X magnification under a oil light microscope until clusters of platelets can be visualized. The magnification can then be increased to 100X while centering the cluster of platelets to further examine clusters of platelets to identify platelet clumping.

On the morning of Day 2 of admission, a CBC obtained via EDTA collection tube showed platelet count of 10×10^9/L, while blood collection at the same time obtained in a tube containing citrate showed a platelet count of 53×10^9/L.

Table 1: Patient's CBC and platelet values during hospital presentation.

Day and time of hospital visit	Platelet count (10^9/L)	WBC (10^9/L)	Hb (g/dL)	Additive in collection tube	Collection method
Day 1 at 9:33	11	10.1	15.2	EDTA	Venipuncture
Day 1 at 15:51	10	7.9	13.2	EDTA	Venipuncture
Day 2 at 6:58	10	5.0	12.4	EDTA	Venipuncture
Day 2 at 6:58	53	—	—	Citrate	Venipuncture
Day 2 at 6:58	Unable to report due to platelet clumping	—	—	Heparin	Venipuncture
Day 2 at 12:56	28	—	—	Citrate	Venipuncture

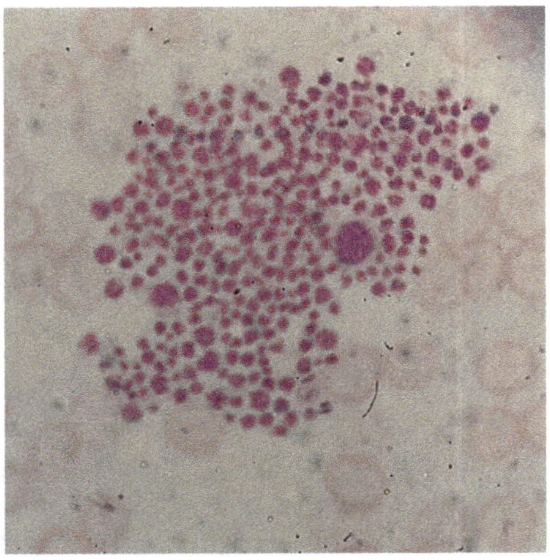

Figure 1: Peripheral smear of CBC drawn in tube containing EDTA (100X/1.30 oil microscope).

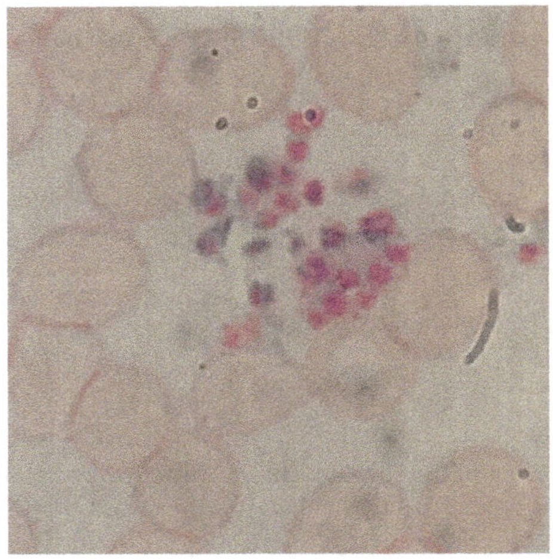

Figure 2: Peripheral smear of CBC drawn in tube containing heparin (100X/1.30 oil microscope).

Repeat blood collection with tube containing citrate later in Day 2 revealed platelet count of 28×10^9/L. A CBC obtained in a collection containing heparin was unable to report a platelet count by the analyzer due to platelet clumping (Table 1). Peripheral smears of blood draw samples containing heparin and citrate both showed platelet clumping when observed under an oil microscope (Figures 2 and 3).

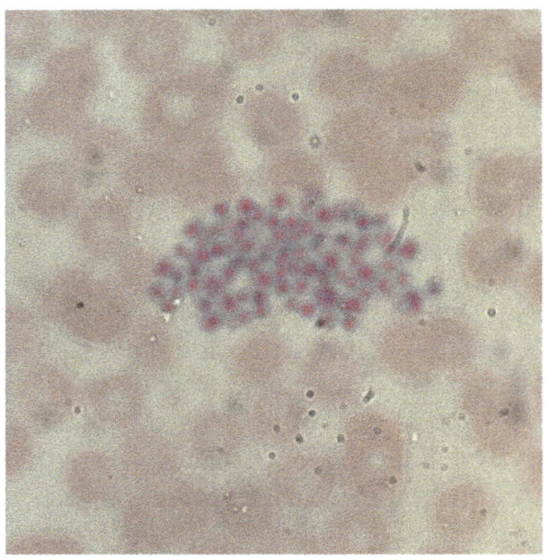

Figure 3: Peripheral smear of CBC drawn in tube containing citrate (100X/1.30 oil microscope).

2. Discussion

Pseudothrombocytopenia (PTCP) is laboratory phenomenon that can occur in hospitalized patients, with approximately 0.1 to 0.2% being EDTA-dependent [1, 2]. The EDTA-dependent mechanism of PTCP occurs due to a conformational change of platelet surface glycoprotein IIb/IIIa (GPIIb/IIIa) caused by EDTA, which allows natural IgM or IgG auto-antibodies to bind to GPIIb/IIIa, leading to platelet agglutination. The phenomenon only occurs *in vitro* and has no known associated clinical significance [3]. However, known risk factors for PTCP due to platelet clumping include active viral infections, capillary or central line blood collection, autoimmune conditions such as rheumatoid arthritis, and medications, such as the GPIIb/IIIa inhibitor abciximab used for the treatment of acute coronary syndrome when undergoing percutaneous coronary intervention [4–7].

A high degree of suspicion is required. PTCP should be on the differential diagnosis for any patient presenting with moderate to severe thrombocytopenia on automated CBC but no clinical signs or symptoms of mucocutaneous bleeding, and a peripheral blood smear be obtained. Otherwise, additional costs and risks associated from further diagnostic testing and treatment for alternate causes of thrombocytopenia may occur. For example, a patient suspected of presenting with ITP may be treated with corticosteroids or even splenectomy, leading to potential iatrogenic injury.

Diagnosis is confirmed by obtaining a blood smear showing platelet clumps. However, PTCP can also be suspected with alerts from an automated hematology analyzer, and a blood smear is thus not always required. Cases of PTCP have been reported in the literature [1–9]. It should be noted that type 2B von Willebrand disease may also lead to platelet clumping that has been misdiagnosed as PTCP. However, the platelet clumps in type 2B von Willebrand disease are generally larger and with more variation in size [8, 10].

In our patient, the most likely precipitating cause of PTCP was a viral infection, given the clinical presentation suggesting acute gastroenteritis. The patient was discharged on Day 2 of her hospital stay in stable condition. However, she was unable to follow-up with us as an outpatient as she returned to her home country. Given the diagnosis of PTCP, oral dexamethasone, which was initially given for empiric treatment of ITP, was discontinued.

Interestingly, this rare laboratory phenomenon appeared to be highly unique in our patient as platelet clumping and pseudothrombocytopenia were observed not only with EDTA tubes, but also with tubes containing heparin and citrate (Table 1). The lack of resolution of platelet clumping in collection tubes containing either heparin or citrate suggests that heparin or citrate may also cause conformational changes to platelet surface glycoproteins in a similar mechanism as that of EDTA that allows binding of certain auto-antibodies. In such a case, a comprehensive work-up to identify alternate etiologies such as autoimmune etiologies is warranted.

Further confirmatory testing for PTCP can be performed by demonstration of a normal platelet count when repeating the CBC with a blood draw obtained in a collection tube containing citrate or heparin, the lack of platelet clumping on a repeat blood smear, or obtaining a peripheral blood film from a drop of blood from a finger stick showing no platelet clumping. The storage temperature of the collection tube has also been reported to affect the occurrence rate of PTCP. It has been reported the antiplatelet antibodies causing PTCP occur optimally between 0°C and 4°C, and that samples that are kept warm at approximately 37°C are less likely to experience clumping [11].

Prognosis of PTCP often involves full recovery when the underlying precipitating factor is treated, as described in several case reports [6, 12]. For example, in the case report by Hsieh et al. of a patient with PTCP associated with infectious mononucleosis, follow-up laboratory studies two months and 1 year after the initial presentation, after the patient had fully recovered from infectious mononucleosis, showed normalization of platelet counts and with no platelet clumping seen on peripheral blood smear [6]. While our patient was unable to follow-up with us, full recovery of PTCP would also be expected as the acute viral gastroenteritis resolved.

References

[1] M. Nagler, P. Keller, D. Siegrist, and L. Alberio, "A case of EDTA-dependent pseudothrombocytopenia: simple recognition of an underdiagnosed and misleading phenomenon," *BMC Clinical Pathology*, vol. 14, no. 1, p. 19, 2014.

[2] A. Vicari, G. Banfi, and P. A. Bonini, "EDTA-dependent pseudothrombocytopaenia: a 12-month epidemiological study," *Scandinavian Journal of Clinical and Laboratory Investigation*, vol. 48, no. 6, pp. 537–542, 1988.

[3] N. Bizzaro and M. Brandalise, "EDTA-dependent pseudothrombocytopenia:association with antiplatelet and antiphospholipid antibodies," *American Journal of Clinical Pathology*, vol. 50, no. 2, pp. 103–109, 1995.

[4] W.-H. Choe, Y.-U. Cho, J.-D. Chae, and S.-H. Kim, "Pseudothrombocytopenia or platelet clumping as a possible cause of low platelet count in patients with viral infection: a case series from single institution focusing on hepatitis A virus infection," *International Journal of Laboratory Hematology*, vol. 35, no. 1, pp. 70–76, 2013.

[5] O. Onder, A. Weinstein, and L. Hoyer, "Pseudothrombocytopenia caused by platelet agglutinins that are reactive in blood anticoagulated with chelating agents," *Blood*, vol. 56, no. 2, pp. 177–182, 1980.

[6] A. T. Hsieh, T. Y. Chao, and Y. C. Chen, "Pseudothrombocytopenia associated with infectious mononucleosis," *Archives of Pathology & Laboratory Medicine*, vol. 127, no. 1, pp. e17–e18, 2003.

[7] D. C. Sane, L. V. Damaraju, E. J. Topol et al., "Occurrence and clinical significance of pseudothrombocytopenia during abciximab therapy," *Journal of the American College of Cardiology*, vol. 36, no. 1, pp. 75–83, 2000.

[8] G. C. Tan, M. Stalling, G. Dennis, M. Nunez, and S. B. Kahwash, "Pseudothrombocytopenia due to platelet clumping: a case report and brief review of the literature," *Case Reports in Hematology*, vol. 2016, Article ID 3036476, 4 pages, 2016.

[9] H. L. Ahn, Y. I. Jo, Y. S. Choi et al., "EDTA-dependent pseudothrombocytopenia confirmed by supplementation of kanamycin ; A case report," *The Korean Journal of Internal Medicine*, vol. 17, no. 1, pp. 65–68, 2002.

[10] R. Kumar, S. Creary, E. A. Varga, and S. B. Kahwash, "Thrombocytopenia pitfalls: misdiagnosing type 2B von Willebrand disease as ethylenediaminetetraacetic acid–dependent pseudothrombocytopenia," *The Journal of Pediatrics*, vol. 175, p. 238, 2016.

[11] G. Lippi and M. Plebani, "EDTA-dependent pseudothrombocytopenia: further insights and recommendations for prevention of a clinically threatening artifact," *Clinical Chemistry and Laboratory Medicine*, vol. 50, no. 8, pp. 1281–1285, 2012.

[12] P. Vaidya and R. Venkataraman, "Pseudothrombocytopenia in a child with dengue," *The Indian Journal of Pediatrics*, vol. 81, no. 12, pp. 1395-1396, 2014.

5

Marked Rebound of Platelet Count in the Early Postpartum Period in a Patient with Essential Thrombocythemia

Yoshinori Hashimoto, Rina Hosoda, Hiromi Omura, and Takayuki Tanaka

Department of Hematology, Tottori Prefectural Central Hospital, Tottori, Japan

Correspondence should be addressed to Yoshinori Hashimoto; 98069yh@jichi.ac.jp

Academic Editor: Gergely Feher

Essential thrombocythemia (ET) occurs predominantly in the elderly, but approximately 20% of patients are <40 years old. Unlike other myeloproliferative neoplasms, ET occurs more commonly in women. We encountered a 38-year-old women diagnosed with ET who exhibited elevated platelet count in early pregnancy. Her platelet count exceeded 1500×10^9/L by late pregnancy; interferon α was administered but failed to induce an adequate response. She underwent emergency cesarean delivery at 37 weeks of gestation. Although her platelet count was 1000×10^9/L immediately after delivery, it markedly increased to 3271×10^9/L approximately 2 weeks later. Cytoreductive therapy was resumed; the subsequent course was free from complications. Several review articles have indicated that because platelet counts of patients may again increase to the pregnancy level or rebound after delivery, cytoreductive therapy should be administered if necessary. However, there is insufficient information on when therapeutic interventions are necessary and how they should be performed. It remains unknown whether the platelet count will decrease after some time without treatment if it rebounds. We hope management guidelines will be established by collecting detailed data on the postpartum course as well as during pregnancy.

1. Introduction

Essential thrombocythemia (ET) occurs predominantly in the elderly, but approximately 20% of patients are <40 years old [1]. Unlike other myeloproliferative neoplasms (MPNs), ET occurs more commonly in women. Consequently, encountering ET in women of reproductive age is not a rare occurrence. Pregnancy and delivery may promote thromboembolism; thus, the perinatal management of patients with ET is becoming an important issue. Although expert consensus and several guidelines describing the management of these patients have been reported [2–6], there are currently no clear guidelines in Japan [7]. Some of the aforementioned guidelines recommend interferon (IFN) therapy for pregnant women with ET who are at a high risk of pregnancy loss. However, IFN is not approved for patients with ET in Japan. Furthermore, because ET is likely to cause thrombotic events, particularly in the postpartum period, low-molecular-weight heparin is commonly administered for 6 weeks after delivery in Europe and the United States. However, it is not indicated for such use in Japan, either. According to aforementioned and other guidelines, the platelet counts of patients with ET increase after delivery [3–6], but many aspects regarding the timing and degree of rebound remain unknown. Few guidelines, including Japanese guidelines [7], mention the optimal blood test interval and therapeutic strategies.

We present a case in which IFN therapy was administered when the platelet count exceeded 1500×10^9/L during late pregnancy. In the present case, the platelet count decreased to approximately 1000×10^9/L immediately after delivery, and cytoreductive therapy was discontinued. However, approximately 2 weeks later, the platelet count markedly rebounded.

2. Case Presentation

The patient was a 38-year-old woman who was referred to our hospital at approximately 7 weeks of gestation for an elevated platelet count detected during a prenatal checkup. She had vaginally delivered her first child at 40 weeks of gestation 8 years earlier and her second child at 39 weeks of gestation 5 years earlier. No abnormalities were observed during the perinatal periods of both pregnancies, and both the patient and her infants were healthy. She had no history of thrombosis or cardiovascular risk factors, such as diabetes mellitus, hypertension, or dyslipidemia, and was a non-smoker. At her visit, the physical examination failed to identify any abnormal findings or splenomegaly. Blood tests indicated a white blood cell count of 11.4×10^9/L, a hemoglobin level of 14.0 g/dL, a hematocrit level of 40.3%, a platelet count of 1074×10^9/L, and a von Willebrand factor ristocetin cofactor activity (vWFRCo) of 49% (Table 1). At 9 weeks of gestation, a bone marrow biopsy was performed that revealed normocellular bone marrow with an increased number of large to giant megakaryocytes and absence of evidence of reactive thrombocytosis; a diagnosis of ET was made. The presence of driver gene mutations was evaluated, and the patient was negative for all Janus kinase 2 (JAK2V617F), calreticulin (CALR), and myeloproliferative leukemia (MPL) mutations, which suggested that she had the so-called triple-negative ET.

Low-dose aspirin was initiated. Her platelet count decreased as the pregnancy progressed. At 30 weeks of gestation, her platelet count had decreased to 432×10^9/L. Subsequently, her platelet count rapidly rebounded. At 34 weeks of gestation, it exceeded 1500×10^9/L, which suggested that she was at a high risk (Figure 1). We provided sufficient explanation to the patient and obtained informed consent from her. After the approval of the ethics committee of our hospital, IFNα (Sumiferon® Dainippon Sumitomo, Osaka, Japan) was administered at 34 weeks and 2 days of gestation. IFNα was administered at a dose of 3 million units 3 times/week at 34 weeks of gestation and at a dose of 6 million units 3 times/week at 35 weeks. The decrease in the platelet count was insufficient; thus, IFNα was administered at a dose of 6 million units daily beginning at 36 weeks, and the daily dose was subsequently increased to 9 million units. Although no adverse events associated with IFNα were observed, her platelet count decreased to only 1229×10^9/L. Ultimately, the patient underwent emergency cesarean delivery at 37 weeks and 1 day of gestation (low-dose aspirin was switched to unfractionated heparin at 36 weeks of gestation).

The infant weighed 2581 g and had Apgar scores of 7 points at 1 min and 8 points at 5 min. Although the infant exhibited transient tachypnea and was temporarily admitted to the neonatal intensive care unit, there were no apparent complications, and the infant was discharged from our hospital. The platelet count of the infant at birth was 317×10^9/L. After delivery, low-molecular-weight heparin was initiated for the mother, and low-dose aspirin was also resumed. Her platelet count was approximately 1000×10^9/L. Cytoreductive therapy was discontinued temporarily, and we allowed her to breastfeed as per her request. At 18 days after delivery, her platelet count had markedly increased to 3271×10^9/L, and her vWFRCo decreased to 31%. She appeared to have acquired von Willebrand syndrome; thus, we determined that she was at a high risk of bleeding. Administration of low-molecular-weight heparin and low-dose aspirin and breastfeeding were discontinued, and hydroxyurea was initiated as a cytoreductive therapy. Approximately 2 months after delivery when her platelet count reached controllable levels, anagrelide was added. Her platelet count was well controlled; thus, hydroxyurea was discontinued after approximately 3 months of use. At present, her platelet count is controlled at approximately 400×10^9/L with 1.0 mg/day of anagrelide. The results of the gene mutation test after cytoreductive therapy were negative for TET oncogene family number 2 (TET2), additional sex combs like 1 (ASXL1), isocitrate dehydrogenase ½ (IDH1/2), and tumor protein p53 (TP53) mutations.

Table 1: Laboratory findings on admission.

Peripheral blood	
WBC	11.4×10^9/L
Neu	76.5%
Lym	17.1%
Mon	4.9%
Eos	1.4%
Bas	1.0%
RBC	4.6×10^{12}/L
Hb	14.0 g/dL
Hct	40.3%
MCV	86.9 fL
Ret	1.8×10^{12}/L
Plt	1074×10^9/L
Chemistry	
TP	7.5 g/dL
Alb	4.8 g/dL
T-bil	0.6 mg/dL
AST	18 U/lL
ALT	25 U/L
ALP	117 U/L
LDH	163 U/L
BUN	7.2 mg/dL
Cr	0.4 mg/dL
UA	3.2 mg/dL
Na	135 mEq/L
K	4.3 mEq/L
Coagulation	
PT-INR	0.95
APTT	30.2 sec
vWFRCo	49%
Serology	
CRP	0.04 mg/dL
Other findings	
JAK2V617F	<1.0%
MPLW515L	(−)
MPLW515K	(−)
CALR type1	<1.0%
CALR type2	<1.0%
ABO/Rh	A/+

Ret, reticulocyte; VWFRCo, von Willebrand factor ristocetin cofactor activity; JAK2, Janus kinase 2; MPL, myeloproliferative leukemia protein; CALR, calreticulin, ABO/Rh, ABO blood group/Rhesus blood group.

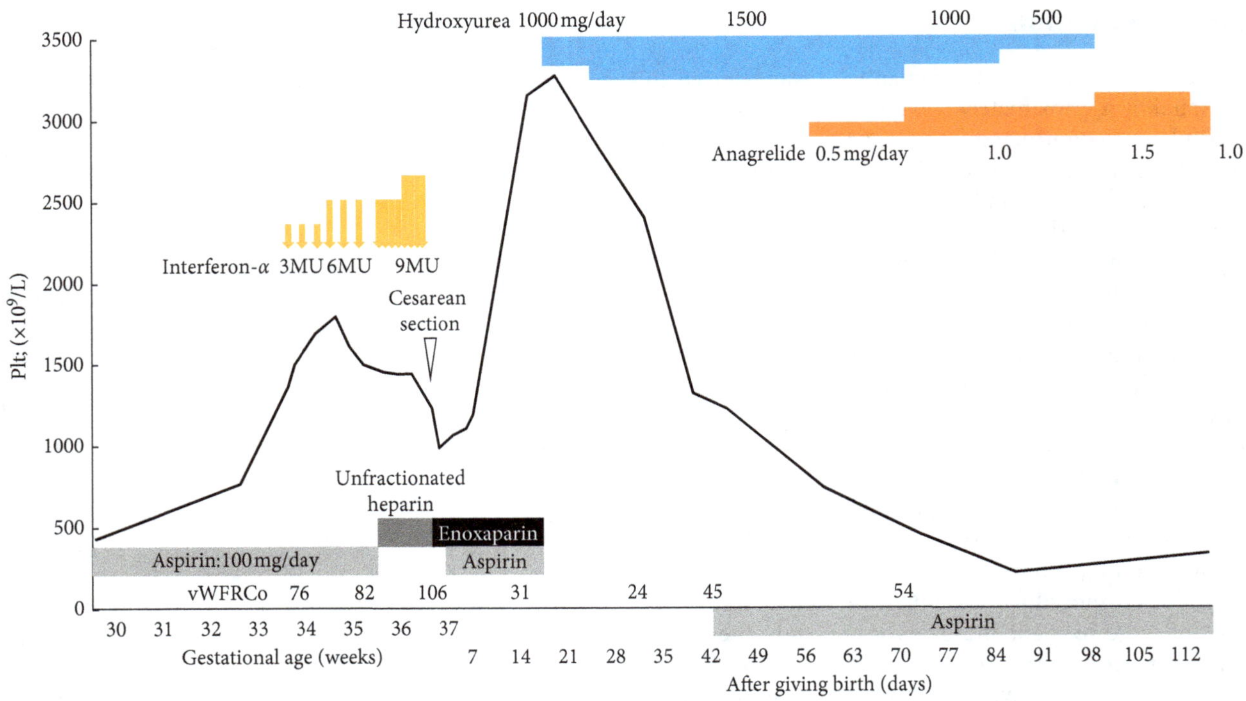

FIGURE 1: Clinical course and serial changes in the platelet count. MU, million units; VWFRCo, von Willebrand factor ristocetin cofactor activity.

3. Discussion

Both pregnancy and ET contribute to the risk of thrombosis; thus, pregnant women with ET may be at a higher risk of thrombosis. Additionally, various complications, such as placental infarction, fetal growth restriction, and fetal wastage, can affect not only the mother but also the fetus. Greiesshammer et al. identified case reports of ≥9 pregnancies in ≥4 patients with ET that were published in and after 2000 and analyzed 10 case reports describing pregnancy outcomes [4]. According to their analysis, the live birth rate in pregnant women with ET was almost 70%; the full-term normal delivery rate was lower in pregnant women with ET than in healthy pregnant women, and the rates of spontaneous abortion and stillbirth were higher. These findings cannot be disregarded. High-risk pregnancies in patients with MPN are often defined based on the definitions developed by Greiesshammer et al. [4] and the European LeukemiaNet [2]. Additionally, expert consensus and several guidelines recommend the use of IFNα for high-risk pregnancy [2–6], and the Japanese guidelines also indicate that the use of IFNα should be considered although it is not covered by the National Health Insurance [7]. A previous retrospective study reported that the use of IFNα is an independent factor affecting the live birth rate [8], and a recent systematic review and meta-analysis of pregnant women with MPN also showed that the use of IFN is associated with a high live birth rate [9].

Based on the above discussion, IFNα was used in our patient with due ethical considerations; unfortunately, its effect was insufficient. Her platelet count rapidly increased around 34 weeks of gestation despite increasing the IFNα dose; hence, the IFNα administration period might have been insufficient. Edahiro et al. reported that the median platelet count decreased by approximately 37% from 910×10^9 to 573×10^9/L in seven patients after 2 months of IFNα therapy that was started after the discovery of pregnancy [10]. As our patient received the drug for approximately 1 month, its effect might have been insufficient. Generally, IFNα is thought to exert favorable molecular genetic effects because it can target cells positive for not only JAK2V617F mutations but also CALR and other mutations [11]. However, a report of the use of pegylated IFNα in patients positive for CALR mutations showed that its molecular genetic effects were lower in patients with CALR mutations and in those with mutations of additional genes such as TET2, ASXL1, IDH2, and TP53 [12]. In other words, the sensitivity of IFNα may differ among mutated clones. Moreover, a small-scale study suggests that patients with triple-negative ET may be more resistant to IFNα than patients with JAK2V617F or CALR mutations [10]. According to our tests, our patient did not have any abnormalities of the aforementioned additional genes, but she did have triple-negative ET. Consequently, the effects of IFNα might have been limited.

Finally, we would like to discuss the postpartum rebound of platelet count in our patient. Several review articles have indicated that because platelet counts of patients may again increase to the prepregnancy level [13] or rebound after delivery, cytoreductive therapy should be administered if necessary [3–6]. However, there is insufficient information on when therapeutic interventions are necessary and how they should be performed. It remains unknown whether the platelet count will decrease after some time without treatment if it rebounds. According to our searches in the English literature, some reports indicate that no particular cytoreductive therapy was required after delivery, whereas other reports describe cases in which patients were treated for a rebound of platelet count [14–18]. Sakai et al. reported a case in which the platelet count increased to $\geq 1000 \times 10^9/L$ within 3 months after delivery and another case in which the platelet count increased to $\geq 800 \times 10^9/L$ within 2 months after delivery. Cytoreductive therapy was resumed in the former case [14]. Iwashita et al. reported a case of a woman, para 2, whose platelet count increased to $\geq 2000 \times 10^9/L$ within 1-2 months after delivery in both pregnancies but decreased to approximately 800×10^9 to $900 \times 10^9/L$ several months later [15]. Although the prepregnancy platelet count affects the postpartum count, one report cited a platelet count increase to a maximum of $3000 \times 10^9/L$ after delivery [19]. However, we did not identify any patients in the literature with a postpartum platelet count increasing as high as that of our patient. After pregnancy, cytoreductive therapy is rarely required because young women are often at a low risk based on the conventional risk classification for thrombosis [20]. Furthermore, the decision to perform cytoreductive therapy is expected to differ depending on whether the patient will breastfeed their infant after delivery. Thus, individualized treatment should be considered. While we assume that treatment varies depending on the postpartum status of the patients, a certain expert consensus indicates that blood tests should be counted at 6 weeks after delivery [3]. However, caution should be exercised because some women exhibit a rebound of platelet count within 2–4 weeks after delivery, as with our patient and the aforementioned cases [16, 17].

In conclusion, we encountered a patient who exhibited a marked rebound of platelet count soon after delivery. She resumed cytoreductive therapy; the subsequent course was uneventful without any complications. The evidence for the treatment of pregnant women with ET is limited. We hope that management guidelines will be established through the collection of data both during pregnancy and detailed data on the postpartum course.

References

[1] R. J. Q. McNally, E. Roman, and R. A. Cartwright, "Leukemias and lymphomas: time trends in the UK, 1984-93," *Cancer Causes & Control*, vol. 10, no. 1, pp. 35–42, 1999.

[2] T. Barbui, A. Tefferi, A. M. Vannucchi et al., "Philadelphia chromosome-negative classical myeloproliferative neoplasms: revised management recommendations from European LeukemiaNet," *Leukemia*, vol. 32, no. 5, pp. 1057–1069, 2018.

[3] S. E. Robinson and C. N. Harrison, "How we manage Philadelphia-negative myeloproliferative neoplasms in pregnancy," *British Journal of Haematology*, vol. 189, no. 4, pp. 625–634, 2020.

[4] M. Griesshammer, P. Sadjadian, and K. Wille, "Contemporary management of patients with BCR-ABL1-negative myeloproliferative neoplasms during pregnancy," *Expert Review of Hematology*, vol. 11, no. 9, pp. 697–706, 2018.

[5] M. Griesshammer, S. Struve, and T. Barbui, "Management of Philadelphia negative chronic myeloproliferative disorders in pregnancy," *Blood Reviews*, vol. 22, no. 5, pp. 235–245, 2008.

[6] C. Harrison, "Pregnancy and its management in the Philadelphia negative myeloproliferative diseases," *British Journal of Haematology*, vol. 129, no. 3, pp. 293–306, 2005.

[7] K. Shimoda, N. Takahashi, K. Kirito, N. Iriyama, T. Kawaguchi, and M. Kizaki, "JSH practical guidelines for hematological malignancies, 2018: I. leukemia-4. chronic myeloid leukemia (CML)/myeloproliferative neoplasms (MPN)," *International Journal of Hematology*, vol. 112, no. 3, pp. 268–291, 2020.

[8] L. Melillo, A. Tieghi, A. Candoni et al., "Outcome of 122 pregnancies in essential thrombocythemia patients: a report from the Italian registry," *American Journal of Hematology*, vol. 84, no. 10, pp. 636–640, 2009.

[9] D. Maze, S. Kazi, V. Gupta et al., "Association of treatments for myeloproliferative neoplasms during pregnancy with birth rates and maternal outcomes: a systematic review and meta-analysis," *JAMA Network Open*, vol. 2, no. 10, Article ID e1912666, 2019.

[10] Y. Edahiro, H. Yasuda, A. Gotoh et al., "Interferon therapy for pregnant patients with essential thrombocythemia in Japan," *International Journal of Hematology*, vol. 113, no. 1, p. 106, 2020.

[11] A. Quintás-Cardama, O. Abdel-Wahab, T. Manshouri et al., "Molecular analysis of patients with polycythemia vera or essential thrombocythemia receiving pegylated interferon α-2a," *Blood*, vol. 122, no. 6, pp. 893–901, 2013.

[12] E. Verger, B. Cassinat, A. Chauveau et al., "Clinical and molecular response to interferon-α therapy in essential thrombocythemia patients with CALR mutations," *Blood*, vol. 126, no. 24, pp. 2585–2591, 2015.

[13] J. Lapoirie, A. Contis, A. Guy et al., "Management and outcomes of 27 pregnancies in women with myeloproliferative neoplasms," *The Journal of Maternal-Fetal & Neonatal Medicine*, vol. 33, no. 1, pp. 49–56, 2020.

[14] K. Sakai, A. Ueda, M. Hasegawa, and Y. Ueda, "Efficacy and safety of interferon alpha for essential thrombocythemia during pregnancy: two cases and a literature review," *International Journal of Hematology*, vol. 108, no. 2, pp. 203–207, 2018.

[15] T. Iwashita, M. Fujitani, Y. Yamamoto, T. Katsurada, and Y. Yoshida, "Interferon-alfa treatment of essential thrombocythemia during pregnancy," *Internal Medicine*, vol. 45, no. 20, pp. 1161–1164, 2006.

[16] N. Singh, S. Kumar, K. K. Roy, V. Sharma, and A. Jalak, "Successful maternal and fetal outcome in a rare case of essential thrombocythemia with pregnancy using interferon alpha," *Platelets*, vol. 23, no. 4, pp. 319–321, 2012.

[17] P. Martinelli, V. Martinelli, A. Agangi et al., "interferon alfa treatment for pregnant women affected by essential thrombocythemia: case reports and a review," *American Journal of Obstetrics and Gynecology*, vol. 191, no. 6, pp. 2016–2020, 2004.

[18] Y. Kanda, S. Chiba, Y. Tanaka et al., "Serial serum thrombopoietin levels in a pregnant woman with essential thrombocythaemia," *British Journal of Haematology*, vol. 105, no. 1, pp. 271–273, 1999.

[19] C. A. Wright and A. Tefferi, "A single institutional experience with 43 pregnancies in essential thrombocythemia," *European Journal of Haematology*, vol. 66, no. 3, pp. 152–159, 2001.

[20] Y. Hashimoto, H. Nakamae, T. Tanaka et al., "Validation of previous prognostic models for thrombosis and exploration of modified models in patients with essential thrombocythemia," *European Journal of Haematology*, vol. 101, no. 4, pp. 508–513, 2018.

6

A Case of Autoimmune Hemolytic Anemia after the First Dose of COVID-19 mRNA-1273 Vaccine with Undetected Pernicious Anemia

Fnu Jaydev,[1] Vinod Kumar,[1] Jaikumar Khatri,[1] Shobha Shahani,[1] and Sead Beganovic[2]

[1]*Division of Internal Medicine and Geriatrics, Indiana University School of Medicine, Indianapolis, IN, USA*
[2]*Indiana University Health Central Indiana Cancer Center, Indianapolis, IN, USA*

Correspondence should be addressed to Fnu Jaydev; fjaydev@iu.edu

Academic Editor: Håkon Reikvam

By this time, multiple vaccines have been approved to limit the spread of SARS-CoV-2 worldwide. These include new-generation vaccines that contain mRNA of the target organism. Some common side effects were identified and reported during phase 3 clinical trials of vaccination, but more rare adverse events were reported in the literature. One such concern is autoimmune conditions that SARS-CoV-2 viral antigens could have possibly incited. We are presenting here a case of a young female with no known autoimmune diseases, diagnosed with autoimmune hemolytic anemia about a week after receiving her first dose of the COVID-19 mRNA vaccine. We discuss the possible culprit for precipitation of autoimmune hemolytic anemia after the SARS-CoV-2 mRNA vaccine, which encodes virus spike protein. This case highlights the importance of being vigilant for identifying rare adverse events that could appear during mass vaccination.

1. Introduction

Since the beginning, the SARS-CoV-2 pandemic has claimed many lives worldwide and caused significant morbidity in many patients [1]. Besides the usual systemic symptoms and signs of COVID-19 infection, some rare medical conditions have been reported in the literature. One such rare phenomenon which has been reported in the literature is autoimmune conditions such as Guillain–Barré syndrome [2], immune thrombocytopenic purpura [3], antiphospholipid antibody syndrome [4], and autoimmune hemolytic anemia, both warm antibody type and cold agglutinin type [4–7]. The first effective approved vaccines against the SARS-CoV-2 virus were the mRNA vaccines from two major pharmaceutical companies, to be followed by mass vaccination programs in many parts of the world [8]. Some of the common side effects of these vaccines include local injection site inflammation, fever, chills, fatigue, myalgia, arthralgia, and headache [9], which are primarily self-resolving within a couple of days. Some relatively rare side effects were reported as medically attended adverse events (MAAEs); for example, Bell's palsy and severe adverse events (SAEs) were reported during clinical trials of the COVID-19 mRNA-1273 vaccine. Despite the numerical difference in frequency of these events, no causal relationship could be established, given the small number of cases. We present a case of warm antibody autoimmune hemolytic anemia in a female with the onset of symptoms about a week after receiving her first COVID-19 mRNA-1273 vaccine shot, who was later found to have undetected pernicious anemia as well.

2. Case

The case was a 42-year-old female with a past medical history of hypertension, congenitally deaf and mute (uses sign language for communication), iron deficiency anemia due to menorrhagia, and history of provoked venous sinus thrombosis in 2015 treated with anticoagulation, but this had to be stopped due to worsening menorrhagia, without recurrence of venous sinus thrombosis. We obtained history with the help of a sign language interpreter. She was admitted to our hospital with a two-week history of worsening dizziness and lightheadedness, progressive shortness of breath with activity, palpitations, mild spells of blurred vision, generalized weakness, lack of energy, and easy fatigue with her activities at home and her workplace. The patient reported the onset of these symptoms was a week after getting her first dose of the COVID-19 mRNA-1273 vaccine on April 7, 2021. Since then, her symptoms had been progressive and got severe enough to limit her physical activity in the last few days. She reported no cough, fever, nausea, vomiting, abdominal pain, melena, blood in the stools, hematemesis, or urinary symptoms. The patient has been on oral iron supplementation, to which she has been very compliant. As recently checked by her primary physician, her iron level had been stable (ferritin: 32.2 ng/mL in 2016 and 355.4 ng/mL on this admission with serum iron 95 μg/dL and iron saturation of 41%). Her menorrhagia has been stable; her periods last for seven days, with the first four days being a little heavier. Her hemoglobin on admission was found to be 4.5 g/dL, MCV was 90 fL, and absolute reticulocyte count was 19.9×10^9/L (see Table 1 for detailed lab results). Creatinine was within the normal range. She had mildly elevated indirect bilirubin. A peripheral blood smear was reported to show a few schistocytes, polychromasia, and anisocytosis. Haptoglobin was <6 mg/dL. LDH was 4332 IU/L, and the indirect Coombs' test was reported positive. We performed a direct Coombs' test, which was reported positive for IgG and C3 with identification of warm autoantibodies. COVID-19 PCR test was found to be negative.

On further investigations, she was noted to have normal serum iron and iron saturation but mildly elevated ferritin, normal folate, and severely low vitamin B12 level <50 pg/mL. Further testing showed positive gastric parietal cell IgG antibodies and intrinsic factor antibodies. Given the hemodynamic stability of the patient and the patient's preference, she did not receive a blood transfusion. The patient was monitored inpatient and started on intravenous steroids, methylprednisolone (2 mg/Kg daily), and intramuscular cyanocobalamin injections daily. Hemoglobin improved from 4.5 g/dL on admission to 6.0 g/dL on day 7 of admission, and on day 10 (Figure 1: trend of hemoglobin during and after hospitalization), which was the day of her discharge, hemoglobin had improved to 7.9 g/dL with schistocytes still present. Her symptoms and hemoglobin level slowly improved, and she was discharged on a long taper of oral prednisone and continued parenteral cyanocobalamin replacement. On the first follow-up about a week after her discharge, labs showed hemoglobin improvement to 8.9 g/dL with no schistocytes on the peripheral smear. LDH improved to 540 IU/L and absolute reticulocyte to 88.2×10^9/L. On the second follow-up, two weeks later, her hemoglobin improved to 9.6 g/dL (see Table 1).

3. Discussion

Autoimmune hemolytic anemia is associated with IgG or IgM antibodies against the intrinsic RBC surface antigens. It causes hemolysis via complement and reticuloendothelial cells, resulting in the extravascular hemolytic process. Our patient was noted to have features of hemolysis (Table 1); both indirect and direct Coombs' tests were positive for warm autoantibodies IgG and C3d. Peripheral blood smear in extravascular hemolysis usually shows spherocytosis, but in this patient, peripheral smear showed moderate to many microcytes and few to moderate macrocytes along with few schistocytes. In autoimmune hemolytic anemia, intravascular hemolysis can be seen depending on the type and concentration of IgG antibodies [10]. We suspect that, in our patient, there could have been a component of intravascular hemolysis along with a predominant extravascular process as evidenced by the presence of few schistocytes and a very high LDH level. The high LDH level, in this case, could also be contributed by the presence of intramedullary hemolytic process secondary to severe vitamin B12 deficiency. Warm antibody AIHA is more commonly associated with lymphoproliferative disorders (e.g., chronic lymphocytic leukemia) and autoimmune disorders (e.g., systemic lupus erythematosus) [11]. Interestingly, our patient was found to have a severe vitamin B12 deficiency; we tested and found her positive for intrinsic factor antibodies and gastric parietal cell antibodies (Table 1), raising the possibility of previously undetected pernicious anemia.

Hemolysis in patients with vitamin B12 deficiency is rare [12] and reported to be 1.5% in a study of hematologic manifestations with vitamin B12 deficiency in 201 patients [13], but the combination of pernicious anemia and autoimmune hemolytic anemia is also an infrequent occurrence. Yeruva et al. reported a case with this rare combination and, from their literature search, found 14 other cases between 1951 and 2010 [14]. In an extensive 18-year study of AIHA in 865 patients, an association of warm antibody AIHA was noted in only 3 cases [15]. Our patient was treated with parenteral cyanocobalamin injection and steroids, resulting in rapid response in hemoglobin, improving from 4.5 g/dl to 9.6 g/dl in less than a month without any red cell transfusion. AIHA in patients with pernicious anemia does not respond to vitamin B12 injections alone but will require steroids [14, 16].

With active hemolysis, one would expect a rapid rise in the reticulocyte count, but our patient's initial reticulocyte count was normal despite signs of severe hemolysis, and we posit that this could be due to intramedullary hemolysis related to vitamin B12 deficiency. Besides intravascular hemolysis, intramedullary hemolysis or ineffective erythropoiesis results in the destruction of red blood cells within the bone marrow and has been recognized as another phenomenon responsible for decreasing red cell counts and anemia. While the exact mechanism is still not well understood, some role of elevated homocysteine level has been postulated as contributing to intramedullary hemolysis based on in vitro experiments and reported in case reports [17–19].

After mass vaccination has rolled out, some rare adverse events have been reported, such as DVT after the BTN162b2 mRNA vaccine [20]. To our knowledge, our case is one of the first few cases of autoimmune hemolytic anemia after the COVID-19 mRNA vaccine, which could have a possible and

Table 1: Laboratory test result during and after hospitalization.

Laboratory results	Admission	Discharge	Follow-up 1 (1 week after discharge)	Follow-up 2 (3 weeks after discharge)	Reference range
WBC (×10^9/L)	3.5	9.0	11.4	12.2	3.6–10.6
Neutrophils (%)	27	93	86	90	
Lymphocytes (%)	68	7	10	8	
Monocytes (%)	3	0	4	1	
Eosinophils (%)	0	0	0	1	
Basophils (%)	0	0	0	0	
Myelocytes (%)	2				
Absolute neutrophils (×10^9/L)	0.9	8.4	9.6	11.2	1.7–7.0
Absolute lymphocytes (×10^9/L)	2.2	0.6	1.1	1.0	1–3.2
Absolute monocytes (×10^9/L)	0.1	0	0.4	0.1	0.1–1.3
Absolute eosinophils (×10^9/L)	0	0	0	0.1	0.0–0.3
Absolute basophils (×10^9/L)	0	0	0	0	0.0–0.2
Absolute myelocytes (×10^9/L)	0.1				
Hemoglobin (g/dL)	4.5	7.9	8.9	9.6	12–15
Hematocrit (%)	12.7	24.1	27.9	31.2	35–49
MCV (fL)	90	95	93	92	81–99
RDW (%)	>40	39.6	29.2	21.6	11.5–14.5
Platelets (×10^9/L)	148	401	628	243	150–450
Schistocytes	Few (1+)	Many (3+)	None seen	None seen	None
Polychromasia	Slight	Marked (3+)	Moderate (2+)	Slight	
Microcytes	Many (3+)	Moderate (2+)	Few (1+)		
Macrocytes	Few (1+)	Moderate (2+)	Moderate (2+)	Few (1+)	
ALT (units/L)	36				7–52
AST (units/L)	71				13–39
Total bilirubin (mg/dL)	2.1			0.5	0.0–1.0
Indirect bilirubin (mg/dL)	1.7			0.4	0.0–0.8
LDH (units/L)	4332	2628	540	257	140–271
Haptoglobin (mg/dL)	<6	<6			30–200
Serum iron (μg/dL)	95				50–212
Iron saturation (%)	41				15–55
TIBC (μg/dL)	231				250–400
Ferritin (ng/mL)	355.4				10–106
Serum B12 level (pg/mL)	<50				200–1,000
Serum folate (ng/mL)	>23.0				>5.9
Reticulocyte count (%)	1.4		2.8	2.0	0.5–2.5
Absolute reticulocyte number (× 10^9/L)	19.9		88.2	69.1	21–115
Gastric parietal cell IgG (units)	18.8				0.0–24.9
Intrinsic factor antibodies	Positive				Negative
Indirect Coombs' test	Positive				Negative
Direct Coombs' test	Positive IgG and C3				Negative
Antibody ID	Warm autoantibodies				Negative
Antibody eluted	Eluate positive with all cells				
Coronavirus SARS-CoV-2 PCR	Not detected				

biologically plausible association with the vaccine. Given the rarity of such disorders, it is hard to make a conclusive argument in favor of the cause-and-effect relationship between the mRNA COVID-19 vaccine and autoimmune hemolytic anemia, but given the previous case reports of AIHA in patients with SARS-CoV-2 infection and recently reported molecular mimicry as a possible culprit in the AIHA-affecting patients with COVID-19 disease, Angileri

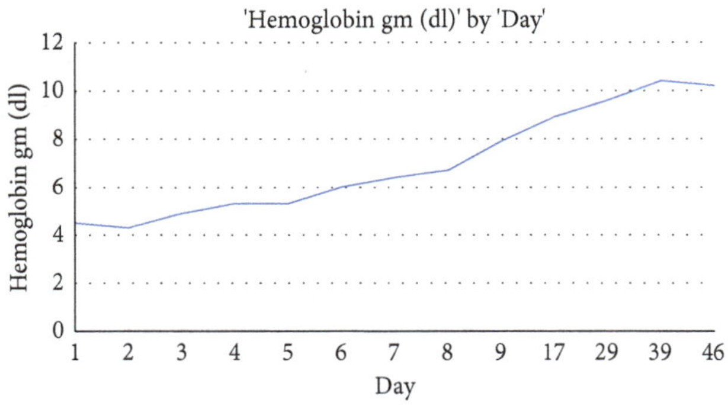

FIGURE 1: Hemoglobin trend during hospitalization and after discharge.

et al., in their correspondence to the British Journal of Hematology [21], postulated such molecular mimicry between ankyrin-1 (ANK-1), a red cell membrane protein, and SARS-CoV-2 viral spike protein. Using the immune epitope database (IEDB, https://www.iedb.org/), they found a 100% identity between the ANK-1 putative immunogenic-antigenic epitope (amino acids LLLQY) and the spike protein's predicted immunogenic epitope 750-SNLLLQYGSFCTQL-763 for B cells. ANK-1 provides a primary linkage between the membrane skeleton and plasma membrane and, if genetically defective, can result in hemolytic anemia such as hereditary spherocytosis [21, 22]. Since this molecular similarity has been hypothesized as the pathogenic basis for AIHA in patients with SARS-CoV-2, we postulate that the same cross-reactivity can be contributing to AIHA after receiving the COVID-19 mRNA-1273 dose in our case. COVID-19 mRNA-1273 vaccine contains a synthetic messenger ribonucleic acid (mRNA) encoding the prefusion stabilized spike glycoprotein (S) of SARS-CoV-2 virus (2) and induces production of spike protein by human cells, which then results in the production of antibodies against spike protein. These antibodies then cross-react with ANK-1 RBC protein, resulting in autoimmune hemolytic anemia.

Per our literature review, we have found two other reported cases of autoimmune hemolytic anemia associated with the mRNA COVID-19 vaccine [23, 24]. One of these patients [24] had a known history of cold agglutinin disease, which had been stable and got exacerbated by the administration of the COVID-19 vaccine. As per the VRBPAC Briefing Document of the FDA on the COVID-19 mRNA-1273 vaccine, the FDA recommended two months' median follow-up after completion of vaccination which may allow for identification of potential immune-mediated adverse events that began within six weeks of vaccination and could be plausibly linked to vaccination [25].

4. Conclusion

The process of warm antibody autoimmune hemolysis in our patient could have an association with underlying undetected pernicious anemia and vitamin B12 deficiency, which in itself is a rare occurrence. Given the timing of presentation of this case and previously reported cases of autoimmune pathologies in association with COVID-19 and with mRNA vaccines, we cannot exclude the possibility of the patient's mRNA vaccination as an inciting or precipitating factor for warm antibody autoimmune hemolysis in this patient. As more and more people worldwide are getting the COVID-19 mRNA vaccine, rare side effects such as autoimmune hemolytic anemia are being reported. Even though rare, these can cause significant morbidity and mortality. This requires high vigilance on the part of the care providers to detect these rare side effects at an earlier stage.

References

[1] C. A. Pollard, M. P. Morran, and A. L. Nestor-Kalinoski, "The COVID-19 pandemic: a global health crisis," *Physiological Genomics*, vol. 52, no. 11, pp. 549–557, 2020.

[2] G. Toscano, F. Palmerini, S. Ravaglia et al., "Guillain-barré syndrome associated with SARS-CoV-2," *New England Journal of Medicine*, vol. 382, no. 26, pp. 2574–2576, 2020.

[3] A.-A. Zulfiqar, N. Lorenzo-Villalba, P. Hassler, and E. Andrès, "Immune thrombocytopenic purpura in a patient with covid-19," *New England Journal of Medicine*, vol. 382, no. 18, p. e43, 2020.

[4] Y. Zhang, M. Xiao, S. Zhang et al., "Coagulopathy and antiphospholipid antibodies in patients with covid-19," *New England Journal of Medicine*, vol. 382, no. 7, p. e38, 2020.

[5] F. Hindilerden, I. Yonal-Hindilerden, E. Akar, Z. Yesilbag, and K. Kart-Yasar, "Severe autoimmune hemolytic anemia in Covid-19 infection," *Mediterranean Journal of Hematology and Infectious Diseases*, vol. 12, no. 1, Article ID e2020053, 2020.

[6] G. Lazarian, A. Quinquenel, M. Bellal et al., "Autoimmune haemolytic anaemia associated with COVID-19 infection," *British Journal of Haematology*, vol. 190, no. 1, pp. 29–31, 2020.

[7] V. Salle, "Coronavirus-induced autoimmunity," *Clinical Immunology*, vol. 226, Article ID 108694, 2021.

[8] Y. H. Chung, V. Beiss, S. N. Fiering, and N. F. Steinmetz, "COVID-19 vaccine frontrunners and their nanotechnology design," *ACS Nano*, vol. 14, no. 10, pp. 12522–12537, 2020.

[9] F. P. Polack, S. J. Thomas, N. Kitchin et al., "Safety and efficacy of the BNT162b2 mRNA covid-19 vaccine," *New England Journal of Medicine*, vol. 383, no. 27, pp. 2603–2615, 2020.

[10] H. A. Liebman and I. C. Weitz, "Autoimmune hemolytic anemia," *Medical Clinics of North America*, vol. 101, no. 2, pp. 351–359, 2017.

[11] U. Jäger, W. Barcellini, C. M. Broome et al., "Diagnosis and treatment of autoimmune hemolytic anemia in adults: recommendations from the first international consensus meeting," *Blood Reviews*, vol. 41, Article ID 100648, 2020.

[12] E. Andrès, N. H. Loukili, E. Noel et al., "Vitamin B12 (cobalamin) deficiency in elderly patients," *Canadian Medical Association Journal*, vol. 171, no. 3, pp. 251–259, 2004.

[13] E. Andrès, S. Affenberger, J. Zimmer et al., "Current hematological findings in cobalamin deficiency. A study of 201 consecutive patients with documented cobalamin deficiency," *Clinical and Laboratory Haematology*, vol. 28, no. 1, pp. 50–56, 2006.

[14] S. L. Yeruva, R. P. Manchandani, and P. Oneal, "Pernicious anemia with autoimmune hemolytic anemia: a case report and literature review," *Case Reports in Hematology*, vol. 2016, Article ID 7231503, 2016.

[15] R. J. Sokol, S. Hewitt, and B. K. Stamps, "Autoimmune haemolysis: an 18-year study of 865 cases referred to a regional transfusion centre," in *BMJ*, C. Res, Ed., vol. 282, no. 6281, pp. 2023–2027, 1981.

[16] A. P. Rabinowitz, Y. Sacks, and R. Carmel, "Autoimmune cytopenias in pernicious anemia: a report of four cases and review of the literature," *European Journal of Haematology*, vol. 44, no. 1, pp. 18–23, 1990.

[17] R. Olinescu, F. A. Kummerow, B. Handler, and L. Fleischer, "The hemolytic activity of homocysteine is increased by the activated polymorphonuclear leukocytes," *Biochemical and Biophysical Research Communications*, vol. 226, no. 3, pp. 912–916, 1996.

[18] P. Ventura, R. Panini, S. Tremosini, and G. Salvioli, "A role for homocysteine increase in haemolysis of megaloblastic anaemias due to vitamin B12 and folate deficiency: results from an in vitro experience," *Biochimica et Biophysica Acta (BBA)-Molecular Basis of Disease*, vol. 1739, no. 1, pp. 33–42, 2004.

[19] U. Acharya, J.-T. Gau, W. Horvath, P. Ventura, C.-T. Hsueh, and W. Carlsen, "Hemolysis and hyperhomocysteinemia caused by cobalamin deficiency: three case reports and review of the literature," *Journal of Hematology & Oncology*, vol. 1, no. 1, p. 26, 2008.

[20] G. Carli, I. Nichele, M. Ruggeri, S. Barra, and A. Tosetto, "Deep vein thrombosis (DVT) occurring shortly after the second dose of mRNA SARS-CoV-2 vaccine," *Internal and Emergency Medicine*, vol. 16, no. 3, pp. 803-804, 2021.

[21] F. Angileri, S. . Légaré, A. M. Gammazza, E. C. de Macario, A. J. L Macario, and F. Cappello, "Is molecular mimicry the culprit in the autoimmune haemolytic anaemia affecting patients with COVID-19?" *British Journal of Haematology*, vol. 190, no. 2, pp. e92–e93, 2020.

[22] P. G. Gallagher, W. T. Tse, A. L. Scarpa, S. E. Lux, and B. G. Forget, "Structure and organization of the human ankyrin-1 gene," *Journal of Biological Chemistry*, vol. 272, no. 31, pp. 19220–19228, 1997.

[23] S. Brito, N. Ferreira, S. Mateus et al., "A case of autoimmune hemolytic anemia following COVID-19 messenger ribonucleic acid vaccination," *Cureus*, vol. 13, no. 5, Article ID e15035, 2021.

[24] L. Pérez-Lamas, G. Moreno-Jiménez, M. C. Tenorio-Núñez et al., "Hemolytic crisis due to Covid-19 vaccination in a woman with cold agglutinin disease," *American Journal of Hematology*, vol. 96, no. 8, 2021.

[25] Vaccines and related biological products advisory committee meeting December 17, 2020. FDA Briefing Document Moderna COVID-19 Vaccine.

7

Recurrence of Thrombotic Thrombocytopenic Purpura after mRNA-1273 COVID-19 Vaccine Administered Shortly after COVID-19

Korin Karabulut,[1] **Ana Andronikashvili**,[1] **and Ahmet Hakki Kapici**[2]

[1]*Steward Carney Hospital, 2100 Dorchester Avenue, Boston, MA 02124, USA*
[2]*Robert Wood Johnson University Hospital, 1 Robert Wood Johnson Place, New Brunswick, NJ 08901, USA*

Correspondence should be addressed to Korin Karabulut; korin.karabulut@steward.org

Academic Editor: Kostas Konstantopoulos

Thrombotic thrombocytopenic purpura (TTP) is a potentially life-threatening consumptive coagulopathy requiring emergent diagnosis and timely treatment. It is characterized by microangiopathic hemolytic anemia and thrombocytopenia with the development of microthrombi caused by inherited or acquired deficiency of the von Willebrand factor-cleaving protease ADAMTS13 and resulting end-organ damage. Most of the cases are the result of acquired deficiency of ADAMTS13, for which the exact etiology is unknown but reported to be related to various autoimmune disorders, infections, and medications. Our case report features of a patient with a history of idiopathic thrombocytopenic purpura and thrombotic thrombocytopenic purpura, who developed a recurrence of TTP 5 days after his first dose of the mRNA Coronavirus disease 2019 (COVID-19) vaccine (mRNA-1273 vaccine) in the setting of recent COVID-19. The close temporal association between vaccine administration, recent COVID-19, and relapse of remitted TTP raises concern for an enhanced immune reaction to COVID-19 vaccine in the setting of recent COVID-19 and underlying autoimmune disease. The association is not absolute, but given the novelty of COVID-19 and the mRNA COVID-19 vaccine and the relapse timing, it leads us to pose this hypothesis. Vaccine distribution to a larger and more diverse population will allow for an increased rate of adverse event reporting. This case report exemplifies potential safety issues that may be encountered with new vaccine administration in patients with recent COVID-19 and underlying autoimmune disease. There are no specific recommendations for COVID-19 vaccine administration in such patients.

1. Introduction

Thrombotic thrombocytopenic purpura (TTP) is a potentially life-threatening consumptive coagulopathy requiring emergent diagnosis and timely treatment. It is characterized by microangiopathic hemolytic anemia and thrombocytopenia with the development of microthrombi caused by severely reduced activity of the von Willebrand factor-cleaving protease ADAMTS13 and resulting end-organ damage. The central nervous system is commonly affected and may manifest with mental status or functional neurologic changes. Renal involvement may lead to cardiac manifestations associated with volume overload or arrhythmogenic electrolyte abnormalities. TTP is a result of an inherited or acquired quantitative or functional deficiency of ADAMTS13. Our case report features a patient with a history of idiopathic thrombocytopenic purpura and thrombotic thrombocytopenic purpura, who developed a recurrence of TTP 5 days after his first dose of the Moderna mRNA COVID-19 vaccine (mRNA-1273 vaccine). The FDA issued an Emergency Use Authorization for the Moderna mRNA COVID-19 vaccine on December 18, 2020. It is a novel vaccine type that has demonstrated 94.1% efficacy at preventing COVID-19 in an ongoing phase 3 clinical trial. Vaccine distribution to a more extensive and more diverse population will allow for an increased rate of adverse event reporting.

2. Case Description

The patient is a 48-year-old Caucasian male who presented complaining of acute-onset, transient right-sided weakness and slurred speech lasting approximately 30 minutes in addition to paresthesia five days after his first dose of COVID-19 mRNA vaccine (Moderna mRNA-1273 vaccine). The patient did not have headache, dyspnea, fever, or visual changes. Vitals were within the normal range. The patient had a normal cardiopulmonary exam, and his neurological exam was intact with complete recovery of transient symptoms. Examination of the skin and mucosa did not show any petechiae, purpura, or active bleeding. He denied any recent medication use, illness, or chemical exposure. The patient's past medical history was significant for diabetes mellitus type 2 on insulin, refractory thrombotic thrombocytopenic purpura (TTP), idiopathic thrombocytopenic purpura (ITP), and COVID-19 2 months before his presentation, which did not require hospitalization. His medical records elucidated that he had a diagnosis of TTP for eight years, a total of 4 episodes in the past for which he was treated with plasmapheresis, steroids, and rituximab. Further treatment options were not initiated since the patient was lost to follow-up in between his relapses. He was also diagnosed with ITP 5 years ago, which was treated with steroids and rituximab. The patient was reported to have normal platelet counts (130.000/uL) approximately three months before the presentation. Family history was nonpertinent. He denied consumption of alcohol, tobacco, or recreational drugs. The patient denied taking any home medications.

On the day of presentation, laboratory results were significant for hemolytic anemia with hemoglobin 8.8 g/dL, 2–3 schistocytes/hpf on peripheral blood smear, haptoglobin<10 mg/dL, total bilirubin 5.0 with indirect bilirubin predominance, lactate dehydrogenase (LDH) 884 U/L, D-dimer 1.45 ug/mFEU, fibrinogen 417 mg/dL, and platelet count 10 × 103/dL (baseline platelet count of 130 × 103/dL). Noncontrast head CT was performed given acute transient neurologic symptoms which did not reveal any hemorrhage, mass effect, or ischemic process. The constellation of hemolytic anemia, thrombocytopenia, and transient neurological symptoms was concerning for a TTP relapse. The PLASMIC score used to predict ADAMTS13 deficiency in suspected TTP patients was 7 points showing that the patient is at high risk of having severe ADAMTS13 deficiency, thus requiring emergent plasmapheresis. ADAMTS13 activity later resulted as <3%, while ADAMTS13 inhibitor was 6.6 BEU (normal <0.4). Meanwhile, the patient's COVID-19 PCR test was negative. High-dose glucocorticoids were immediately administered, and fresh frozen plasma was used for bridging to urgent plasmapheresis. The patient had a full recovery after a 10-day course of plasmapheresis in addition to glucocorticoids and rituximab. The patient was to complete outpatient rituximab therapy and steroid tapering with hematology follow-up on discharge. His platelet and hemoglobin count was normalized on the day of discharge. The second dose of the COVID-19 vaccine was deferred.

3. Discussion

TTP is a result of an inherited or acquired quantitative or functional deficiency of ADAMTS13. Acquired TTP is characterized by severe ADAMTS13 deficiency (typically, activity <10 percent) due to an inhibitor (autoantibody) directed against ADAMTS13; patients with inherited ADAMTS13 mutations are referred to as having hereditary TTP. Reduction in ADAMTS13 activity leads to the accumulation of von Willebrand factor multimers followed by an increase in platelet aggregation and thrombotic microangiopathy. The disease manifests with thrombocytopenia, mechanical hemolysis, anemia, renal failure, neurologic impairment, and fever. Acquired TTP diagnosis is confirmed when ADAMTS13 activity is <10%. ADAMTS13 assay typically requires days and, thus, is not an actionable measure and instead acts as a confirmatory test. Acute diagnosis relies on clinical presentation and laboratory data. Laboratory data demonstrate thrombocytopenia, microangiopathic hemolytic anemia (anemia in conjunction with lab values of cell lysis: elevated LDH, decreased haptoglobin, and indirect hyperbilirubinemia), reticulocytosis, and peripheral smear with schistocytes. The platelet-rich microvascular thrombi lead to organ hypoperfusion. In our case, as we had a high suspicion for TTP initially given the past medical history of TTP, hemolytic anemia with thrombocytopenia with neurologic symptoms, we initiated plasmapheresis without waiting ADAMTS13 levels. We confirmed the diagnosis with low ADAMTS13 levels which were withdrawn before plasmapheresis. MRI of the brain was not obtained as the neurologic symptoms were transient and resolved entirely once the underlying etiology improved. Of note, per documentation, our patient had past medical history of ITP, which was not deemed as the etiology of his presentation at this time given hallmarks of thrombotic microangiopathic anemia and low levels of ADAMTS13 levels. Concomitant ITP with TTP is a rare phenomenon, per the patient's external medical records, and he had ITP in the past; however, we did not have adequate data to confirm.

The timing of TTP identification and treatment determines disease mortality. The PLASMIC score predicts disease severity and potential response to plasmapheresis [1]. Treatment primarily involves plasmapheresis, steroids, and rituximab. Plasmapheresis removes circulating autoantibodies while also supplying functionally active ADAMTS13. Steroids suppress the immune system. Relapsing TTP is defined as thrombocytopenia and increased LDH that persists despite 5–7 plasmapheresis sessions [2]. Rituximab, a monoclonal anti-CD20 antibody, results in B-cell depletion and has been shown to reduce the rate of TTP recurrence. Caplacizumab is an anti-VWF antibody fragment that has been shown to normalize platelet count faster with shorter hospitalization, fewer plasmapheresis sessions, and lower rates of composite death, recurrence, and major thromboembolic events compared with placebo [2].

Although the exact etiology is unknown, acquired TTP can be triggered by bacterial and viral infections, pregnancy, malignancy, and medications (including quinine, cyclosporine, and mitomycin C). In the literature, only few publications reported vaccination-induced TTP [3–8]. Vaccinations can rarely induce autoimmune reactions including acquired TTP. According to these case reports, TTP occurred within 2 weeks after vaccination, mostly with influenza vaccination ($n = 3$), followed by vaccines against pneumococcus ($n = 1$), rabies ($n = 1$), and H1N1 ($n = 1$). To date, COVID-19 vaccination associated is present in the literature. Literature is evolving for COVID-19 coagulopathy; although the mechanism is still unclear, COVID-19 promotes a hypercoagulable state with wide-spectrum clinical manifestations. According to a recent literature review, four cases of TTP related to COVID-19 were described [9]. Three of the four patients had plasmapheresis with steroids. However, one of them could not have plasmapheresis due to logistics but responded well to fresh frozen plasma and IVIG therapy. Two of the cases required rituximab therapy as full recovery was not achieved with plasmapheresis. The literature review demonstrated two TTP cases related to mRNA COVID-19 vaccine administration without any hematologic disorders and a possible trigger for TTP occurrence. A case of TTP with a 62-year-old female without any hematologic disease was identified after 37 days of Ad26.COV2-S administration was seen, treated with plasmapheresis and high-dose steroids, and the outcome was not reported. Another case was a 38-year-old woman with a de novo iTTP, two weeks after exposure to BNT-162b2, who was successfully treated with plasma exchange, corticosteroids, rituximab, and caplacizumab.

Our patient's COVID-19 test resulted positive via nasopharyngeal swab PCR, two months before COVID-19 vaccination. At the time of the COVID-19 infection, he was asymptomatic and quarantined for 14 days. In the COVID mRNA-1273 trial [10], 2.3% in the mRNA-1273 group demonstrated serologic and/or virologic evidence of SARS-CoV-2 infection prior to vaccination. The primary endpoint of the study was to determine efficacy in preventing symptomatic COVID-19 in those without prior infection. Although neutralizing antibody titers (SARS-CoV-2 spike IgG) have been measured after vaccination to assess appropriate response, B and T (CD4+ and CD8+) memory cells may be more important in those with previous infection [11, 12]. Participants with prior infection who received mRNA vaccine tended to have a more robust and uniform antibody response to the first dose [13]. In contrast, there was no increase in antibody response to the second dose. The intensity of antibody production in previously infected individuals seems to reflect heightened reactogenicity to the mRNA vaccine. Reactogenicity was higher in those with preexisting immunity, as systemic side effects (fatigue, headache, chills, muscle pain, fever, and joint pain) occurred more frequently [13]. In TTP, this level of immune system stimulation may have led to anti-ADAMTS13 autoantibody production. The interval between infection and vaccination was approximately two months in this case. Most studies have started vaccine administration 30 to 60 days after seropositive status. Measuring antibody titer before vaccination may help inform vaccine schedule, as immunogenic potential may depend on this. However, immunologic response to infection may vary based on viral load and other individual factors and, thus, is unpredictable. Our patient exemplifies recurrence of TTP after COVID-19 mRNA vaccination in the setting of recent COVID-19. Given the lack of any other possible trigger, including sepsis, HIV, malignancy, and medications, we pose that COVID-19 vaccination shortly after COVID-19 caused a relapse of TTP. Considering the patient's COVID-19 two months before vaccination, enhanced immune response after the vaccination might have resulted in a relapse of the underlying autoimmune disorder.

Widespread vaccination against COVID-19 will be playing a key role in fighting the ongoing pandemic. Meanwhile, vaccine administration to a more extensive and more diverse population will allow for adverse event reporting. This case report exemplifies potential safety issues encountered with new vaccine administration in patients, especially shortly after COVID-19 with underlying autoimmune disease.

Consent

The patient's written consent was obtained for publication.

References

[1] P. K. Bendapudi, S. Hurwitz, A. Fry et al., "Derivation and external validation of the PLASMIC score for rapid assessment of adults with thrombotic microangiopathies: a cohort study," *The Lancet Haematology*, vol. 4, no. 4, pp. e157–e164, 2017.

[2] R. Kalpatthi and J. E. Kiss, "Thrombotic thrombocytopenic purpura, heparin-induced thrombocytopenia, and disseminated intravascular coagulation," *Critical Care Clinics*, vol. 36, no. 2, pp. 357–377, 2020.

[3] G. Kadikoylu, I. Yavasoglu, and Z. Bolaman, "Rabies vaccine-associated thrombotic thrombocytopenic purpura," *Transfusion Medicine*, vol. 24, no. 6, pp. 428-429, 2014.

[4] Y. Kojima, H. Ohashi, T. Nakamura et al., "Acute thrombotic thrombocytopenic purpura after pneumococcal vaccination," *Blood Coagulation and Fibrinolysis*, vol. 25, no. 5, pp. 512–514, 2014.

[5] N. Ramakrishnan and L. P. Parker, "Thrombotic thrombocytopenic purpura following influenza vaccination—a brief case report," *Connecticut Medicine*, vol. 62, no. 10, pp. 587-588, 1998.

[6] P. J. Dias and S. Gopal, "Refractory thrombotic thrombocytopenic purpura following influenza vaccination," *Anaesthesia*, vol. 64, no. 4, pp. 444–446, 2009.

[7] R. Hermann, A. Pfeil, M. Busch et al., "Schwerste thrombotisch-thrombozytopenische Purpura (TTP) nach H1N1-Vakzinierung," *Medizinische Klinik*, vol. 105, no. 9, pp. 663–668, 2010.

[8] R. C. Brown, T. E. Blecher, E. A. French, and P. J. Toghill, "Thrombotic thrombocytopenic purpura after influenza vaccination," *BMJ*, vol. 2, no. 5861, p. 303, 1973.

[9] H. A. Tehrani, M. Darnahal, M. Vaezi, and S. Haghighi, "COVID-19 associated thrombotic thrombocytopenic purpura (TTP); A case series and mini-review," *International Immunopharmacology*, vol. 93, Article ID 107397, 2021.

[10] L. R. Baden, H. M. El Sahly, B. Essink et al., "Efficacy and safety of the mRNA-1273 SARS-CoV-2 vaccine," *New England Journal of Medicine*, vol. 384, no. 5, pp. 403–416, 2021.
[11] A. Sette and S. Crotty, "Adaptive immunity to SARS-CoV-2 and COVID-19," *Cell*, vol. 184, no. 4, pp. 861–880, 2021.
[12] F. Krammer, K. Srivastava, H. Alshammary et al., "Antibody responses in seropositive persons after a single dose of SARS-CoV-2 mRNA vaccine," *New England Journal of Medicine*, vol. 384, no. 14, pp. 1372–1374, 2021.
[13] A. T. Widge, N. G. Rouphael, L. A. Jackson et al., "Durability of responses after SARS-CoV-2 mRNA-1273 vaccination," *New England Journal of Medicine*, vol. 384, no. 1, pp. 80–82, 2021.

8

A Rapid and Satisfactory Outcome with Combined Immunosuppressive Therapy in Acquired Haemophilia A with Underlying Tuberculosis

G. A. C. Gamakaranage,[1] C. Kulathilake,[1] P. G. N. Nadeeshani,[2] K. H. B. P. Fernandopulle,[1] C. S. Moonesinghe,[1] D. Gunawardena,[1] R. S. Gamage,[1] N. Perera,[3] and J. Indrakumar[3]

[1]*Department of Pathology, Faculty of Medical Sciences, University of Sri Jayewardenepura, Nugegoda, Sri Lanka*
[2]*Professorial Medical Unit, Colombo South Teaching Hospital, Dehiwala-Mount Lavinia, Sri Lanka*
[3]*Department of Medicine, Faculty of Medical Sciences, University of Sri Jayewardenepura, Nugegoda, Sri Lanka*

Correspondence should be addressed to G. A. C. Gamakaranage; chamani@med.sab.ac.lk

Academic Editor: Kostas Konstantopoulos

Acquired haemophilia A (AHA) is a rare disorder with an incidence of 1.5 cases per million per year in the United Kingdom. The incidence could be underestimated due to difficulty in diagnosis and also due to the fact that people with low titre inhibitor levels are asymptomatic. It is usually a disease affecting elderly but a disease peak in the younger population is known. The common underlying diseases are autoimmune disorders, malignancies, infections, and drugs. However, approximately 50% of the cases do not have a specific aetiology and about 10% will not have bleeding manifestations. Therefore, an isolated prolongation of APTT should be evaluated, especially prior to any haemostatic challenges. We report a case of a middle-aged man who presented with bleeding due to AHA associated with high inhibitory titres and active pulmonary tuberculosis. He was treated with both antituberculous and combined-aggressive immunosuppressive therapy which resulted in satisfactory disease remission.

1. Introduction

Acquired haemophilia A (AHA) is a rare disorder with an incidence of 1.5 per million per year in the United Kingdom [1]. The incidence of these cases in Sri Lanka is not known. The number of reported cases could be underestimated due to difficulty in diagnosis and the fact that people with low titre inhibitor levels do not have bleeding manifestations. It is usually a disease affecting the elderly population. However, a peak incidence in the younger population is recognized. The main underlying aetiologies are autoimmune disorders, malignancies, infections, and drugs [1]. AHA can be very rarely seen during the initial postpartum period [1, 2]. Approximately 50% of the cases do not have a specific aetiology and about 10% will not have bleeding manifestations [1]. Therefore, an isolated prolongation of APTT should be evaluated, especially prior to any haemostatic challenges.

Acquired haemophilia occurs due to acquired coagulation inhibitors resulting in an immune-mediated depletion or inhibition of a coagulation factor, most commonly directed against coagulation factor VIII (FVIII) [1]. Unlike FVIII inhibitors formed in congenital haemophilia A (alloantibodies against factor VIII concentrates), acquired inhibitors (auto antibodies) show complex second order kinetics with incomplete inhibition which results in some level of residual FVIII activity, which can be detected in the laboratory but does not correlate with severity of clinical bleeding [3]. AHA has a significant mortality of 8%–42%, and 3–12% of deaths are caused by effects of immunosuppression resulting in infection and 3–8% due to bleeding [1].

Bruising, retroperitoneal, muscle, gastrointestinal, and urogenital bleeding are common in AHA, but haemarthrosis is uncommon in contrast to congenital haemophilia A [1]. The management of AHA includes effective control of bleeding manifestations, elimination of the inhibitor, and treatment of any underlying aetiology to cure the disease. As such, AHA requires an individualized therapeutic approach [1].

2. Case History

A 46 year old man presented with a 7 month history of episodic pain and swelling of left knee joint, nocturnal fever, productive cough, loss of appetite, and on and off painful erythematous skin nodules on arms and legs. He was a known patient with type 2 diabetes mellitus who was not receiving proper treatment. He was a smoker and admitted to excessive alcohol consumption. He was not taking any long-term medication. On examination, he was averagely built with a swollen, warm, and tender left knee joint with restricted movements. There were tender subcutaneous nodules over the left arm and right thigh, compatible with a clinical diagnosis of erythema nodosum. He also had finger clubbing and bilateral cervical and axillary lymphadenopathy but no hepatosplenomegaly or organomegaly, and the rest of the examination was essentially normal.

His initial investigations revealed a normochromic normocytic anaemia with haemoglobin of 84 g/L, moderate rouleaux formation, normal platelet, and white cell count with neutrophil predominance. The blood picture showed evidence of an infective or inflammatory process. His inflammatory markers were elevated, with a CRP of 42 mg/L and an erythrocyte sedimentation rate (ESR) of 138 mm/1st hour.

Renal and liver profiles were normal apart from hypoalbuminaemia with reversed albumin globulin ratio. Lactate dehydrogenase level (LDH) was elevated (398.4 U/L). His chest radiograph revealed prominent bilateral hilar lymphadenopathy. Contrast-enhanced computed tomography (CECT) of the abdomen and chest revealed multiple discrete lymphadenopathy in the bilateral axillae, cervical, hilar, paratracheal, subcarinal, and para-aortic regions. Additionally, the high-resolution computed tomography chest revealed paraseptal emphysema, fibrosis, a thick-walled cavity in the right upper lobe apical segment with a ground glass appearance, and a patchy consolidation in the left lingual region. Findings were more suggestive of an infective pathology than sarcoidosis. Mantoux test was 13 mm and sputum was thrice negative for acid fast bacilli initially. At this point, the patient defaulted on follow-up for 3 months until he presented to the medical casualty with severe pain and swelling of the left knee joint and painful subcutaneous nodules on the legs and arms. The joint aspirate was blood stained and subsequently diagnosed as haemarthrosis. A skin biopsy was done for the skin nodules as well, for which he developed delayed bleeding from the biopsy site.

A coagulation screen was performed, which revealed an isolated prolongation of activated partial thromboplastin time (APTT) of 139 seconds with normal prothrombin time, thrombin time, and fibrinogen levels. Further inquiry revealed no family history of bleeding tendency, but his episodic left knee joint swelling over the past few months was suggestive of recurrent haemarthrosis.

A detailed coagulation work-up was done at this time. APTT mixing test with pooled normal plasma (PNP) revealed uncorrected APTT and that the FVIII and factor IX levels were markedly low at 0.3% and 0.006%, respectively. Factor XI was undetectable. The inhibitor assay showed a very high titre of FVIII inhibitor of >1000 Bethesda units (BU).

A diagnosis of AHA was made, and a possible aetiology was sought. An autoimmune screen revealed weakly positive antinuclear antibodies, but double-stranded DNA and rheumatoid factor were negative.

With a strong suspicion of active tuberculosis, the CECT chest and abdomen were repeated which revealed a cavity with a tree in bud appearance in the right upper lobe with a progressive right hilar lymphadenopathy suggestive of active pulmonary tuberculosis with bronchogenic spread. His fourth and fifth sputum samples were positive for acid-fast bacilli which confirmed pulmonary tuberculosis. An APL antibody screen was done which revealed weakly positive DRVVT, moderately positive antibeta 2 glycoprotein IgM (53.8 U/L), and a weakly positive anticardiolipin IgM levels. Repeat testing after 3-months confirmed the persistence of APL antibodies with a moderately positive DRVVT.

A final diagnosis of AHA due to a possible underlying autoimmune disease in the background of active pulmonary tuberculosis was made. It was not clear whether pulmonary tuberculosis contributed to autoimmunity. However, the coexistence of secondary APS was still considered due to the persistence of APL antibodies.

Patient had several bleeding episodes involving the left knee joint and the right elbow joint. He also developed a gluteal muscle haematoma and all bleeding manifestations were successfully managed with recombinant factor VIIa (r FVIIa) infusions and tranexamic acid. Following a multidisciplinary meeting, antituberculous drugs (ATD) for pulmonary tuberculosis were started. Concurrent immunosuppression therapy commenced with high dose steroids including initial intravenous methyl prednisolone followed by oral prednisolone. After a period of 10 weeks, oral cyclophosphamide 100 mg daily was added while tapering off oral steroids as the APTT was persistently prolonged with poor response. With cyclophosphamide, APTT was reduced to 50 s and the inhibitor titre came down to 700 BU. He responded well to ATD, with clinical improvement, a declining ESR, and clearance of the initial findings on his repeat CECTs.

Unfortunately, the patient developed transaminitis during this time of high-dose cyclophosphamide therapy and ATD therapy requiring drug withdrawal. Interruption of cyclophosphamide therapy resulted in several episodes of bleeding (haemarthrosis and epistaxis) which required aggressive factor replacement therapy. As he had almost completed 11 months of therapy, ATD was also discontinued at the same time.

At this point, a combined-aggressive immunosuppression therapy was started with rituximab, high-dose oral prednisolone and low-dose cyclophosphamide, with close monitoring of liver functions aimed at disease remission.

He showed a dramatic response just after the third dose of rituximab with normalization of APTT with both lupus sensitive and insensitive reagents and normalization of ESR after completion of rituximab 4 doses.

He was given low-dose (50 mg daily) therapy with cyclophosphamide which was continued for another 6 months, and prednisolone was tailed off slowly with monthly monitoring of APTT, ESR, and liver functions.

Subsequent regular assessments showed persistently normal APTT with both lupus-sensitive and insensitive reagents and normalized ESR with a normal FVIII level (70%) and factor IX (90%). But we could not perform the Factor XI levels due to resource constraints at that time.

A repeat APL screen with DRVVT was still positive which confirmed the persistence of APL antibodies. We considered this could more likely to be due to secondary APS with an underlying, undetermined autoimmune disorder than tuberculosis which had been completely treated by that time.

3. Discussion

We present a complicated case of AHA with concurrent active tuberculosis and the persistent presence of APL antibodies. We suspected that these autoantibodies could be due to tuberculosis or an underlying autoimmune disorder.

The occurrence of autoantibodies in active tuberculosis has been described. A randomized case-control study done in Taiwan found that a significant proportion of patients (32%) with active TB in endemic areas have elevated autoantibody titres, especially anticardiolipin IgG and anti-Scl70 which do not associate with the typical manifestations of the particular autoimmune disease. As these autoantibodies decrease or normalize in titres with the control of TB, it is suggested that they do not require any immunosuppressant therapy [4]. There are reported cases of AHA in patients with tuberculosis in the literature where the acquired inhibitor has been successfully eradiated with ATD alone [4, 5, 9, 10]. With the presence of an abnormally high titre of inhibitory levels with a recurrent bleeding in this patient, he required strong combined immunosuppression therapy from the beginning [12].

An unusually high titre of inhibitor of FVIII detected in the Bethesda assay and a very low FVIII level despite no spontaneous bleeding initially could be due to the assay interference of these APL antibodies. This could have been overcome if we used a lupus insensitive reagent to perform the Bethesda assay and a lupus insensitive reagent or a chromogenic assay to do the factor assay. The presence of active TB and uncontrolled diabetes were significant concerns to start strong immunosuppressive therapy in our patient initially. However, regardless of many challenges such as interrupted immunosuppressive therapy due to hepatotoxicity, the continuation of uninterrupted ATD for 11 months cured his TB. But the inhibitory status and the APL antibodies persisted, indicating that autoimmunity was probably not due to tuberculosis.

He was a good candidate for combined immunosuppressive therapy with rituximab, as he had a very high inhibitory titre [12, 13]. With the completion of 4 doses of rituximab, he showed a good response having a normalized APTT with both lupus sensitive and insensitive reagents and a good clinical improvement as well.

We did not consider thromboprophylaxis for him considering the presence of APL antibodies during remission due to several reasons. His FVIII level was not high initially (70%), and he was not compliant in taking anticoagulants. He will be further assessed with a repeat factor assay and DRVVT along with risk assessment for thrombosis during follow-up.

4. Conclusion

Even though AHA is a rare disease, it is challenging to manage affected patients who have high mortality and morbidity. Management is further difficult in a low-resource country as AHA requires costly haemostatic therapy and laboratory investigations.

Prompt evaluation, diagnosis, effective timely management of bleeding episodes, and appropriate individualized therapy to eradicate the inhibitor are essential to achieve a good outcome. This case needed a multidisciplinary approach with the involvement of a haematologist, physician, respiratory specialist, radiologist, and laboratory expertise for timely decision-making and to deliver an effective and comprehensive treatment for a successful story.

The dramatic response seen with combined immunosuppressive therapy with rituximab highlights that prompt and appropriate therapy is lifesaving in this rare disease.

Abbreviations

AHA: Acquired haemophilia A
APTT: Activated partial thromboplastin time
ATD: Antituberculous drugs
BU: Bethesda unit
CECT: Contrast-enhanced computed tomogram
HRCT: High-resolution computed tomogram
MDT: Multidisciplinary team.

Consent

The authors have obtained the informed written consent from the patient to report and publish the clinical details anonymously.

Authors' Contributions

Gamakaranage G.A.C was involved in diagnosing, managing, monitoring of the patient, and writing the manuscript.

Kulathilake C, Moonesinghe CS, NP, and JI were involved in diagnosing, managing, monitoring the patient, and preparing the manuscript for publication. Fernandopulle KHBP, Gunawardena D, Gamage RS and Nadeeshani PGN were involved in diagnosing, managing, monitoring of the patient, and editing the manuscript. All authors read and approved the final manuscript.

Acknowledgments

Coagulation laboratory services provided by -Haematology Laboratory–National Hospital of Sri Lanka (NHSL) and Medical Research Institute (MRI) Sri Lanka. Respiratory physician at Colombo South Teaching Hospital (Dr M.N.M. Masaima) and the team for their contribution in diagnostic work up and management.

References

[1] P. W. Collins, E. Chalmers, D. Hart et al., "Diagnosis and management of acquired coagulation inhibitors: a guideline from UKHCDO," *British Journal of Haematology*, vol. 162, 2013.

[2] Medscape, "Medscape reference," 2022, https://reference.medscape.com/.

[3] S. Kitchen, A. McCraw, and M. Echenagucia, *Diagnosis of Hemophilia and Other Bleeding Disorders A LABORATORY MANUAL*, World Federation of Hemophilia, Montreal, Canada, 2010.

[4] C. Y. Shen, S. C. Hsieh, C. L. Yu, J. Y. Wang, L. N. Lee, and C. J. Yu, "Autoantibody prevalence in active tuberculosis: reactive or pathognomonic?" *BMJ Open*, vol. 3, no. 7, Article ID e002665, 2013.

[5] F. Yang, Y. S. Zhou, and Y. Jia, "[Systemic lupus erythematosus with acquired hemophilia A: a case report]," *Beijing Da Xue Xue Bao*, vol. 50, no. 6, pp. 1108–1111, 2018.

[6] S. Seethala, N. P. J. Collins, and G. J. Comerci, "An unusual etiology for elevation of activated partial thromboplastin time (aPTT) in SLE: acquired hemophilia and lupus anticoagulant," *Case Reports in Hematology*, vol. 2013, pp. 1–3, 2013.

[7] Z. Khodamoradi, M. A. Nazarinia, and S. Bazdar, "Acquired hemophilia as initial presentation in a patient with systemic lupus erythematosus," *Current Rheumatology Reviews*, vol. 13, no. 3, pp. 236–238, 2017.

[8] A. R. Z. Zaidi, M. AlSheef, I. H. Motabi, S. Z. A. Zaidi, and I. K. Tailor, "Systemic lupus erythematosus presenting as hematoma of the hand due to acquired inhibitors to factor VIII: early and prolonged remission achieved with upfront rituximab," *Cureus*, vol. 11, Article ID e4786, 2019.

[9] O. Elkayam, D. Bendayan, R. Segal et al., "The effect of antituberculosis treatment on levels of anti-phospholipid and anti-neutrophil cytoplasmatic antibodies in patients with active tuberculosis," *Rheumatology International*, vol. 33, pp. 949–953, 2012.

[10] J. G. Duque Ortega and J. G. Ortega, "Acquired hemophilia and tuberculosis: case report and literature review," *Hematology & Transfusion International Journal*, vol. 5, no. 5, pp. 315–317, 2017.

[11] I. Takenami, C. C. de Oliveira, J. D. Petrilli, A. Machado, L. W. Riley, and S. Arruda, "Serum antiphospholipid antibody levels as biomarkers for diagnosis of pulmonary tuberculosis patients," *International Journal of Tuberculosis & Lung Disease*, vol. 22, no. 9, pp. 1063–1070, 2018.

[12] A. Tiede, P. Collins, P. Knoebl et al., "International recommendations on the diagnosis and treatment of acquired hemophilia A," *Haematologica*, vol. 105, no. 7, pp. 1791–1801, 2020.

[13] R. Kruse-Jarres, C. L. Kempton, F. Baudo et al., "Acquired hemophilia A: updated review of evidence and treatment guidance," *American Journal of Hematology Hematol*, vol. 92, no. 7, pp. 695–705, 2017.

9

A Curious Case of Hemolytic Anemia with Pseudoreticulopenia

Scott Mayer,[1] **Nikhilesh Srinivasan**,[1] **Jenny Nguyen**,[2] **Ryan Spilman**,[1] **and Dmitriy Scherbak**[1]

[1]*HCA HealthONE, Lone Tree, CO, USA*
[2]*Rocky Vista University School of Osteopathic Medicine, Lone Tree, CO, USA*

Correspondence should be addressed to Scott Mayer; scott.mayer736@gmail.com

Academic Editor: Kostas Konstantopoulos

Herein, we present a unique case of a Coombs-negative, steroid-refractory autoimmune hemolytic anemia (AIHA) complicated by pseudoreticulopenia, describe its clinical presentation, histopathologic findings, and management, and review the salient literature. Coombs-negative, steroid-refractory AIHAs represent fewer than 1% of all AIHAs. Diagnosis of the disease is difficult and often delayed due to the pursuit of alternate diagnoses following a negative Coombs test. However, when suspicion remains high for an autoimmune process, the super-Coombs test may be utilized for the diagnosis of AIHA that the traditional Coombs test fails to detect. A majority of cases respond to rituximab as the indicated second-line therapy, but delays in diagnosis and subsequent treatment may increase morbidity. Reticulopenia may be associated with AIHAs secondary to bone marrow dysfunction, but this patient had a normal function marrow confirmed on biopsy. Indeed, reticulopenia in this case was a diagnostic conundrum that further obscured the diagnosis and delayed treatment. Ultimately, reticulopenia was determined to be pseudoreticulopenia secondary to an alteration in the maturation of the erythroid lineage due to an independent, newly diagnosed pernicious anemia. The interaction of these multiple coexisting disease processes is not previously described in the literature. Increased physician awareness of steroid-refractory, Coombs-negative AIHA, and the development of pseudoreticulopenia as a laboratory finding in pernicious anemia may help to improve patient outcomes.

1. Introduction

Coombs-negative, steroid-refractory autoimmune hemolytic anemias (AIHAs) are rare, accounting for fewer than 1% of AIHAs. We present a case that meets these criteria and is further complicated by a reduced reticulocyte index despite a functioning bone marrow secondary to newly diagnosed pernicious anemia. A total of 20 cases of simultaneous AIHA and PA are reported in the literature [1]. To our knowledge, this is the first reported case of Coombs-negative, steroid-refractory AIHA with a simultaneous PA.

2. Case Presentation

A previously healthy 28-year-old male with the medical history of hypothyroidism presented to an outside hospital with progressive nausea, vomiting, fatigue, exercise intolerance, jaundice, and dark urine for the previous 10 days. Hgb was 3.8 g/dL, and the patient was transferred to an HCA Healthcare Facility in Denver, Colorado, for hematology consultation.

Initial laboratory values were consistent with normocytic hemolytic anemia. Total bilirubin was elevated with a normal direct bilirubin. Haptoglobin was less than 1.0 mg/dL. Lactate dehydrogenase was greater than 600 U/L. MCV was 94.6 fL. Reticulocyte was 3.5% with a reticulocyte index equal to 0.35. Multiple direct and indirect Coombs tests were negative. Peripheral blood smear was reviewed by pathology without pertinent abnormalities. Vitamin B12 was 301 pg/mL. Methylmalonic acid was 187 nmol/L. Homocysteine was 11.3 μmol/L. Three fecal occult blood tests returned negative, and computed tomography imaging was negative for any signs of bleeding. Viral serologies including hepatitis A, B, and C, CMV, EBV, HSV, HIV, and parvovirus were negative. Immunologic work-up including IgG subtype levels, cryoglobulins, rheumatoid factor, cyclic citrullinated peptide, CD55 and CD59, double-stranded DNA, and complement C3 and C4 were all within normal limits. The patient's antiintrinsic factor antibody returned positive. The remainder of the laboratory values was unremarkable. Abdominal ultrasound revealed splenomegaly to 17.6 cm.

Concurrently, the patient was hemolyzing rapidly requiring 1-2 units of packed red blood cells per day. The patient's reduced reticulocyte index prompted investigation for a marrow-mediated process. Abdominal positron emission tomography/computed tomography was negative for focal areas of tracer uptake, and bone marrow biopsy was mildly hypercellular with erythroid hyperplasia and <1% blasts and no overt dysplasia. On hospital day 13, the patient's super-Coombs test returned positive and he was diagnosed with AIHA.

Whereas, the patient was initially treated with high-dose corticosteroids with no improvement. Upon diagnosis of AIHA via the super-Coombs test, the patient was started on 5 consecutive days of intravenous immunoglobulin and weekly infusions of rituximab for 4 weeks. The patient became transfusion-independent following his second dose of rituximab, and he completed his remaining infusions as an outpatient.

3. Discussion

AIHA is diagnosed traditionally with a direct antiglobulin Coombs test. At least 90% of AIHAs are Coombs-positive and another 90% will respond to steroids as the first-line treatment [2–5]. The patient of interest demonstrated all of the classic clinical characteristics of AIHA, but his condition was Coombs-negative, steroid-refractory, and had an unexplained reduced reticulocyte index.

The direct antiglobulin test (DAT) "Coombs test" used to confirm AIHA uses a commercial reagent to detect IgG and C3d on the surface of red blood cells [3, 6–9]. Negative tests may be triggered for several reasons, including IgG levels below threshold, an IgA mediated process, or a lack of complement fixation [3–5]. Coombs-negative AIHAs may be evaluated by further serologic testing or treated empirically if suspicion is high enough [5, 7].

Several studies have evaluated the use of flow cytometry (colloquially known as the super-Coombs test) in evaluating DAT-negative cases [6, 7, 10–12]. Flow cytometry-direct antiglobulin testing has a higher sensitivity than the column agglutination technique, the traditional method of conducting a Coombs test [4, 9–11]. A 2012 study found that flow cytometry could detect as few as 30–40 antibody molecules per red blood cell, which is significantly more sensitive than traditional column agglutination DAT that cannot detect values below 500 molecules [3, 10–12].

Despite an eventual diagnosis of AIHA using the super-Coombs test, this case remained a diagnostic conundrum due to an unexplained reduced reticulocyte index. Reduced reticulocyte indexes are associated with AIHAs due to marrow-mediated processes such as leukemias, lymphomas, and aplastic crisis [2, 6]. However, the patient's bone marrow biopsy confirmed appropriate erythroplasia and <1% blasts, consistent with a properly functioning marrow. The disconnection between the central and peripheral findings in the erythroid lineage could not be reconciled with a simple diagnosis of AIHA. Near discharge, an antiintrinsic factor antibody test returned positive. The presence of a simultaneous, newly diagnosed, pernicious anemia (PA) offers as a possible reconciliation for the patient's reduced reticulocyte index in setting of a functioning bone marrow [13, 14]. Of note, the patient's vitamin B12 levels were repleted empirically with no clinical improvement. He also had no history of anemia and did not present with a macrocytosis.

In a state of active hemolysis, the bone marrow releases reticulum-laden reticulocytes to replace lost RBCs. PA marks an exception to this rule; despite an appropriate erythroblastic response of the marrow, the reticulocyte index may remain low [13]. This is due to an alteration in the maturation process of young erythroid cells, such that the ample reticulum is lost prior to exiting the marrow [13]. Consequently, the erythroid cells released by the marrow are not reticulocytes and thus cannot be detected by standard laboratory reticulocyte assays. This altered maturation of red blood cells provides an explanation why, despite his properly functioning bone marrow, this patient had a reduced reticulocyte index [13].

Coexisting PA and AIHA may be stratified into two distinct categories: PA with a transiently positive AIHA and simultaneous primary AIHA and PA. PA with transiently positive AIHA is relatively common and marks low levels hemolysis due to ineffective hematopoiesis in patients with PA [1, 14, 15]. While a Coombs test is often negative, the AIHA will resolve with repletion of vitamin B12 deficiency, and the Coombs test, if initially positive, will turn negative with treatment [13, 14]. Our patient's hemolysis was persistent despite empiric repletion of vitamin B12 on presentation. In AIHA with simultaneous PA, the two processes are independent and the hemoglobin will not recover with vitamin B12 repletion, as it does not address the separate AIHA [14, 15]. Instead, immunosuppression is required for treatment [14]. The autoimmune connection between AIHA and PA is poorly understood. As is typical with other autoimmune disorders, individuals with one autoimmune disorder have a greater susceptibility to develop other autoimmune disorders [1].

Coombs-negative, steroid-refractory AIHAs represent <1% of AIHAs; this finding coupled with a simultaneous, newly diagnosed PA is not previously described in the literature. Key takeaways are that the super-Coombs test should be ordered when suspicion for AIHA remains high despite a negative Coombs test, and a reduced reticulocyte index in the setting of AIHA may not represent inadequacy of erythroid production if there is concomitant PA.

Acknowledgments

The authors would like to thank the HCA Healthcare Department of Graduate Medical Education for supporting research endeavors. This research was supported (in whole or in part) by HCA Healthcare and/or an HCA Healthcare affiliated entity.

References

[1] S. L. H. Yeruva, R. P. Manchandani, and P. Oneal, "Pernicious anemia with autoimmune hemolytic anemia: a case report and literature review," *Case Reports in Hematology*, vol. 2016, Article ID 7231503, 4 pages, 2016.

[2] U. Jäger, W. Barcellini, C. M. Broome et al., "Diagnosis and treatment of autoimmune hemolytic anemia in adults: recommendations from the first international consensus meeting," *Blood Reviews*, vol. 41, Article ID 100648, 2020.

[3] R. Kerr, P. S. M. Rawlinson, and P. G. Cachia, "Direct antiglobulin test negative, non spherocytic autoimmune haemolytic anaemia," *Clinical and Laboratory Haematology*, vol. 22, no. 6, pp. 365–367, 2000.

[4] G. B. Segel and M. A. Lichtman, "Direct antiglobulin ("Coombs") test-negative autoimmune hemolytic anemia: a review," *Blood Cells, Molecules, and Diseases*, vol. 52, no. 4, pp. 152–160, 2014.

[5] B. C. Gehrs and R. C. Friedberg, "Autoimmune hemolytic anemia," *American Journal of Hematology*, vol. 69, no. 4, pp. 258–271, 2002.

[6] Z. Wang, J. Shi, Y. Zhou, and C. Ruan, "Detection of red blood cell-bound immunoglobulin G by flow cytometry and its application in the diagnosis of autoimmune hemolytic anemia," *International Journal of Hematology*, vol. 73, no. 2, pp. 188–193, 2001.

[7] J. S. Lin, T. C. Hao, J. Y. Lyou et al., "Clinical application of a flow cytometric direct antiglobulin test," *Transfusion*, vol. 49, no. 7, pp. 1335–1346, 2009.

[8] R. J. Sokol, S. Hewitt, and B. K. Stamps, "Autoimmune haemolysis: an 18-year study of 865 cases referred to a regional transfusion centre," *British Medical Journal*, vol. 282, no. 6281, pp. 2023–2027, 1981.

[9] D. F. Stroncek, J. M. Njoroge, J. L. Procter, R. W. Childs, and J. Miller, "A preliminary comparison of flow cytometry and tube agglutination assays in detecting red blood cell associated C3d," *Transfusion Medicine*, vol. 13, no. 1, pp. 35–42, 2003.

[10] A. Thedsawad, O. Taka, and W. Wanachiwanawin, "Development of flow cytometry for detection and quantitation of red cell bound immunoglobulin G in autoimmune hemolytic anemia with negative direct Coombs test," *Asian Pacific Journal of Allergy & Immunology*, vol. 29, no. 4, pp. 364–367, 2011.

[11] M. H. Fayek, A. A. Saad, D. G. Eissa, L. M. Tawfik, and G. Kamal, "Role of gel test and flow cytometry in diagnosis of Coombs' negative autoimmune haemolytic anaemia," *International Journal of Literary Humanities*, vol. 34, no. 3, pp. 311–319, 2012.

[12] R. Chaudhary, S. S. Das, R. Gupta, and D. Khetan, "Application of flow cytometry in detection of red-cell-bound IgG in Coombs-negative AIHA," *Hematology*, vol. 11, no. 4, pp. 295–300, 2006.

[13] W. H. Crosby and H. Rappaport, "Reticulocytopenia in autoimmune hemolytic anemia," *Blood*, vol. 11, no. 10, pp. 929–936, 1956.

[14] A. P. Rabinowitz, Y. Sacks, and R. Carmel, "Autoimmune cytopenias in pernicious anemia: a report of four cases and review of the literature," *European Journal of Haematology*, vol. 44, no. 1, pp. 18–23, 2009.

[15] S. Zafad, A. Madani, M. Harif, A. Quessar, and S. Benchekroun, "Pernicious anemia associated with autoimmune hemolytic anemia and alopecia areata," *Pediatric Blood and Cancer*, vol. 49, no. 7, pp. 1017-1018, 2007.

10

Atypical Hemolytic Uremic Syndrome following Acute Type A Aortic Dissection

Eigo Ikushima,[1] **Manabu Hisahara**,[1] **Takuya Nishijima**,[1] **Hikaru Uchiyama**,[1] **Tatsushi Onzuka**,[1] **Yoshie Ochiai**,[1] **Tsuyoshi Muta**,[2] **and Shigehiko Tokunaga**[1]

[1]*Department of Cardiovascular Surgery, Japan Community Healthcare Organization (JCHO) Kyushu Hospital, 1-8-1, Kishinoura, Yahatanishi-ku, Kitakyushu, Fukuoka 806-8501, Japan*
[2]*Department of Hematology/Oncology, Japan Community Healthcare Organization (JCHO) Kyushu Hospital, 1-8-1, Kishinoura, Yahatanishi-ku, Kitakyushu, Fukuoka 806-8501, Japan*

Correspondence should be addressed to Eigo Ikushima; eigo@clnc.uoeh-u.ac.jp

Academic Editor: Marie-Christine Kyrtsonis

Atypical hemolytic uremic syndrome (aHUS) is a thrombotic microangiopathy (TMA)-related disease that manifests as a triad of microangiopathic hemolytic anemia, thrombocytopenia, and acute kidney injury (AKI) and is caused by uncontrolled activation of the complement system. We report the case of a 61-year-old woman with acute type A aortic dissection that subsequently developed into aHUS. The hematologic disorders underlying aHUS improved after treatment with the complement inhibitor eculizumab. It is important to consider aHUS when a patient clinically develops a triad of microangiopathic hemolytic anemia, thrombocytopenia, and an increasing creatinine level following cardiovascular surgery.

1. Introduction

Atypical hemolytic uremic syndrome (aHUS) is related to thrombotic microangiopathy (TMA) and is diagnosed by clinical presentation of a triad of microangiopathic hemolytic anemia, thrombocytopenia, and acute kidney injury (AKI) with negative results for Shiga-toxin-producing *Escherichia coli* (STEC), thrombotic thrombocytopenic purpura (TTP), and other TMA-related diseases, such as autoimmune diseases [1].

Aortic dissection develops due to tearing of the intima of the aorta and bleeding within the aortic wall, resulting in its dissection. The risk factors for aortic dissection are hypertension, dyslipidemia, or connective tissue disorder, such as Marfan syndrome. According to the Stanford classification, it is classified into type A and type B based on whether the ascending aorta is involved. Acute type A aortic dissection (ATAAD) is life-threatening and needs emergency open surgical repair. Despite emergency surgery, early mortality is approximately 20% [2]. Because ATAAD itself and surgical treatment, including cardiopulmonary bypass, induced hypothermia, or the lower body circulatory arrest technique, are highly invasive, bleeding could provoke anemia and thrombocytopenia, while malperfusion or surgical stress could provoke AKI. However, aHUS following ATAAD has not been reported. We report the first case of a 61-year-old woman with ATTAD who subsequently developed aHUS.

2. Case Presentation

A 61-year-old woman with a history of untreated hypertension presented to a local physician with sudden back pain. She was diagnosed with ATAAD using enhanced computed tomography (CT), which revealed the presence of a widespread patent false lumen from the sinus of Valsalva to the terminal abdominal aorta and poor enhancement of the left kidney (Figure 1). Transthoracic echocardiography revealed moderate aortic valve regurgitation (AR). She was transferred to our hospital. We performed total arch replacement

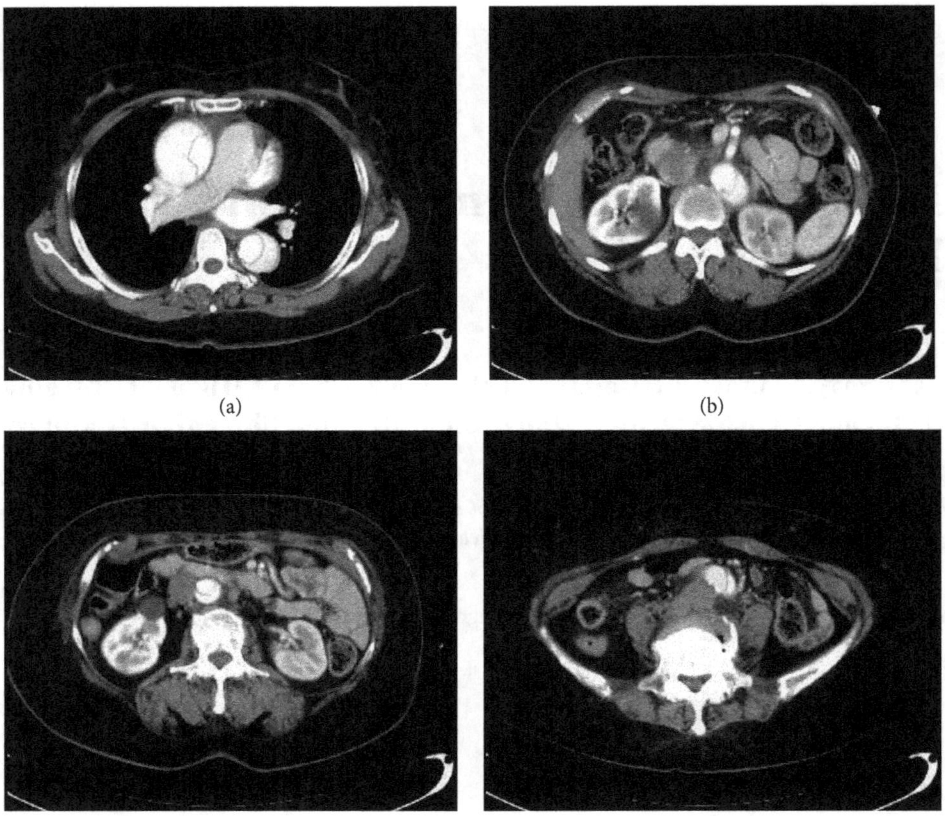

(a) (b) (c) (d)

FIGURE 1: Preoperative enhanced computed tomography (CT) image shows (a) acute type A aortic dissection, (b) superior mesenteric artery perfusion from the true lumen, (c) left kidney not well enhanced, and (d) dissected lumen extending to the terminal aorta.

and resuspension of the aortic valve commissures under hypothermia (lowest rectal temperature was 25.7°C) and the lower body circulatory arrest using cardiopulmonary bypass and selective cerebral perfusion. We transfused 6 units of red blood cells (RBC), 26 units of fresh frozen plasma (FFP), and 20 units of platelet concentrates (PC) during the surgery.

On postoperative day 1, the platelet count decreased from $116 \times 10^3/\mu l$ to $28 \times 10^3/\mu l$, and we transfused 20 units of PC. On postoperative day 2, her platelet count did not increase. On postoperative day 3, her platelet count further dropped to $8 \times 10^3/\mu l$, and her renal function worsened. On the same day, we confirmed schistocytes in her blood smear. Immediate consultations with the hematology team yielded a diagnosis of thrombotic microangiopathy (TMA), and we initiated plasma exchange (PE) and hemodialysis (HD). Therefore, we investigated for HUS and TTP as the major causes of TMA. Although PE increased the platelet count, renal function did not improve, and the schistocytes continued to increase. The tests for HUS and TTP were negative, and both these conditions were excluded. Furthermore, her medical history, physical examination, and laboratory data were not suggestive of other TMA-related diseases (Table 1). We diagnosed her with aHUS on postoperative day 14 and immediately started eculizumab treatment, following which, hemolytic anemia and thrombocytopenia improved without the need for further eculizumab or transfusion support. However, renal function did not recover, and maintenance hemodialysis was needed. Figure 2 shows the postoperative clinical course. Subsequently, the patient was transferred to another hospital for rehabilitation. One year postoperatively, she died of multiorgan failure.

3. Discussion and Conclusion

Patients presenting with triad of TMA, such as microangiopathic hemolytic anemia, thrombocytopenia, and AKI, and tests positive for STEC infection are diagnosed with HUS [3]. Conversely, patients presenting with TMA and <10% of the normal activity of a disintegrin-like and metalloproteinase with thrombospondin type 1 motifs 13 (ADAMTS-13) or positive for anti-ADAMTS-13 antibodies are diagnosed with TTP. Further, patients with TMA tests negative for STEC infection, TTP, and other known causes of TMA, such as calcineurin inhibitors, sirolimus, anti-VEGF agents, transplantation, cobalamin deficiency, and autoimmune diseases, are clinically diagnosed with aHUS [1]. aHUS is caused by uncontrolled activation of the complement system in the alternative pathway, causing microvascular thrombosis and vascular endothelial injury, and subsequently, microangiopathic hemolytic anemia, thrombocytopenia, and AKI. Gene mutations in complement system proteins such as *CFH*, *C3*, *CFI*, *MCP*, *CFB*, and *THBD* are documented in aHUS patients [4]. aHUS is a rare disease with an estimated incidence of 0.2–2 cases per million [5]. Several definitions for

Table 1: Diagnostic tests for TMA-related disease.

Parameters	Results	Normal range
Shiga-toxin-producing *Escherichia coli* infection		
Stool culture	Negative	Negative
O-157 LPS Ab	Not detected	Not detected
Diagnostic tests for TTP		
ADAMTS-13 activity (%)	69.1	70–120
Anti-ADAMTS-13 antibody (BU/mL)	<0.5	<0.5
Diagnostic tests for secondary TMA		
C3 (mg/dL)	96	65–135
C4 (mg/dL)	11	13–35
CH50 (IU/ml)	42.2	30–46
Direct Coombs test	Negative	Negative
Indirect Coombs test	Negative	Negative
Anti-nuclear antibody (titer)	<1 : 20	<1 : 40
PR3-ANCA (IU/ml)	Not detected	<3.5
MPO-ANCA (IU/ml)	Not detected	<3.5
Lupus anticoagulant	Negative	Negative
CLβ2GPI (IU/ml)	Not detected	<10

O-157 LPS Ab: O-157 lipopolysaccharide antibody, TTP: thrombocytopenic purpura, ADAMTS-13: a disintegrin-like and metalloproteinase with thrombospondin type 1 motifs *13*, PR-3 ANCA: proteinase 3 anti-neutrophil cytoplasmic antibody, MPO-ANCA: myeloperoxidase anti-neutrophil cytoplasmic antibody CLβ2GPI: anti-cardiolipin β2-glycoprotein I complex antibody.

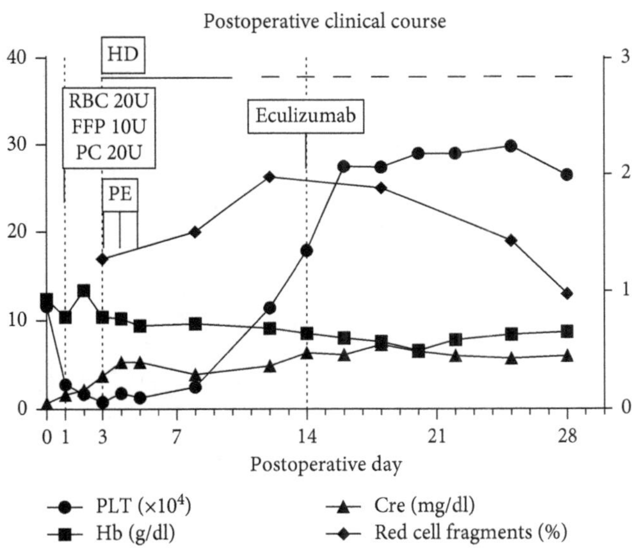

Figure 2: Graph shows the postoperative clinical course. Hb: haemoglobin, PLT: platelet count, Cre: creatinine, RBC: red blood cell, FFP: fresh frozen plasma, PC: platelet concentrates, HD: hemodialysis, and PE: plasma exchange.

TMA and aHUS have been published. In brief, the diagnosis of aHUS is made based on the triad of TMA and negative results for STEC-HUS, TTP, and other TMA-related diseases, such as autoimmune diseases.

Published reports show poor prognosis, with 33%–40% of aHUS patients dying or progressing to end-stage renal disease (ESRD) during the acute phase and up to 65% of cases progressing to ESRD or dying within 1 year.

Table 2: Analysis of the responsible gene for aHUS.

Responsible gene	Mutation	Comment
CFH	+	Polymorphism
C3	+	Polymorphism
CFI	−	—
MCP	−	—
CFB	+	Variation seen within normal 2% in Japanese
THBD	+	Polymorphism

Traditionally, the treatment for aHUS has been PE. However, recently, a study showed successful treatment of aHUS with eculizumab, a humanised monoclonal antibody that binds to C5 and inhibits the generation of proinflammatory C5a and C5b-9 in the alternative pathway. Eculizumab has been established as the first-line treatment for aHUS [6].

In this case, multiple factors, such as the disease itself and surgical stress, including hypothermia, cardiopulmonary bypass and lower body circulatory arrest, could have triggered the uncontrolled complement activation. Despite immediate treatment with PE following the manifestation of the TMA triad, thrombocytopenia improved, but the progression of schistocytes was not resolved. Further, eculizumab treatment 10 days after PE initiation without additional transfusion suppressed the progression of hemolytic anemia; however, her renal function did not recover enough. An investigation into gene mutations of aHUS is needed for the definitive diagnosis of aHUS when the patient has been clinically diagnosed with aHUS; however, specific mutations in the complement genes are not determined in 40% of patients clinically diagnosed with aHUS [5]. In this case, no significant gene mutations in *CFH*, *C3*, *CFI*, *MCP*, *CFB*, and *THBD* associated with aHUS were detected (Table 2).

Some cases of aHUS have been reported following transplantation surgery, including heart transplantation [7]. Conversely, only two cases of aHUS developing after non-transplantation cardiac surgery have been reported [8,9]. Although Saltzman et al. reported five cases of TTP following open heart surgery, ADAMTS-13 levels in four of those five cases were >10%, and anti-ADAMTS-13 antibody levels were within the normal level [10]. According to the current diagnostic criteria, these four cases might have developed aHUS.

This is the first case report of aHUS following ATAAD. aHUS must be suspected if the patient manifests the triad of TMA during treatment of acute aortic dissection, and the relevant diagnostic workup must be performed.

Acknowledgments

The authors would like to thank Editage (http://www.editage.com) for editing and reviewing this manuscript for English language.

References

[1] M. Scully and T. Goodship, "How I treat thrombotic thrombocytopenic purpura and atypical haemolytic uraemic syndrome," *British Journal of Haematology*, vol. 164, no. 6, pp. 759–766, 2014.
[2] A. Evangelista, E. M. Isselbacher, E. Bossone et al., "Insights from the International Registry of acute aortic dissection: 20-year experience of collaborative clinical research," *Circulation*, vol. 137, no. 17, pp. 1846–1860, 2018.
[3] R. K. Mody, R. E. Luna-Gierke, T. F. Jones et al., "Infections in pediatric postdiarrheal hemolytic uremic syndrome: factors associated with identifying shiga toxin-producing *Escherichia coli*," *Archives of Pediatrics & Adolescent Medicine*, vol. 166, no. 10, pp. 902–909, 2012.
[4] M. Noris, J. Caprioli, E. Bresin et al., "Relative role of genetic complement abnormalities in sporadic and familial aHUS and their impact on clinical phenotype," *Clinical Journal of the American Society of Nephrology*, vol. 5, no. 10, pp. 1844–1859, 2010.
[5] V. Fremeaux-Bacchi, F. Fakhouri, A. Garnier et al., "Genetics and outcome of atypical hemolytic uremic syndrome: a nationwide French series comparing children and adults," *Clinical Journal of the American Society of Nephrology*, vol. 8, no. 4, pp. 554–562, 2013.
[6] C. M. Legendre, C. Licht, P. Muus et al., "Terminal complement inhibitor eculizumab in atypical hemolytic-uremic syndrome," *New England Journal of Medicine*, vol. 368, no. 23, pp. 2169–2181, 2013.
[7] P. N. Vardas, Z. A. Hashmi, and M. A. Hadi, "Identification and management of atypical hemolytic uremic syndrome immediately post-heart transplantation," *Journal of Cardiac Surgery*, vol. 30, no. 4, pp. 373–375, 2015.
[8] E. Matsukuma, A. Imamura, Y. Iwata et al., "Postoperative atypical hemolytic uremic syndrome associated with complement C3 mutation," *Case Reports in Nephrology*, vol. 2014, Article ID 784943, 5 pages, 2014.
[9] K. Markakis, T. H. Westhoff, and N. Pagonas, "Aortic valve replacement as a trigger of atypical hemolytic uremic syndrome," *The Annals of Thoracic Surgery*, vol. 104, no. 3, pp. 255-256, 2017.
[10] D. J. Saltzman, J. C. Chang, J. C. Jimenez et al., "Postoperative thrombotic thrombocytopenic purpura after open heart operations," *The Annals of Thoracic Surgery*, vol. 89, no. 1, pp. 119–123, 2010.

11

Entecavir-Associated Thrombocytopenia: A Case Report and Review of the Pathophysiology, Diagnosis and Treatment of a Rare but Reversible Cause of Thrombocytopenia

Binoy Yohannan[1] **Dai Chu N. Luu,**[2] **and Mark Feldman**[1]

[1]*Department of Internal Medicine, Texas Health Presbyterian Hospital, Dallas, Texas 75231, USA*
[2]*Department of Internal Medicine, Division of Hematology and Oncology, Texas Health Presbyterian Hospital, Dallas, Texas 75231, USA*

Correspondence should be addressed to Mark Feldman; markfeldman@texashealth.org

Academic Editor: Marie-Christine Kyrtsonis

Drug-associated thrombocytopenia is often unrecognized. We report a 76-year-old female with lymphoma who presented with easy bruising and oral bleeding. She had undergone screening for hepatitis B virus (HBV) prior to starting rituximab and was found to have hepatitis B core serum antibody (IgG anti-HBc). She was therefore treated with prophylactic entecavir 0.5 mg daily to prevent reactivation of HBV. Her initial platelet count was 136,000/mm^3. Five days after starting entecavir, she presented with bruising and oral bleeding and was found to have a platelet count of 7,000/mm^3. A coagulation profile and the rest of the blood parameters (RBC and WBC counts) were normal. Entecavir was stopped, and she was given 3 units of apheresed platelets followed by intravenous immunoglobulin (1 g/kg) for 5 consecutive days. Her platelet counts improved and normalized in one week. She was diagnosed with entecavir-induced thrombocytopenia based on the temporal relationship and after carefully excluding alternate causes of thrombocytopenia. This case highlights the importance of recognizing drug-induced thrombocytopenia (DITP) as a reversible cause of thrombocytopenia.

1. Introduction

The most common side effects of entecavir therapy for hepatitis B virus (HBV) include headache, fatigue, dizziness, nausea, and vomiting. Very rarely, patients can develop lactic acidosis and hepatic steatosis. Although other nucleoside analogues with activity against HBV such as lamivudine [1] and adefovir [2] have been associated with drug-induced thrombocytopenia, the incidence is very low with entecavir. Here, we report a case of an elderly female with serological evidence of past HBV infection who developed severe thrombocytopenia with bleeding after she had received entecavir for 5 days. This is the second case report of entecavir-induced thrombocytopenia.

2. Case Presentation

A 76-year-old female presented with a 2-day history of easy bruising and bleeding from her mouth. She denied epistaxis, melena, hematochezia, hematuria, or other bleeding manifestations. She had estrogen receptor positive stage 1 breast cancer 24 years ago for which she underwent lumpectomy followed by tamoxifen for 5 years. She has had regular mammograms since then, and there has been no evidence of local disease recurrence. Fourteen years ago, she was diagnosed with Waldenstrom's macroglobulinemia for which she was treated with chlorambucil and prednisone for 3 months with significant improvement. Her plasma cell dyscrasia has been quiescent. M-spike on serum protein electrophoresis was minimal. She had intermittent hospitalizations for pneumonia, thought to be related to functional immunoglobulin deficiency. She was on intravenous immunoglobulin replacement for 6 months, but it was discontinued later. Three years ago, she presented with pleural and pericardial effusions, and pleural biopsy showed activated B-cell (ABC) diffuse large B-cell lymphoma (DLBCL). A PET scan showed uptake in the pleural space with no lymphadenopathy. A bone marrow biopsy showed no evidence of DLBCL, and she was treated with rituximab and bendamustine for 3 months and remained in remission for the next three years. Four weeks prior to the current admission, she presented with fatigue, night sweats, and 10-pound weight loss and was found to have retroperitoneal lymphadenopathy. She underwent CT-guided core biopsy of the retroperitoneal nodes that confirmed recurrence of her DLBCL. A repeat bone marrow biopsy showed normocellular bone marrow with progressive trilineage hematopoiesis, but no evidence of DLBCL. She was scheduled to start salvage therapy for DLBCL with rituximab and lenalidomide. Viral hepatitis serologies were performed prior to initiation of rituximab, showing evidence of prior hepatitis B infection (IgG anti-HBc antibody). She was therefore started on prophylactic entecavir 0.5 mg daily 5 days prior to the current admission. Other medical problems included diabetes mellitus, hypertension, atrial fibrillation, gout, hypothyroidism, hyperlipidemia, and osteoporosis. Her other medications besides entecavir included allopurinol, amiodarone, rosuvastatin, diltiazem, pantoprazole, dabigatran, ramipril, and levothyroxine. No recent change in these medications had occurred.

On physical examination, her temperature was 98.3°F with blood pressure 100/68 mmHg, pulse 90 beats per min, and respiratory rate 18 per minute. She looked tired but had no pallor, icterus, or generalized lymphadenopathy. The anterior nares were clear without epistaxis. Mucous membranes were moist, and the oropharynx revealed two scabs in the buccal mucosa with dried blood. She had normal S1 and S2 without any rubs, murmurs or gallops, and normal vesicular breath sounds. Her abdomen was soft and nontender without hepatosplenomegaly or ascites. Skin was warm and dry without petechia, purpura, or ecchymosis. The rest of the physical exam was unremarkable. Complete blood count showed thrombocytopenia with a platelet count of 7000/mm^3. Peripheral blood smear showed no evidence of platelet clumping. The hemoglobin and white blood cell counts were normal. Thyroid function tests and a coagulation profile were essentially normal. Her last recorded platelet count 10 days prior to starting entecavir was 136,000/mm^3. Her baseline platelet count range is between 120,000 and 150,000/mm^3. Entecavir was discontinued, but her other drugs were continued. She received 3 units of platelets followed by intravenous immunoglobulin (1 g/kg) for 5 consecutive days. Her platelet counts improved and normalized in one week (Figure 1). She then received lenalidomide and rituximab for her DLBCL, but did not receive any HBV prophylaxis as it was considered unsafe to expose her to any of the other nucleoside analogues.

3. Discussion

Patients with chronic hepatitis B or serological evidence of past infection are at risk for viral reactivation when treated with immunosuppressive therapy. B-cell depleting agents such as rituximab have the highest risk of HBV reactivation [3, 4]. The nucleos(t)ide analogues such as entecavir (ETV) and tenofovir can be used for HBV prophylactic therapy, and it should be continued for at least 12 months for those

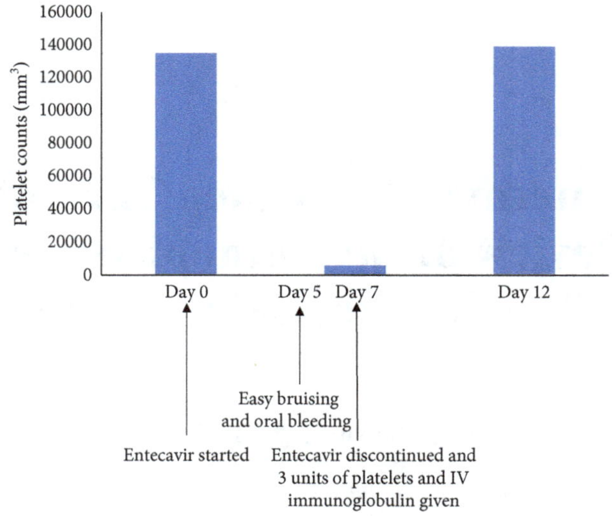

FIGURE 1: Course of drug-induced immune thrombocytopenia in a patient treated with entecavir. Entecavir was prescribed for prophylaxis to prevent HBV reactivation before initiating rituximab therapy. Starting from day 5 of treatment, the patient reported having easy bruising and bleeding from the oral cavity. She came to the office on day 7, and her platelet count was 7000 per cubic millimeter. Entecavir was discontinued immediately, and 3 units of apheresed platelets and IV immunoglobulin were given (days 7–11). The platelet counts improved and normalized in a week.

receiving B-cell depleting agents [5]. ETV, a guanine nucleoside analogue, has been associated with thrombocytopenia in only one case report in which an elderly female with hepatitis B cirrhosis suffered from severe thrombocytopenia after she received ETV therapy; and this was successfully treated by discontinuation of entecavir and intravenous immunoglobulin [6]. Clinicians should consider drug-induced thrombocytopenia (DITP) in the differential diagnosis of a patient on ETV therapy presenting with unexplained isolated thrombocytopenia. DITP can mimic primary immune thrombocytopenia (ITP); however, differentiating these syndromes is important to avoid unnecessary immunosuppressive treatments and to avoid future exposure to the sensitizing drug. Hence, it is important for clinicians to be aware of this adverse drug event and have a general understanding of the common drugs associated with thrombocytopenia. Drugs commonly implicated as triggers of DITP include heparin, quinine, glycoprotein II_b III_a inhibitors, gold salts, antibiotics (e.g., linezolid, rifampin, sulfonamides, and vancomycin), antiepileptics (e.g., carbamazepine, phenytoin, and valproic acid), analgesics (e.g., acetaminophen, diclofenac, and naproxen), diuretics (e.g., hydrochlorothiazide and chlorothiazide), and chemotherapeutic agents including proteasome inhibitors [7, 8]. DITP can be either nonimmune or immune-mediated. Nonimmune DITP can be secondary to bone marrow suppression (e.g., cytotoxic chemotherapy and linezolid) or inhibition of proplatelet formation in megakaryocytes (proteasome inhibitors) [9]. Immune-mediated thrombocytopenia in the presence of certain drugs can be explained by the following mechanisms: (a) classic drug-dependent platelet antibodies (quinine-type); (b) hapten-induced platelet antibodies (e.g., penicillin); (c) fiban-dependent antibodies (e.g., tirofiban); (d) fragments antigen binding monoclonal antibodies (e.g., abciximab); and (e) drug-induced autoantibody formation (e.g., gold). Drug-induced autoantibodies can either attach firmly to the epitopes on the platelet surface and cause accelerated destruction or target the megakaryocyte causing immune-mediated suppression of platelet production [10–12]. These autoantibodies can also affect the other cell lines including neutrophils and red blood cells causing neutropenia and immune hemolytic anemia, respectively [13].

Clinicians should elicit a detailed drug exposure history to establish the diagnosis of DITP, specifically enquiring about prescription drugs, over the counterdrugs, herbal preparations, certain foods, and beverages [7]. There is no definitive diagnostic test for DITP, but instead DITP is usually diagnosed by the temporal association of exposure to a suspected drug with an acute, severe thrombocytopenia, with the nadir platelet counts often less than 20,000/mm^3 [11, 14]. Patients are often exposed to the sensitizing drug for about 5–7 days, but DITP can also occur following intermittent use of a drug over a long time period. Glycoprotein II_b III_a inhibitors such as abciximab can cause severe thrombocytopenia within 1 or 2 days, even with the first exposure to the drug [15]. George et al. [8] proposed 4 clinical criteria and level of evidence to help establish the likelihood that a specific drug is responsible for thrombocytopenia (Table 1). Our patient met 3 of these criteria and thus probably had DITP. Furthermore, she had had a bone marrow biopsy ten days prior to the presentation, the megakaryocyte morphology was normal, and she had no evidence of malignant marrow infiltration. Autoimmune thrombocytopenia is a common hematologic complication of B-cell lymphomas and could potentially confound thrombocytopenia in this patient, but the temporal association with entecavir exposure and quick resolution after discontinuation of the drug favors DITP. Except for heparin, testing for drug-induced autoantibodies is not widely available and hence not helpful in clinical decision-making. Drug metabolites produced in vivo can act as a sensitizing agent, and thus, even in cases of typical DITP, antibody testing against the parent drug can be negative [16]. If the clinical suspicion is strong for DITP, reexposure to the suspected drug can be considered to document drug sensitivity. However, in sensitized individuals, a conventional dose can cause severe thrombocytopenia and bleeding. Therefore, if rechallenge is considered, one should start with a very low dose and closely monitor platelet counts and clinical status [17]. In cases of DITP, once the offending drug is discontinued, symptoms usually resolve quickly, and the platelet count returns to normal in less than a week. Prolonged thrombocytopenia after discontinuation of the suspected drug is evidence against a causal role for that drug.

The clinical presentation of DITP can vary from asymptomatic thrombocytopenia to life-threatening hemorrhage. Patients may have epistaxis, gum bleeding, oral mucous membrane blood blisters, melena, hematochezia, and hematuria when the platelet count drops below 20,000/mm^3, and deaths from bleeding have been reported [14]. Most patients with mild to moderate DITP can be managed conservatively with discontinuation of the offending drugs and closely monitoring the platelet count. When there is uncertainty about the causative drug, all medications should be discontinued [7]. Patients with severe thrombocytopenia and bleeding manifestations are at high risk for life-threatening hemorrhage and should be managed aggressively with platelet transfusions [12]. The role of glucocorticoids in patients with DITP is controversial, and there is no evidence that it improves clinical outcomes. Nevertheless, glucocorticoids are often used in unexplained isolated thrombocytopenia, since ITP cannot be easily excluded. When DITP is strongly suspected, it is appropriate to stop glucocorticoid therapy abruptly after the platelet count returns to normal. In DITP, plasma exchange [18] and intravenous immune globulins [19] have been used in patients with severe thrombocytopenia and bleeding manifestations, but the benefit of these treatments is uncertain [12].

Once drug sensitivity is documented, autoantibodies persist for life, and patients should be advised to avoid the drug in future, and this should be documented in their medical records as a serious "allergy."

Table 1: Clinical criteria and levels of evidence for evaluation of patients with suspected drug-induced thrombocytopenia.

Clinical criteria
(1) Drug administration preceded thrombocytopenia; complete and sustained recovery from thrombocytopenia is noted after drug discontinuation
(2) Other drugs administered prior to thrombocytopenia were continued or reintroduced after discontinuation of the suspected drug
(3) Other etiologies of thrombocytopenia excluded
(4) Reexposure to the drug resulted in recurrent thrombocytopenia
Levels of evidence
(1) Definite: all 4 criteria met
(2) Probable: criteria 1–3 met
(3) Possible: criterion 1 met
(4) Unlikely: criterion 1 not met

Adapted from http://www.ouhsc.edu/platelets and Reference [6].

4. Conclusion

Entecavir-induced thrombocytopenia is a reversible cause of thrombocytopenia potentially mediated via numerous immune and nonimmune mechanisms. Clinicians should maintain a high index of clinical suspicion for DITP in the patient presenting with severe thrombocytopenia soon after starting entecavir and quick resolution after discontinuing the drug. Early recognition and prompt discontinuation of entecavir is critical to avoid life-threatening hemorrhage.

References

[1] D. Lebensztejn and M. Kaczmarski, "Lamivudine-associated thrombocytopenia," *American Journal of Gastroenterology*, vol. 97, no. 10, pp. 2687-2688, 2002.

[2] G. Stornaiuolo, A. Amato, and G. Gaeta, "Adefovir dipivoxil-associated thrombocytopenia in a patient with chronic hep-

atitis B," *Digestive and Liver Disease*, vol. 38, no. 3, pp. 211-212, 2006.
[3] Y. H. Huang, L. T. Hsiao, Y. C. Hong et al., "Randomized controlled trial of entecavir prophylaxis for rituximab-associated hepatitis B virus reactivation in patients with lymphoma and resolved hepatitis B," *Journal of Clinical Oncology*, vol. 31, no. 22, pp. 2765–2772, 2013.
[4] W. Yeo, T. C. Chan, N. W. Y. Leung et al., "Hepatitis B virus reactivation in lymphoma patients with prior resolved hepatitis B undergoing anticancer therapy with or without rituximab," *Journal of Clinical Oncology*, vol. 27, no. 4, pp. 605–611, 2009.
[5] W. K. Seto, T. S. Y. Chan, Y. Y. Hwang et al., "Hepatitis B reactivation in patients with previous hepatitis B virus exposure undergoing rituximab-containing chemotherapy for lymphoma: a prospective study," *Journal of Clinical Oncology*, vol. 32, no. 33, pp. 3736–3743, 2014.
[6] X. Fan, L. Chen, J. Yang, and P. Feng, "Entecavir-associated thrombocytopenia in a decompensated cirrhotic patient," *Medicine*, vol. 95, no. 12, p. e3103, 2016.
[7] R. H. Aster and D. W. Bougie, "Drug-induced immune thrombocytopenia," *New England Journal of Medicine*, vol. 357, no. 6, pp. 580–587, 2007.
[8] J. N. George, G. E. Raskob, S. R. Shah et al., "Drug-induced thrombocytopenia," *Annals of Internal Medicine*, vol. 129, no. 11, pp. 886–90, 1998.
[9] K. Murali and S. Kowata, "Bortezomib induces thrombocytopenia by the inhibition of proplatelet formation of megakaryocytes," *European Journal of Haematology*, vol. 93, no. 4, pp. 290–296, 2014.
[10] J. P. Freiman, "Fatal quinine-induced thrombocytopenia," *Annals of Internal Medicine*, vol. 112, no. 4, pp. 308-309, 1990.
[11] R. H. Aster, B. R. Curtis, J. G. McFarland, and D. W. Bougie, "Drug-induced immune thrombocytopenia: pathogenesis, diagnosis, and management," *Journal of Thrombosis and Haemostasis*, vol. 7, no. 6, pp. 911–918, 2009.
[12] R. Aster, "Drug-induced thrombocytopenia," in *Platelets*, A. D. Michelson, Ed., Academic Press, New York, NY, USA, 2007.
[13] P. A. Arndt and G. Garratty, "The changing spectrum of drug-induced immune hemolytic anemia," *Seminars in Hematology*, vol. 42, no. 3, pp. 137–144, 2005.
[14] B. R. Curtis, "Drug-induced immune thrombocytopenia: incidence, clinical features, laboratory testing, and pathogenic mechanisms," *Immunohematology*, vol. 30, no. 2, pp. 55–65, 2014.
[15] R. H. Aster, "Immune thrombocytopenia caused by glycoprotein IIb/IIIa inhibitors," *Chest*, vol. 127, no. 2, pp. 53S–59S, 2005.
[16] D. Bougie and R. Aster, "Immune thrombocytopenia resulting from sensitivity to metabolites of naproxen and acetaminophen," *Blood*, vol. 97, no. 12, pp. 3846–3850, 2001.
[17] N. R. Shulman, "Immunoreactions involving platelets: IV. Studies on the pathogenesis of thrombocytopenia in drug purpura using test doses of quinidine in sensitized individuals; their implications in idiopathic thrombocytopenic purpura," *Journal of Experimental Medicine*, vol. 107, no. 5, pp. 711–729, 1958.
[18] O. Pourrat, "Treatment of drug-related diseases by plasma exchanges," *Annales de Médecine Interne (Paris)*, vol. 145, pp. 357–60, 1994.
[19] J. B. Ray, W. F. Brereton, and F. R. Nullet, "Intravenous immune globulin for the treatment of presumed quinidine-induced thrombocytopenia," *DICP*, vol. 24, no. 7-8, pp. 693–695, 1990.

12

A Case Report of Premalignant Plasma Cell Dyscrasia-Induced Renal Failure in a 31-Year-Old Female

Ayrton Bangolo,[1] Mahabuba Akhter,[1] Amer Jarri,[1] Manpreet Kaur,[1] Ali Atoot,[2] Parul Jandir,[1] Mahmood Ibrahim,[1] Lochana Manandhar,[3] and Adam Atoot[1]

[1]*Hackensack, Meridian Health Palisades Medical Center, Department of Internal Medicine, North Bergen, NJ, USA*
[2]*Hackensack University Medical Center, Department of Anesthesia, Hackensack, NJ, USA*
[3]*Hackensack Meridian Health Palisades Medical Center, Department of Nephrology, North Bergen, NJ, USA*

Correspondence should be addressed to Ayrton Bangolo; ayrtonbangolo@yahoo.com

Academic Editor: Kostas Konstantopoulos

Monoclonal gammopathy of renal significance (MGRS) is a rare disorder in which monoclonal immunoglobulin secreted by nonmalignant B cell or plasma cell clone causes kidney damage. Although MGRS is a premalignant condition, it can cause severe kidney disease and end-stage renal disease (ESRD) at any age. Herein, we present a 31-year-old female with past medical history of lupus nephritis who presented with signs of volume overload and worsening renal function despite adequate immunosuppressive therapy. Renal biopsy revealed heavy and light chain deposition consistent with MGRS. This case report demonstrates the importance of including MGRS in the differential diagnosis of worsening renal function despite adequate treatment, raising awareness of this premalignant yet morbid condition.

1. Introduction

Monoclonal gammopathy of undetermined significance (MGUS) consists of a premalignant clonal plasma cell or lymphoplasmacytic proliferative disorder. MGUS is characterized by the absence of end organ damage [1]. However, some patients, meeting diagnosis criteria of MGUS can develop significant kidney injury, and the condition is then termed monoclonal gammopathy of renal significance (MGRS) [2]. MGRS is associated with high morbidity due to the severity of renal lesions. Suppression of monoclonal immunoglobulins (MIg) often improves outcome [3]. Here, we report the case of a 31-year-old female with stage 4 lupus nephritis and worsening renal function despite adequate treatment, found to have MIg on renal biopsy. With this case report we aim to encourage physicians to include MGRS in the differential diagnosis of rapidly progressing renal failure, as early detection and intervention will improve the outcome.

2. Case Presentation

This is a 31-year-old female with past medical history significant for stage IV lupus nephritis who presented for evaluation of a 2-day history of worsening face and extremities swelling. The patient denied any recent insect bite, joint pain, hematuria, or recent upper respiratory tract infection. Of note, the patient was evaluated a year ago for the same symptoms and was found to have severe renal dysfunction. A renal biopsy at that time revealed stage IV lupus nephritis. The patient was discharged on prednisone and mycophenolate. However, she reports noncompliance to the regimen.

Physical exam was notable for facial swelling, bilateral jugular venous distention, and 3+ bilateral lower extremity edema. Laboratory results revealed a creatinine of 7.58 (0.6–1.2) milligram per deciliter (mg/dL), Creatinine a year ago upon discharge was 1.21 mg/dL. She was also found to be hyponatremic, with low serum protein, elevated serum free

Table 1: Laboratory values on admission and a year ago.

	Laboratory values
Creatinine upon admission	7.58 (0.6–1.2) milligram per deciliter (mg/dL)
Creatinine a year ago upon discharge	1.21 mg/dL
Blood urea nitrogen	38 (7–25) mg/dL
Total serum protein	4.5 (6.4–8.9) gram per deciliter (g/dL)
Serum albumin	2.2 (3.5–5.7) g/dL
Sodium	129 (136–145) millimole per liter (mmol/L)
Calcium	6.8 (8.6–10.3) mg/dL
24-hours total urine protein	6456 mg/24 hours (<150 mg/24 hours)
Serum complement 3	56 (83–193) mg/dL
Serum complement 4	24 (15–57) mg/dL
Free kappa light chain in the serum	44.9 (3.3–19.4) milligram per liter (mg/L)
Free lambda light chain in the serum	47.1 (5.7–26.3) mg/L
Kappa/lambda light chain free ratio	0.95 (0.26–1.65)
Antinuclear antibody	Negative
Double-stranded DNA antibody	Negative

Table 2: Serum protein electrophoresis with immunofixation.

	Laboratory values
Total protein	3.9 (6.1–8.1) gram per deciliter (g/dL)
Albumin	2 (3.8–4.8)
Alpha 1 globulin	0.3 (0.2–0.3)
Alpha 2 globulin	0.8 (0.5–0.9)
Beta 1 globulin	0.3 (0.4–0.6)
Beta 2 globulin	0.2 (0.2–0.5)
Gamma globulin	0.4 (0.8–1.7)
Abnormal protein band	Faint band visible with overall polyclonal pattern in the gamma region, a developing plasma cell disorder cannot be excluded
Serum immunofixation	A faint band in immunoglobulin G and lambda against a dense polyclonal background. a developing plasma cell disorder cannot be excluded

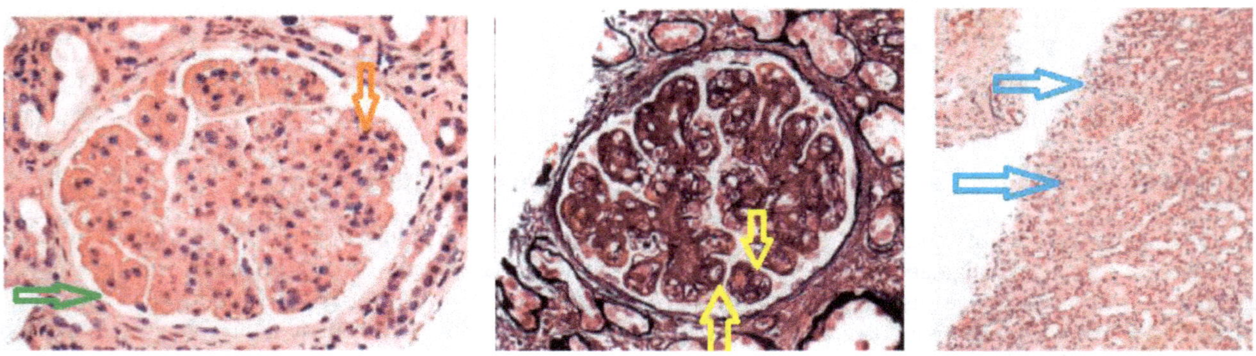

(a) (b) (c)

Figure 1: Image (a) showing diffuse proliferative glomerulonephritis, reduced bowman space (green arow) and increased cellularity in glomeruli (orange arow). Image (b) showing global glomerular basement membrane duplication (yellow arrow). Image (c) showing cortical scarring (blue arow).

kappa and lambda light chains, and normal kappa/lambda ratio as seen in Table 1.

The patient was started back on prednisone and mycophenolate which she had self-discontinued; nephrology was consulted as well. The patient's creatinine further deteriorated despite being on the regimen. A serum electrophoresis revealed a visible faint band with polyclonal pattern in the gamma region, a developing plasma cell disorder could not be excluded as seen in Table 2. A subsequent serum immunofixation revealed a faint band in immunoglobulin G (IgG) and lambda chain against a dense polyclonal background.

The patient was continued on prednisone and mycophenolate, and furosemide was added to the regimen with some improvement of the volume overload. She underwent a renal biopsy which revealed diffuse proliferative

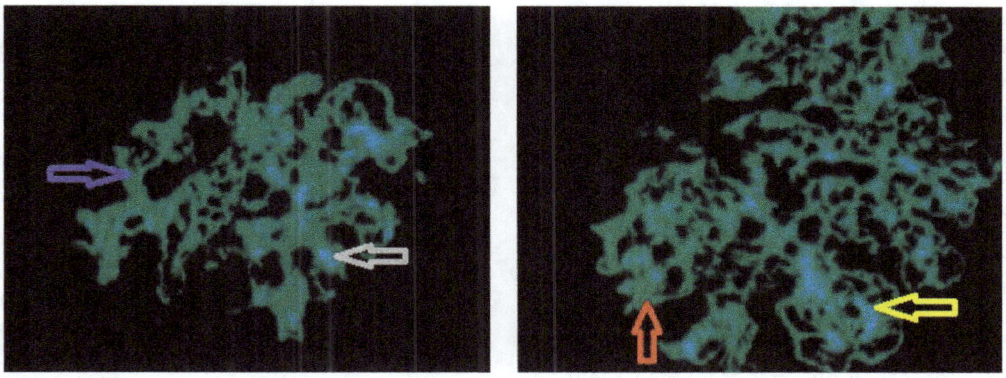

(a) (b)

Figure 2: Image (a) showing immunofluorescence (IF) staining for immunoglobulin G 3 (IG3), green representing the signal for IG3 (blue arow), with the nuclei in blue pointed with the gray arow. Image (b) showing IF staining for lambda, green representing the signal (red arow), with the nuclei in blue pointed with the yellow arow.

glomerulonephritis with prominent membranoproliferative features as seen on Figure 1. Immunofluorescence revealed granular, global mesangial, and capillary wall deposits each staining 3 + for IgG-3, complement 3, complement 1, and lambda as seen on Figure 2. Findings were consistent with proliferative glomerulonephritis with monoclonal IgG deposits, and a diagnosis of monoclonal gammopathy of renal significance was then made. The patient was started on bortezomib, cyclophosphamide, and prednisone was switched to dexamethasone, and mycophenolate was discontinued.

3. Discussion

Monoclonal gammopathy of renal significance (MGRS) encompasses patients who would otherwise meet the criteria for monoclonal gammopathy of undetermined significance (MGUS) but demonstrate kidney injury attributable to the underlying monoclonal protein [2]. Monoclonal gammopathy is more frequent in systemic lupus erythematosus (SLE) patients than in the general population [4]. SLE may present with nephritis as the sole disease manifestation [5]. In one study by Giavinti et al. in which nephritis was the initial manifestation of SLE, antinuclear (ANA) and anti-double-stranded DNA antibodies were positive up to 10 years after the original presentation [6]. Our patient was diagnosed, a year ago, with lupus nephritis. However, she did not have any clinical manifestations of SLE, and the ANA and anti-double-stranded DNA antibodies were negative. Given her history of lupus nephritis, the patient was at higher risk of developing MGRS.

In monoclonal gammopathy of renal significance (MGRS), the kidney lesions are primarily caused by the abnormal deposition or activity of monoclonal proteins in the kidney [7]. Monoclonal proteins can also act as autoantibodies directed against complement components, leading to uncontrolled activation of the alternative complement pathway, and causing complement 3 (C3) glomerulopathy [8]. Cases of monoclonal anti-glomerular basement membrane (GBM) disease due to circulating monoclonal antibodies have been reported [9, 10]. Monoclonal deposits must be restricted to a single class of light and/or heavy chain based on immunofluorescence to make the diagnosis of MGRS [11]. For unclear reasons, most patients with proliferative glomerulonephritis with monoclonal immunoglobulin deposits (PGNMID) do not have detectable circulating monoclonal gammopathy by serum and urine monoclonal protein testing [12]. Our patient's renal biopsy revealed monoclonal deposits of a single class of light chain (lambda) and a single class of heavy chain (immunoglobulin G) consistent with MGRS. The biopsy also revealed C3 deposit, consistent with C3 glomerulopathy, and a duplication of GBM was also reported. The patient's biopsy was consistent with proliferative glomerulonephritis with prominent membranoproliferative features and the serum electrophoresis did not reveal a monoclonal spike, and the immunofixation only revealed a faint immunoglobulin G and lambda. These findings are adequate with the literature.

Patients with monoclonal gammopathy-associated proliferative glomerulonephritis (PGNMID or C3 glomerulopathy with monoclonal gammopathy) are at risk for progressive kidney disease and should be treated to prevent further kidney injury and deterioration of kidney function. The treatment focuses upon eradication of the pathologic clone [13]. In patients with a detectable plasma cell clone, a treatment regimen similar to that used to treat multiple myeloma (MM) is recommended [13]. Treatment should be continued for up to six months if there is evidence of a hematologic response and no toxicity [13]. Our patient's biopsy expressed plasma cell monoclonal protein, with a heavy chain (immunoglobulin G) complexed with a light chain (lambda). She qualified for a treatment regimen similar to that used in MM. The patient will be reevaluated for response to treatment at regular intervals.

4. Conclusion

Monoclonal gammopathy of renal significance (MGRS) is a premalignant clonal plasma cell or lymphoplasmacytic proliferative disorder. Although MGRS is a premalignant condition, it is associated with high morbidity due the rapidly progressive nature of kidney disease. Early detection is essential, as suppression of immunoglobulin improves the outcome. With this case report, we hope to encourage clinicians to include MGRS in the differential diagnosis of unexplained worsening kidney function and raise awareness of this premalignant yet morbid condition.

Consent

Written informed consent was obtained from the patient for publication of this case report and any accompanying images.

Authors' Contributions

Ayrton Bangolo searched the literature, wrote, and revised the manuscript. Mahabuba Akhter, Amer Jarri, Manpreet Kaur, Parul Jandir, Ali Atoot, and Mahmood Ibrahim revised and edited the manuscript. Adam Atoot and Lochna Manandhar revised and approved the final version and are the article's guarantors. All authors certify that they contributed sufficiently to the intellectual content and data analysis. Each author has reviewed the final version of the manuscript and approves it for publication.

References

[1] S. V. Rajkumar, M. A. Dimopoulos, A. Palumbo et al., "International Myeloma working group updated criteria for the diagnosis of multiple myeloma," *The Lancet Oncology*, vol. 15, no. 12, pp. e538–e548, 2014.

[2] N. Leung, F. Bridoux, C. A. Hutchison et al., "Monoclonal gammopathy of renal significance: when MGUS is no longer undetermined or insignificant," *Blood*, vol. 120, no. 22, pp. 4292–4295, 2012.

[3] F. Bridoux, N. Leung, N. Leung et al., "Diagnosis of monoclonal gammopathy of renal significance," *Kidney International*, vol. 87, no. 4, pp. 698–711, 2015.

[4] Y. M. Ali, M. B. Urowitz, D. Ibanez, and D. D. Gladman, "Monoclonal gammopathy in systemic lupus erythematosus," *Lupus*, vol. 16, no. 6, pp. 426–429, 2007.

[5] D. Adu, D. G. Williams, D. Taube et al., "Late onset systemic lupus erythematosus and lupus-like disease in patients with apparent idiopathic glomerulonephritis," *Quarterly Journal of Medicine*, vol. 52, no. 208, pp. 471–487, 1983.

[6] A. Gianviti, P. Barsotti, V. Barbera, T. Faraggiana, and G. Rizzoni, "Delayed onset of systemic lupus erythematosus in patients with "full-house" nephropathy," *Pediatric Nephrology*, vol. 13, no. 8, pp. 683–687, 1999.

[7] R. H. Sayed, A. D. Wechalekar, J. A. Gilbertson et al., "Natural history and outcome of light chain deposition disease," *Blood*, vol. 126, no. 26, pp. 2805–2810, 2015.

[8] S. Meri, V. Koistinen, A. Miettinen, T. Törnroth, and I. J. Seppälä, "Activation of the alternative pathway of complement by monoclonal lambda light chains in membranoproliferative glomerulonephritis," *Journal of Experimental Medicine*, vol. 175, no. 4, pp. 939–950, 1992.

[9] M. Turner, A. Crawford, C. Winterbottom et al., "Heavy chain deposition disease presenting with raised anti-GBM antibody levels; a case report," *BMC Nephrology*, vol. 21, no. 1, 2020.

[10] S. M. Coley, S. Shirazian, J. Radhakrishnan, and V. D. D'Agati, "Monoclonal IgG1κ anti-glomerular basement membrane disease: a case report," *American Journal of Kidney Diseases*, vol. 65, no. 2, pp. 322–326, 2015.

[11] N. Klomjit, N. Leung, F. Fervenza, S. Sethi, and L. Zand, "Rate and predictors of finding monoclonal gammopathy of renal significance (MGRS) lesions on kidney biopsy in patients with monoclonal gammopathy," *Journal of the American Society of Nephrology*, vol. 31, no. 10, pp. 2400–2411, 2020.

[12] R. Fish, J. Pinney, P. Jain et al., "The incidence of major hemorrhagic complications after renal biopsies in patients with monoclonal gammopathies," *Clinical Journal of the American Society of Nephrology*, vol. 5, no. 11, pp. 1977–1980, 2010.

[13] S. Sethi and S. V. Rajkumar, "Monoclonal gammopathy-associated proliferative glomerulonephritis," *Mayo Clinic Proceedings*, vol. 88, no. 11, pp. 1284–1293, 2013.

13

Management of Chronic Disseminated Intravascular Coagulation Associated with Aortic Aneurysm/Dissection

Shigeru Koba,[1] Tomoya Yamaguchi,[1] Kenji Miki,[1] Hiroshi Makihara,[1] and Shinsaku Imashuku[2]

[1]*Department of Internal Medicine, Uji-Tokushukai Medical Center, Uji 611-0041, Japan*
[2]*Department of Laboratory Medicine, Uji-Tokushukai Medical Center, Uji 611-0041, Japan*

Correspondence should be addressed to Shinsaku Imashuku; shinim95@mbox.kyoto-inet.or.jp

Academic Editor: Gergely Feher

Disseminated intravascular coagulation (DIC) is a systemic life-threatening process that can cause thrombosis and hemorrhage. Chronic DIC has been associated with aortic aneurysm/dissection. Aortic aneurysm/dissection should be included in the differential diagnosis of elderly patients with hemorrhagic diathesis due to DIC of uncertain etiology. Treatment depends on various factors, including the severity of underlying disease, extent of DIC, and patient comorbidities, as well as the ability of the patient to maintain activities of daily living once discharged from the hospital. This report describes the clinical characteristics of four elderly patients with chronic DIC associated with aortic aneurysm/dissection who were treated in our institution. We also offer the recommendations around most appropriate nonsurgical treatment of these patients.

1. Introduction

Disseminated intravascular coagulation (DIC) is an acquired disorder that occurs in patients with a wide variety of clinical conditions, including leukemia, other cancers, and sepsis. Patients with DIC also experience secondary fibrinolysis, with the degree of activation of the fibrinolytic system dependent on the underlying disease [1, 2]. Chronic DIC is a rare but life-threatening complication of aortic aneurysm/dissection [3, 4], which was first described in 1967 [5]. However, compensatory mechanisms in aortic chronic DIC may result in mild or even occult clinical symptoms [6, 7], leading to a delayed diagnosis. Case reports have described various treatments in patients with chronic DIC associated with aortic aneurysm/dissection [3,4,8–15], but the optimal type of treatment has not yet been determined.

Two types of treatment are available for patients with chronic aortic DIC: surgery or nonsurgical treatment by using systemic anticoagulation. Although open or endovascular surgery can result in a radical cure, there is a risk of bleeding; moreover, surgical methods are not suitable for some patients, depending on their age, health conditions, and disease backgrounds [3, 4]. Three major nonsurgical strategies are available for patients with aortic DIC: anticoagulation therapy [8–10], antifibrinolytic therapy [11], and a combination of both [12]. The main purpose of these treatments is to halt the cycle of thrombus formation and destruction, by blocking the consumption of systemic coagulation factors, fibrinogen and platelets and by halting further bleeding. This report describes the clinical course, treatment, and outcomes of four elderly patients with chronic DIC accompanied with aortic aneurysm/dissection, all of whom developed excessive fibrinolytic activity.

1.1. Case Reports. The summary of the four patients is given in Table 1.

Patient 1 was an 84-year-old woman who had undergone thoracic endovascular aortic repair (TEVAR) for an aortic dissected aneurysm (Figure 1(a)) and was hospitalized for thrombocytopenia and abnormal coagulation. Her laboratory data showed hemoglobin (Hb) 7.9 (reference; 11–16)

Table 1: Clinical features of 4 cases of chronic DIC in association with aortic aneurysm/dissection.

	Case 1	Case 2	Case 3	Case 4
Age/sex	84/F	87/M	91/F	83/F
Causes of DIC	AA	AD	CIAA/IIAA	AA
Surgical procedures (EVAR)	Yes (pre-)	Yes (pre-)	Yes (post-)	None
Site(s)/event(s) of bleeding	Subcutaneous	Tooth extraction	Gingiva	GI tract
Data on DIC				
Platelet counts (/μL)	64,000	73,000	100,000	62,000
Fibrinogen (mg/dL)	98	73	72	79
FDP/D-dimer (μg/mL)	101/49.8	96.8/24	109/51.4	177/81.7
TAT/PIC (ng, μg/mL)	40.5/12.7	58/17.6	49/NA	69.2/12.6
DIC score*	11	7	6	7
Treatment				
Supportive	None	PRBC	PRBC, FFP	PRBC, FFP, PC
Treatment for coagulopathy				
Initial	Heparin (DIV) + TA (DIV)	Heparin (SC) + TA (PO)	TA (DIV)	Heparin (DIV) + TA(DIV)
Later	Heparin (SC) + TA (PO)	Heparin (SC) + TA (PO)	Surgical (EVAR)	
Maintenance	Rivaroxaban (PO)	Rivaroxaban (PO)		
Outcome				
DIC	Well controlled	Well controlled	Well controlled	Delayed control
Alive/dead	Alive	Alive	Alive	Dead**

DIC = disseminated intravascular coagulation, AA = aortic aneurysm, AD = aortic dissection, FDP = fibrin degradation product, TAT = thrombin-antithrombin complex, PIC = plasmin-α2 plasmin inhibitor complex, GI = gastrointestinal, PRBC = packed red blood cell, FFP = fresh frozen plasma, PC = platelet concentrates, TA = tranexamic acid, EVAR = endovascular aortic repair, pre- = prior to DIC development, post- = after DIC development, DIV = drip infusion, SC = subcutaneous injection, PO = per oral, CIAA = common iliac artery aneurysm, and IIAA = internal iliac artery aneurysm. *Based on the DIC criteria of the Ministry of Health and Welfare of Japan; **died of aspiration pneumonia.

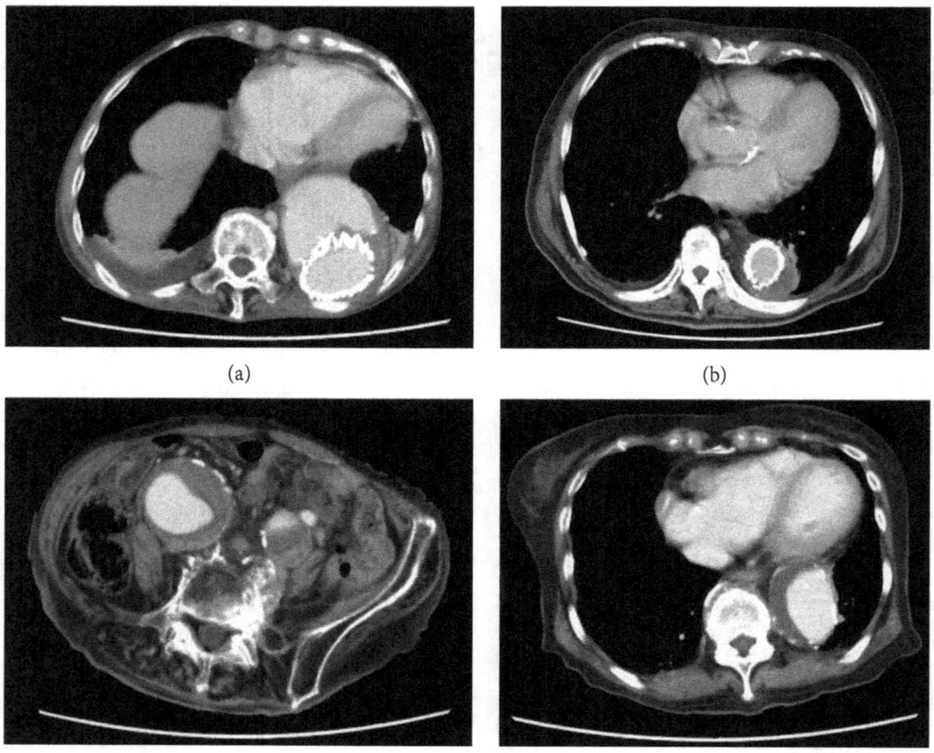

(a) (b) (c) (d)

Figure 1: Contrast-enhanced axial CT findings showing aortic aneurysm/dissection in (a) Patient 1, showing a stent graft in the descending aorta; (b) Patient 2, showing a stent graft in the descending aorta; (c) Patient 3, showing aneurysms in the bilateral common and internal iliac arteries; and (d) Patient 4, showing an aneurysm in the descending aorta.

g/dl, platelet count 79,000 (reference; 150,000–360,000)/μl, fibrinogen degradation product (FDP) of 101.5 (reference; <5) μg/ml, D-dimer of 49.8 (reference; <1.0) μg/ml, fibrinogen 98 (reference; 200–400) mg/dl, thrombin-antithrombin complex (TAT) 40.5 (reference; <3) ng/ml, and plasmin-α2 plasmin inhibitor complex (PIC) 12.7

(reference; <0.8) μg/ml. Prior to admission, she had been treated with warfarin. Our vascular surgeons regarded her aneurysm condition after TEVAR as inoperable. She was started on a continuous intravenous infusion of 10,000 units/day heparin and 250 mg twice daily intravenous tranexamic acid. This combination treatment was effective as her plasma FDP and D-dimer concentrations decreased while her fibrinogen level and platelet count increased (Figure 2). To facilitate her discharge, she was switched from intravenous to oral tranexamic acid (750 mg/day) and from intravenous to subcutaneous administration of heparin calcium (5,000 units twice daily), and warfarin was stopped. Although this combination was effective, the patient was intolerant of subcutaneous heparin calcium because of pain, and she was transitioned to oral rivaroxaban 15 mg/day for discharge from hospital.

Patient 2 was an 87-year-old man who had undergone TEVAR for a Stanford type B aortic dissection 7 months earlier (Figure 1(b)). Thereafter, he was sent to a rehabilitation center, where his plasma FDP and D-dimer increased gradually, while fibrinogen and platelet count decreased, and anemia progressed. He received transfusions of packed red blood cell (PRBC) and platelet concentrate (PC) several times (precise units unknown), although the cause of his abnormal coagulopathy was not adequately assessed. Following persistent gingival bleeding for 2 weeks, he was transferred to our hospital for evaluation. His laboratory data showed Hb 7.9 g/dl, platelet count 73,000/μl, FDP 96.8 μg/ml, D-dimer 24 μg/ml, fibrinogen 73 mg/dl, TAT 58 ng/ml, and PIC 17.6 μg/ml. Following PRBC (4 units) infusion, he was treated with subcutaneous heparin calcium (5,000 units twice daily) and oral tranexamic acid (1,500 mg/day). After 1 week, his laboratory data improved, with Hb 9.1 g/dl, platelet count 146,000/μl, FDP 10.9 μg/ml, D-dimer 6.3 μg/ml, and fibrinogen 186 mg/dl. Later, he was successfully switched to oral rivaroxaban (15 mg/day) as maintenance treatment at the outpatient clinic (Figure 3).

Patient 3 was a 91-year-old woman, who was hospitalized for gingival bleeding. Her laboratory data showed Hb 8.4 g/dl, platelet count 100,000/μl, FDP 109 μg/ml, D-dimer 51.4 μg/ml, and fibrinogen 72 mg/dl. Enhanced CT revealed bilateral iliac aneurysms, with the right and left aneurysms having maximum diameters of 60.5 mm and 43.7 mm, respectively (Figure 1(c)). She was initially treated with PRBC (6 units) and fresh frozen plasma (FFP; 10 units), followed by intravenous tranexamic acid (250 mg four times daily) for 3 days. However, because these aneurysms were thought to be responsible for her coagulopathy and the patient was regarded eligible for surgery, EVAR operation was performed, after which her DIC resolved.

Patient 4 was an 83-year-old woman, who was hospitalized with gastrointestinal (GI) bleeding and dyspnea due to persistent chronic obstructive pulmonary disease. Her laboratory data showed Hb 3.0 g/dl, platelet count 62,000/μl, mean corpuscular volume 82.9 (reference; 83–100) fl, serum blood urea nitrogen 98.0 (reference; 7.8–18.9) mg/dl, and creatinine 1.41 (reference; 0.45–0.82) mg/dl. Upper GI endoscopy showed bleeding in the duodenum which continued after admission, and it was found to be DIC-related. Her plasma FDP was 177 μg/ml, D-dimer 81.7 μg/ml, TAT 69.2 ng/ml, and PIC 12.6 μg/ml. Eventually, she was identified with an aortic aneurysm (Figure 1(d)), and hemostasis laboratory abnormalities were attributed to be related to her aortic aneurysm. Surgical treatment of her aortic aneurysm was discussed; however, her general condition was poor, and because of repeat GI bleedings, she required upper GI endoscopy 13 times over 23 days for emergency hemostasis and with incomplete and persistent DIC. During the period, she received PRBC (36 units), FFP (70 units), and PC (50 units) transfusions. On day 38, she was started on systemic treatment for DIC, consisting of intravenous heparin (12,000 U/day) and intravenous tranexamic acid (250 mg twice daily), which resulted in rapid improvement of laboratory data. Unfortunately, the patient died of aspiration pneumonia 2 days later.

2. Discussion

Chronic DIC associated with aortic aneurysm/dissection is a primary cause of hemorrhagic diathesis in elderly patients. In aortic aneurysms, endothelial disruption associated with either dissection or atheromatous plaque rupture leads to the exposure of collagen and tissue factor, triggering the coagulation cascade, including the activation of FX, and leading to excess consumption of clotting factors and the induction of DIC [13]. Similarly, in aortic dissection, chronic expansion of the false lumen activates extrinsic tissue factors and intrinsic coagulation factors, leading to the exposure of subendothelial collagen tissue and the pooling of a high volume of blood in the false lumen. This pooled blood forms a thrombus, resulting in the continuous consumption of numerous coagulation factors [12]. As a result, DIC caused by aortic aneurysm/dissection is often classified as enhanced fibrinolytic type. DIC in these patients may therefore be controllable by inhibiting fibrinolysis.

Although the mechanism of DIC in aortic aneurysm/dissection mimics that of giant hemangioma, the incidence of clinically overt DIC ranges from 0.5% to 5.7% in patients with large aortic aneurysms compared with 25% among patients with giant hemangiomas [5, 16]. Some patients with aortic aneurysm-/dissection-related chronic DIC develop hemorrhagic diathesis, first detected when trauma or an invasive procedure such as tooth extraction triggers a sudden difficulty in achieving hemostasis. However, without such triggers, these patients may be asymptomatic, and chronic DIC may go unnoticed despite coagulation-fibrinolytic activation, in part because of compensatory mechanisms resulting in mild or even occult clinical symptoms [6, 7]. When bleeding was first identified in our four patients, two (Patients 1 and 2) had already been diagnosed with aortic aneurysm/dissection, whereas in the other two (Patients 3 and 4), aortic aneurysm/dissection was identified after bleeding developed. DIC control was immediately possible in Patients 1 and 2, delayed slightly in

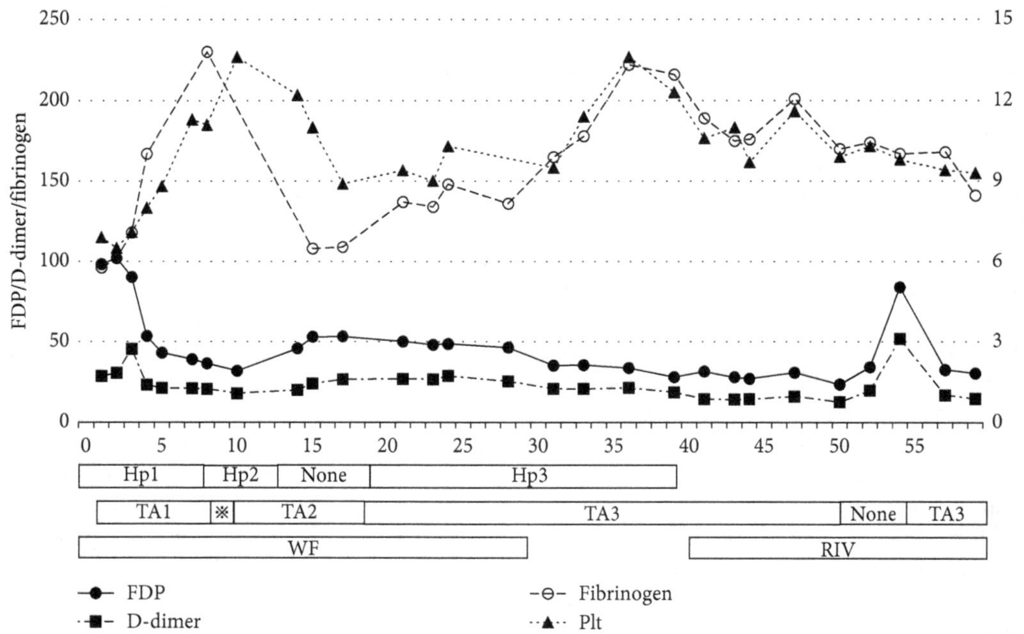

Figure 2: Clinical course correlation of treatment and improvement of DIC-related data in Patient 1. (Vertical axis) FDP = fibrin degradation product (μg/ml); D-dimer (μg/ml); fibrinogen (mg/dl); Plt = platelet count (x10e4/μl). (Horizontal axis) days; Hp = heparin: Hp1 = continuous intravenous infusion (10,000 U/day), Hp2 = continuous intravenous infusion (8,000 U/day), and Hp3 = subcutaneous administration (5,000 U twice daily); TA = tranexamic acid: TA1 = intravenous infusion (250 mg twice daily), ※ = intravenous TA (250 mg twice daily) + oral TA (750 mg/day), TA2 = oral (750 mg/day), and TA3 = oral (1500 mg/day); WF = warfarin oral; RIV = rivaroxaban oral (15 mg/day).

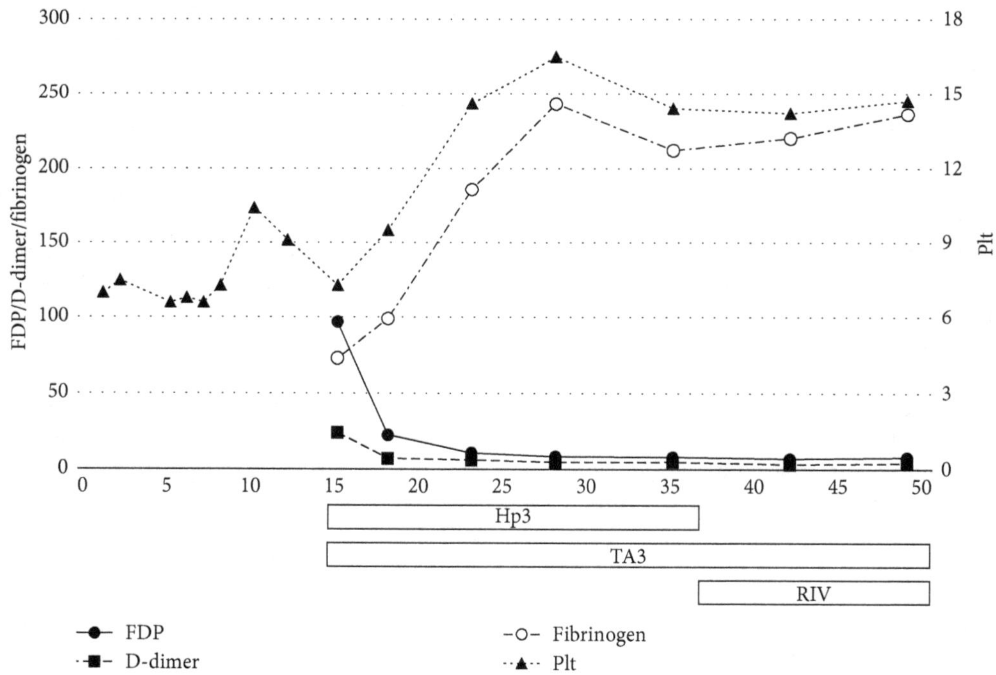

Figure 3: Clinical course correlation of treatment and improvement of DIC-related data in Patient 2. (Vertical axis) FDP = fibrin degradation product (μg/ml); D-dimer (μg/ml); fibrinogen (mg/dl); Plt = platelet count (x10e4/μl). (Horizontal axis) days; Hp = heparin: Hp3 = subcutaneous administration (5,000 U twice daily); TA3 = oral (1500 mg/day); RIV = rivaroxaban oral (15 mg/day).

Patient 3, and delayed significantly in Patient 4 because of emergency care of her profuse GI bleedings in association of her poor general condition.

Hemorrhagic diathesis due to chronic DIC caused by aortic aneurysm/dissection may be corrected by surgical intervention (e.g., replacement surgery and stent grafting) or medical treatment. When possible, surgical or interventional radiology correction of the aneurysm is the primary treatment; however, this study focused on the medical treatment of chronic DIC, which requires long-term management.

Three systemic therapeutic strategies for aortic DIC are available: anticoagulation therapy with heparin [8–10], antifibrinolytic therapy [11], and a combination of both [12]. The main purpose of treatment is to halt the consumption of systemic coagulation factors, fibrinogen, and platelets, as well as stop bleeding by blocking the cycle of thrombus formation and destruction. These treatments have opposite effects, preventing while generating thrombi. To date, heparin [8–10], camostat or nafamostat mesilate [17, 18], tranexamic acid [11], combinations of these medications [12], as well as rivaroxaban, a direct oral anticoagulant (DOAC) [13–15], have been reported as beneficial or successful, mostly in case reports and case series. Warfarin, on the contrary, may be less effective because it may worsen coagulopathy by reducing the expression of protein C and protein S (a cofactor of protein C) in patients with chronic DIC associated with aneurysm [14]. Stopping warfarin improved DIC parameters in Patient 1, perhaps for the reason.

In practice, patients with DIC showing severe anemia (Hb < 7.0 g/dl), low fibrinogen (<100 mg/dl), and low platelet counts (<20,000/μl) should initially receive transfusions of PRBC, FFP, and PC. At the same time, patients should be started on IV or SC heparin, and its favorable pharmacokinetic profile and low cost make this an attractive option. Combinations of heparin and tranexamic acid may benefit patients with high fibrinolytic activity [12]. However, the necessity of long-term management beyond hospital stay makes it difficult to continue IV/SC heparin administration. Oral camostat mesilate [17, 18] or rivaroxaban [13–15] may be a good alternative in these patients. Rivaroxaban may suppress DIC progression by inhibiting FXa [13–15]. Patients 1 and 2 were first successfully treated with heparin (IV and/or SC) plus tranexamic acid (IV or PO), followed by oral rivaroxaban after DIC stabilized. Especially, rivaroxaban was employed as maintenance therapy to facilitate discharge from the hospital. Although administration of rivaroxaban was bolstered by several recent case reports in similar contexts [11–15], the drug has not been adapted to DIC. Therefore, its off-label use was approved by the Institutional Review Boards of our hospital in accordance with the Declaration of Helsinki (UTMC approval number #2018–20). DOACs are currently adapted for thrombotic event prophylaxis in cases of nonvalvular atrial fibrillation as well as for treatment of deep vein thrombosis-pulmonary thromboembolism, but not for treatment of aortic thromboembolism which involves the aortic aneurysm-/dissection-related chronic DIC. Considering its effectiveness, it is hoped that DOACs will be adapted for the treatment of aortic thromboembolism in future. In addition, it remains to be confirmed if other DOAC agents, such as edoxaban or apixaban, will also show similar benefits like rivaroxaban in this clinical context.

In summary, elderly patients with hemorrhagic diathesis and unexplained DIC should be assessed for aortic aneurysm/dissection. Patients diagnosed with aortic aneurysm-/dissection-related DIC should be consulted first by the vascular surgeon or interventional radiologist and be considered for systemic medical treatments. The choice of treatment depends on various factors, including underlying diseases, severity of DIC, and patient comorbidities. Nonsurgical management of chronic DIC may require a long treatment period, with use of sufficiently tolerable and effective combination treatments to maintain patients' daily activities, even outside the hospital.

References

[1] M. Levi, C. H. Toh, J. Thachil, and H. G. Watson, "Guidelines for the diagnosis and management of disseminated intravascular coagulation," *British Journal of Haematology*, vol. 145, no. 1, pp. 24–33, 2009.

[2] H. Wada, T. Matsumoto, and Y. Yamashita, "Diagnosis and treatment of disseminated intravascular coagulation (DIC) according to four DIC guidelines," *Journal of Intensive Care*, vol. 2, no. 1, p. 15, 2014.

[3] H. Mukaiyama, S. Shionoya, T. Ikezawa, T. Kamiya, M. Hamaguchi, and H. Saito, "Abdominal aortic aneurysm complicated with chronic disseminated intravascular coagulopathy: a case of surgical treatment," *Journal of Vascular Surgery*, vol. 6, no. 6, pp. 600–604, 1987.

[4] S. Hinata, T. Kawada, N. Andou et al., "Thoracoabdominal aneurysm complicated with disseminated intravascular coagulopathy—a case of surgical treatment following heparin pretreatment," *Nihon Kyobu Geka Gakkai Zasshi*, vol. 39, no. 3, pp. 336–340, 1991, in Japanese.

[5] N. L. Fine, J. Applebaum, A. Elguezabal, and L. Castleman, "Multiple coagulation defects in association with dissecting aneurysm," *Archives of Internal Medicine*, vol. 119, no. 5, pp. 522–526, 1967.

[6] R. L. Bick, "Disseminated intravascular coagulation," *Hematology/Oncology Clinics of North America*, vol. 17, no. 1, pp. 149–176, 2003.

[7] H. Wada, E. C. Gabazza, H. Asakura et al., "Comparison of diagnostic criteria for disseminated intravascular coagulation (DIC): diagnostic criteria of the International Society of Thrombosis and Hemostasis (ISTH) and of the Japanese Ministry of Health and Welfare for overt DIC," *American Journal of Hematology*, vol. 74, no. 1, pp. 17–22, 2003.

[8] K. Takahashi, Y. Ichikawa, and S. Arimori, "Disseminated intravascular coagulation related to atherosclerosis and aneurysm of aorta: successful management with subcutaneous self-injection of heparin sodium," *Rinsho Ketsueki*, vol. 30, no. 10, pp. 1820–1825, 1989, in Japanese.

[9] I. Kurihara, Y. Yamaguchi, J. Soma et al., "Two aged patients with chronic renal failure and chronic disseminated intravascular coagulation secondary to aortic aneurysms: effect of continuous subcutaneous heparin infusion therapy," *Nihon Jinzo Gakkai Shi*, vol. 42, no. 7, pp. 603–607, 2000, in Japanese.

[10] K. Togami, Y. Nagai, H. Arima et al., "Successful treatment of chronic disseminated intravascular coagulation syndrome with continuous subcutaneous infusion of heparin using a mobile infusion pump: report of 2 cases," *Rinsho Ketsueki*, vol. 50, no. 12, pp. 1700–1705, 2009, in Japanese.

[11] T. Tsuji, K. Morikawa, T. Hirano et al., "Effective treatment with tranexamic acid for chronic disseminated intravascular coagulation associated with aortic dissection," *Rinsho Ketsueki*, vol. 54, no. 8, pp. 769–771, 2013, in Japanese.

[12] Y. Gatate, N. Masaki, A. Sato et al., "Tranexamic acid controlled chronic disseminated intravascular coagulation associated with aortic dissection and patent false lumen for three years," *Internal Medicine*, vol. 56, no. 8, pp. 925–929, 2017.

[13] H. Kawano, T. Hata, A. Uda, and K. Maemura, "Use of rivaroxaban for the effective management of disseminated intravascular coagulation associated with abdominal aortic aneurysm," *Internal Medicine*, vol. 54, no. 20, pp. 2625–2628, 2015.

[14] Y. Kadohira, S. Yamada, E. Matsuura et al., "Aortic aneurysm-associated disseminated intravascular coagulation that responded well to a switch from warfarin to rivaroxaban," *Internal Medicine*, vol. 56, no. 21, pp. 2913–2917, 2017.

[15] T. Hayashi, N. Nakagawa, Y. Kadohira, E. Morishita, and H. Asakura, "Rivaroxaban in a patient with disseminated intravascular coagulation associated with an aortic aneurysm: a case report," *Annals of Internal Medicine*, vol. 161, no. 2, pp. 158-159, 2014.

[16] D. M. Aboulafia and E. D. Aboulafia, "Aortic aneurysm-induced disseminated intravascular coagulation," *Annals of Vascular Surgery*, vol. 10, no. 4, pp. 396–405, 1996.

[17] N. Fukuda, Y. Shimohakamada, Y. Nakamori et al., "Thoracic aortic aneurysm with chronic disseminated intravascular coagulation treated successfully with orally administered camostat mesilate, warfarin and aspirin," *Rinsho Ketsueki*, vol. 43, no. 3, pp. 199–203, 2002, in Japanese.

[18] K. Yoneda, I. Amano, H. Tanaka et al., "Effective use of camostat mesilate for chronic disseminated intravascular coagulation complicated by thoracoabdominal aortic aneurysm," *Rinsho Ketsueki*, vol. 42, no. 1, pp. 30–34, 2001, in Japanese.

14

A Case of Warm Autoimmune Hemolytic Anemia and a Pulmonary Embolus in a Patient Treated with Triple Therapy

Gurchetan Randhawa,[1] **Chia-Yu Chiu**,[2] **and Thanunthorn Suban Na Ayutthaya**[2]

[1]*Maimonides Medical Center, Department of Medicine, Brooklyn, NY, USA*
[2]*Lincoln Medical Center, Department of Medicine, The Bronx, NY, USA*

Correspondence should be addressed to Gurchetan Randhawa; grandhawa@maimonidesmed.org

Academic Editor: Gergely Feher

Autoimmune hemolytic anemia (AIHA) can be caused by a variety of etiologies. AIHA is associated with the development of coagulopathy, leading to potentially fatal pulmonary emboli. Here, we present a case of a 66-year-old female with a past medical history of non-Hodgkin's lymphoma and gastritis treated with triple therapy that developed warm AIHA. The patient later succumbed to a suspected pulmonary embolus.

1. Introduction

Approximately one-half of warm AIHAs are idiopathic, while the nonidiopathic etiologies include lymphoproliferative disorders, autoimmune disease, and medication-induced AIHA. Medication-induced AIHA is a syndrome where a medication acts as a hapten on the surface of red blood cells (RBC) causing a sequence of hemolysis. IgG antibodies attach to the medication-RBC complex at body temperature, and the complex is transported to the spleen where it is consumed by macrophages. This, in turn, produces spherocytes, which are then destroyed by the spleen, thus causing hemolysis. This is contrast to cold AIHA, where IgM is the implicated immunoglobulin, and the complex forms at below core body temperature.

The association between non-Hodgkin's lymphoma and AIHA has been well established in the literature. It is possible that non-Hodgkin's lymphoma acts as a paraneoplastic syndrome producing antibodies against the surface of RBCs although the exact pathophysiology remains controversial.

2. Case Presentation

A 66-year-old female with a past medical history of hypertension, stage IIIA diffuse large B-cell lymphoma (DLBCL), and *H. pylori* gastritis presented to the emergency department complaining of epigastric pain for one week. The patient was recently treated for *H. pylori* gastritis (confirmed via esophagogastroduodenoscopy) with triple therapy but returned to the emergency department due to recurrent pain. She denied the presence of blood in her stool. The pain is worse with eating, is associated with a metallic taste, and prevented her from eating for the past ten days. She could only complete ten out of the fourteen days of her triple therapy regimen consisting of: amoxicillin 500 mg twice a day, clarithromycin 500 mg twice a day, and lansoprazole 30 mg twice a day.

The patient was treated for DLBCL three years ago with six cycles of R-CHOP (rituximab, cyclophosphamide, doxorubicin, vincristine, and prednisone) therapy. She attained a complete response and was on surveillance; however, a follow-up chest computed tomography (CT) scan one month prior to her admission indicated the presence of nine bilateral pulmonary nodules. The etiology of the nodules was unknown; however, they were concerning for recurrent lymphoma, primary lung malignancy, and metastatic disease.

Her physical exam was remarkable for dry oral mucosa and epigastric tenderness. Her lab studies were remarkable for leukocytosis (WBC: 18.5 K/μL), macrocytic anemia (Hgb: 5.1 g/dL, Hct: 13.8%, MCV: 122.7 fL), and LDH: 551 U/L. A fecal occult blood test was negative. A direct antiglobulin test (DAT) was IgG positive and C-3 negative. A peripheral smear indicated the presence of spherocytes and hypersegmented neutrophils. She received 3 units of packed RBCs and prednisone 70 mg (1 mg/kg) on the first day of admission.

On her second day of admission, the patient complained of dyspnea with oxygen saturation between 70 and 80% on 2 L nasal cannula. Her vital signs were temperature: 98.7°F, blood pressure: 140/90 mmHg, heart rate: 120 beats/min, and respiratory rate: 25 breaths/min. On physical exam, she had jugular venous distention with bibasilar crackles; however, she denied calf pain and the presence of varicose veins. She was switched to BiPAP with improvement in oxygen saturation to 98%. Due to the patient's rapid deterioration, a bedside point-of-care ultrasound was performed and indicated the presence of a dilated right ventricle (positive D sign with septal flattening) on the parasternal short axis view. A chest X-ray indicated cephalization of the pulmonary vasculature as well as right atrial enlargement. An initial electrocardiogram (EKG) indicated the presence of an S1 Q3 T3 pattern. The patient was intubated due to hypoxia. The clinical suspicion for a pulmonary embolus was high based upon these acute findings. Possible etiologies for the suspected pulmonary embolus include infection, recent blood transfusion, glucocorticoid use, immobility, AIHA, and malignancy.

Approximately ten minutes postintubation, the patient became hypotensive and bradycardic. The patient received a repeat EKG that demonstrated pulseless electrical activity, and she received cardiopulmonary resuscitation. She was given tissue plasminogen activator (tPA), and her oxygen saturation only improved after completing tPA therapy. She continued to receive resuscitation for approximately 35 minutes before regaining a pulse and was transferred to the medicine intensive care unit. Upon arrival to the intensive care unit, the patient went into cardiac arrest once again, and despite medical intervention, the patient expired.

3. Discussion

Warm AIHA is more common than cold AIHA, and it accounts for approximately 75% of all AIHAs in adults. The signs and symptoms of autoimmune hemolytic anemia are nonspecific, and the patient may initially present with weakness, dyspnea, jaundice, and tachycardia.

Laboratory findings of patients with warm AIHA include positive direct antiglobulin testing (Coombs test), spherocytes on peripheral blood smears, reticulocytosis, elevated lactate dehydrogenase (LDH), elevated indirect bilirubin, and decreased haptoglobin. At the behest of the patient's family, an autopsy was not performed; therefore, the true etiology of AIHA and the pulmonary nodules remains unknown. However, we suspect that the AIHA was medication-induced or malignancy-induced.

The most common medications to cause AIHA are antibiotics. The American Red Cross collected data in Southern California from 2000 to 2009 and reported 83 episodes of medication-related warm AIHA. The most commonly implicated agents were cefotetan (36 cases), ceftriaxone (17 cases), and piperacillin (14 cases) [1]. Another review article published in 2015 from a single center in Germany analyzed data from 1996 to 2015. They reported 73 cases of medication-related AIHA. Their most implicated agents were diclofenac (23 cases), followed by piperacillin (13 cases), ceftriaxone (12 cases), and oxaliplatin (10 cases) [2].

The first documented case of amoxicillin-induced autoimmune hemolytic anemia was reported in 1985 [3]. To the best of our knowledge, our case is the first documented case in which a patient developed warm AIHA while being treated with triple therapy (amoxicillin, clarithromycin, and lansaprazole). Although unreported in the literature, antibodies to clarithromycin or lansoprazole should also be considered as potential offending agents implicated in warm AIHA.

The association between venous thromboembolism (VTE) and AIHA has been well established in the literature. One meta-analysis from 2015 indicated that patients with AIHA had a 2.6-fold higher risk of developing VTE when compared with non-AIHA patients. The risk was more pronounced in the first year after diagnosis [4].

The mechanism of coagulation activation in hemolytic anemia is unclear and likely multifactorial. Normally, phosphatidylserine is found in the inner monolayer of the cell membrane. Destruction of the RBC membrane by autoantibodies leads to alteration of RBC membrane organization. This results in a loss of membrane phospholipid asymmetry and increased expression of anionic phospholipids, especially phosphatidylserine. This process causes an increased risk for coagulation and the development of VTE [5, 6].

AIHA are associated with lymphoproliferative disorders, the most common being chronic lymphocytic leukemia (CLL) [7]. In one retrospective study from 2010 involving 960 patients with CLL, 7% had autoimmune cytopenia, of which 19 were detected at diagnosis, 3 before diagnosis, and 48 during the course of the disease. 49 patients had autoimmune hemolytic anemia, 20 patients had immune thrombocytopenic purpura, and 1 patient had both conditions [8]. Both Hodgkin's and non-Hodgkin's lymphoma have also been associated with AIHA [9].

Treatment approaches for warm AIHA include reduction in autoantibody production and effectiveness. Glucocorticoids, cytotoxic agents, and rituximab are used to reduce autoantibody production. To reduce autoantibody effectiveness, splenectomy or intravenous immune globulin are utilized. Intravenous immune globulin acts by decreasing the interaction between splenic macrophages and antibody-coated RBCs [10].

Initial management includes stabilization of the patient (e.g., blood transfusion), administration of glucocorticoids as first-line agents, and searching for secondary causes (e.g., offending medications and contributing disorders). The recommended initial doses of glucocorticoids are 1 to 1.5 mg/kg per day. For patients with rapidly evolving, severe hemolysis, intravenous methylprednisolone 250–1000 mg/day for 1–3 days or 100–200 mg/day for 10–14 days is recommended. Once remission is achieved, the glucocorticoid dose is gradually tapered to find the optimal, lowest dose that maintains remission. Patients with warm AIHA should be treated for a minimum of 3-4 months with prednisone ≤10 mg/day. Bisphosphonates, vitamin D, calcium, and folic acid should also be given with long-term glucocorticoid therapy. Once hemoglobin, haptoglobin, LDH, and the absolute reticulocyte count are normalized, glucocorticoids can be discontinued, even with a positive Coombs test [11].

Second-line therapies include splenectomy and rituximab. Since there are no randomized trials comparing these therapies, the choice of splenectomy vs. rituximab relies upon the healthcare provider. Rituximab, a monoclonal antibody against CD20, has been successfully used in treatment-resistant AIHA as a single agent or in conjunction with glucocorticoids [10].

Third-line agents include immunosuppressive and cytotoxic agents, such as cyclophosphamide and azathioprine. The initial dose of cyclophosphamide is 100 mg/day orally or 500–700 mg intravenously every 3-4 weeks. The initial dose of azathioprine is 100–150 mg/day orally. For cases refractory to prednisone and splenectomy, high doses of intravenous gamma globulin (1000 mg/kg per day for five days) may be utilized [11].

4. Conclusion

In summary, this is a case of a 66-year-old woman with warm AIHA after 10 days of treatment with triple therapy for *H. pylori* gastritis. She also had bilateral pulmonary nodules of unclear etiology, which were concerning for the presence of malignancy, possibly due to a recurrent DLBCL treated 3 years prior. The patient eventually succumbed on the second day of admission with clinical findings consistent with a pulmonary embolus. Although the etiology of this patient's AIHA remains unclear, we hope that our paper can highlight the development of AIHA, as well as its potentially devastating complication of VTE formation.

References

[1] G. Garratty, "Immune hemolytic anemia associated with drug therapy," *Blood Reviews*, vol. 24, no. 4-5, pp. 143–150, 2010.

[2] B. Mayer, T. Bartolmäs, S. Yürek, and A. Salama, "Variability of findings in drug-induced immune haemolytic anaemia: experience over 20 years in a single centre," *Transfusion Medicine and Hemotherapy*, vol. 42, no. 5, pp. 333–339, 2015.

[3] J. Gmür, M. Wälti, and K. A. Neftel, "Amoxicillin-induced immune hemolysis," *Acta Haematologica*, vol. 74, no. 4, pp. 230–233, 1985.

[4] P. Ungprasert, P. Tanratana, and N. Srivali, "Autoimmune hemolytic anemia and venous thromboembolism: a systematic review and meta-analysis," *Thrombosis Research*, vol. 136, no. 5, pp. 1013–1017, 2015.

[5] S. K. Sadashiv, N. Patel, C. Hilton, D. Monga, and R. Kaplan, "A case of fatal pulmonary embolism in a patient with warm autoimmune hemolytic anemia: an under-appreciated thrombotic risk," *Journal of Hematology*, vol. 2, no. 2, pp. 85–88, 2013.

[6] K. I. Ataga, "Hypercoagulability and thrombotic complications in hemolytic anemias," *Haematologica*, vol. 94, no. 11, pp. 1481–1484, 2009.

[7] C. Moreno, K. Hodgson, G. Ferrer et al., "Autoimmune cytopenia in chronic lymphocytic leukemia: prevalence, clinical associations, and prognostic significance," *Blood*, vol. 116, no. 23, pp. 4771–4776, 2010.

[8] F. R. Mauro, R. Foa, R. Cerretti et al., "Autoimmune hemolytic anemia in chronic lymphocytic leukemia: clinical, therapeutic, and prognostic features," *Blood*, vol. 95, no. 9, pp. 2786–2792, 2000.

[9] S. Sallah, G. Sigounas, P. Vos, J. Y. Wan, and N. P. Nguyen, "Autoimmune hemolytic anemia in patients with non-Hodgkin's lymphoma: characteristics and significance," *Annals of Oncology*, vol. 11, no. 12, pp. 1571–1577, 2000.

[10] K. E. King and P. M. Ness, "Treatment of autoimmune hemolytic anemia," *Seminars in Hematology*, vol. 42, no. 3, pp. 131–136, 2005.

[11] A. Zanella and W. Barcellini, "Treatment of autoimmune hemolytic anemias," *Haematologica*, vol. 99, no. 10, pp. 1547–1554, 2014.

15

Danazol: An Effective and Underutilised Treatment Option in Diamond-Blackfan Anaemia

Kern Y. Chai, Cara J. Quijano, and Shingirai Chiruka

Department of Haematology, Dunedin Hospital, 201 Great King Street, Dunedin 9016, New Zealand

Correspondence should be addressed to Kern Y. Chai; kernchai@gmail.com

Academic Editor: Neelam Giri

Diamond-Blackfan anaemia (DBA) is a rare congenital red cell aplasia that presents in infancy. The exact molecular mechanism of ineffective erythropoiesis and red cell aplasia remains unclear, rendering targeted therapy elusive. The mainstay treatment of DBA is with regular blood transfusion and long-term corticosteroids, both of which have long-term side effects. We report a case of DBA successfully treated with danazol, a synthetic androgen, and suggest that danazol be considered as a viable option in patients who become refractory to steroids and are considered high risk or unfit for allogeneic stem cell transplantation.

1. Introduction

Diamond-Blackfan anaemia (DBA) is a rare congenital bone marrow failure syndrome characterised by an isolated macrocytic anaemia that presents in infancy. The mainstay treatment of DBA is with regular blood transfusion with long-term corticosteroids, both of which have long-term side effects. Steroid refractory or intolerant patients may benefit from an allogeneic stem cell transplant, but it is associated with high mortality and morbidity. Danazol has been shown in previous case reports to be a safe treatment option with reasonable efficacy in DBA. We suggest that danazol be considered as an option for patients refractory to steroids or as a steroid-sparing agent in DBA.

2. Case Report

A 33-year-old New Zealand European male was suspected of having DBA when he was two months old. He was taken to his general practitioner for a routine 6-week check, during which he was noted to be pale, and a subsequent full blood count revealed an isolated macrocytic anaemia (Hb 94 g/L). Of relevance, his mother was diagnosed with pure red cell aplasia when she was 14 months old, raising the possibility of a congenital bone marrow failure syndrome. A bone marrow biopsy revealed markedly reduced erythroid precursors consistent with DBA. He was placed on prednisone from two months of age. In addition to treatment with a corticosteroid, he required multiple blood transfusions between the ages of two months and two years. At four and a half years of age, oxymetholone was trailed as adjunctive therapy to prednisone at a total daily dose of 25 mg (2 mg/kg) to allow a steroid taper but was ineffective. A trial of danazol or cyclosporine was considered but was never undertaken due to lack of evidence regarding its efficacy in DBA. The patient's erythropoietin (EPO) levels were evaluated at the age of six and found to be raised at 197 μM/ml (normal range 5–53 μM/ml).

Later in life, it was noted that the patient had several physical malformations associated with DBA. He had dysmorphic features of short stature, micrognathia, small hands with long fingers, and a slightly widened neck. An echocardiogram revealed no cardiac abnormalities. When he was 12 years of age, he required orchidopexy for an undescended testis. Latterly, he was assessed by the endocrine service who concluded he was eugonadal, and his short stature was related to his long-term steroid use. As a result, attempts were made to reduce the prednisone dose slowly to the most tolerated but effective dose. He was stable for a number of years on between 7.5 mg daily and 7.5 mg on alternate days. He was transfusion independent between the ages of 2 and 32.

In November 2017, he presented with a profound hypoproliferative anaemia (Hb 47 g/L, reticulocyte 2×10^9). He denied any new medications or bleeding. At the time, his prednisone dose was 7.5 mg/5 mg on alternate days. Investigations for alternate causes of anaemia were unrevealing, with pertinent negatives including an unremarkable blood film, normal haematinics (B12 263 pmol/L, folate 36.4 nmol/L, and iron 23 μmol/L), negative haemolysis screen, and negative parvovirus, EBV, and CMV serology and PCR. Ferritin and transferrin saturation at the time were slightly elevated (737 μg/L and 92%, respectively), and transferrin was slightly decreased (1 g/L) likely secondary to ineffective erythropoiesis. A repeat bone marrow showed a hypocellular trephine with relatively preserved macronormoblastic erythropoiesis. There was no evidence of dysplasia, disease progression, or transformation. Cytogenetics revealed a normal karyotype. Finally, genetic testing was sent to Oxford University Hospital in the United Kingdom which revealed a point mutation in intron 2 of *RPS19*, confirming the diagnosis of DBA.

One month later, his prednisone was increased up to 2 mg per kg (totalling 110 mg per day) after requiring 7 units of RBCs within the preceding month. He remained on this dose of prednisone for three months, achieving a peak haemoglobin level of 84 g/L, but relapsed into transfusion dependency each time his prednisone was tapered. By this stage, the patient had cumulated many side effects related to his medical therapy. The long-term steroid use led to gastritis, osteoporosis, hypokalaemia, and central serous retinopathy requiring further co-treatment with omeprazole, alendronic acid, and cholecalciferol. He also developed transfusional haemosiderosis with a peak ferritin level of 1946 μg/L and transferrin saturation of 96%, necessitating chelation therapy with deferiprone. This was the first time that the patient had required a chelating drug. Unfortunately, he developed profound neutropenia from the deferiprone which culminated in a prolonged admission with extensive lower limb cellulitis, and the deferiprone was permanently discontinued. A cardiac MRI did not show significant iron overloading.

Given the toxicities, alternate treatment options were rediscussed including danazol, metoclopramide, and allogeneic stem cell transplant (AlloSCT). He was worked up for a transplant but did not have any matched sibling donors, and he was also considered as high risk for allogeneic stem cell transplantation given his age and multiple prior RBC transfusions. Thus, the decision was made to commence danazol 200 mg daily in March 2018. A starting dose of 200 mg was chosen as it is a standard starting dose for most indications. At this time, he was taking 60 mg of prednisone a day. Following the introduction of danazol, his haemoglobin rose, allowing the prednisone dose to be decreased (Figure 1, Table 1). Over the following few months, he had been weaned down to 7.5 mg of prednisone daily which he is taking in addition to the 200 mg of danazol while maintaining a haemoglobin level of 148–160 g/L six months later. The patient has been left on the minimum effective dose of danazol. His liver function tests have remained normal while on danazol.

3. Discussion

3.1. Introduction, Epidemiology, and Clinical Presentation. DBA is a rare congenital ribosomopathy characterised by erythroid hypoplasia, developmental malformations, and an increased risk of malignancy. The vast majority of patients are diagnosed within the first year of life with an incidence rate of 5–7 : 1,000,000 live births [1, 2]. Patients typically present with severe isolated macrocytic anaemia with reticulocytopenia. Bone marrow findings are usually normocellular with absent erythroid precursors [3]. Approximately half of all patients will have maxillofacial, thumb, cardiac, or renal malformations [2, 4]. There is an approximate 20% cumulative incidence of malignancies by the age of 50 [5, 6].

3.2. Pathogenesis and Inheritance. DBA is inherited in autosomal dominant fashion but with incomplete penetrance. Over 50% of DBA cases have somatic mutations or deletions in one of 14 genes encoding for ribosomal proteins, with the *RPS19* gene being the commonest genetic abnormality accounting for a quarter of cases [4, 7–9]. Genotype-phenotype correlations have been observed with *RPL5* and *RPL11* mutations associated with higher rates of physical malformations [8]. The exact molecular mechanism by which ribosomal dysfunction leads to ineffective erythropoiesis and red cell aplasia remains unclear. Dutt et al. found that haploinsufficiency of ribosomal protein genes activates the p53 pathway, culminating in preferential accumulation of p21 in erythroid progenitor cells and consequent cell cycle arrest [10]. Other postulated mechanisms relate to defective erythroblast mRNA generation or altered haeme metabolism [9, 11, 12]. Further empiric proof is evidenced by rescued erythropoiesis with pharmacological inhibition of p53 in both human and mouse models [13, 14].

In relation to our case, the patient was found to be heterozygous for a G to A nucleotide substitution at the first nucleotide in intron 2 of *RPS19* (*RPS19* C. 71 + 1G > A). The testing was undertaken at Oxford University Hospital using a combination of Sanger sequencing and next generation sequencing involving custom design amplicons run on the Illumina MiSeq. This mutation has been previously reported to be associated with DBA [15].

The patient's mother was diagnosed with red cell aplasia when she was 14 months of age. She was treated initially with cortisol and then switched to prednisone at the age of two in addition to multiple blood transfusions. She went into remission between the ages of two and three. The anaemia reoccurred when she was six years old, and she was placed back on prednisone until she once again went into remission at the age of 12. Since her second remission, she has not required further treatment. The other members of the patient's family, including maternal grandparents, have not shown symptoms of DBA. Therefore, this may be a de novo mutation that has arisen in the mother. The mother has not been tested for the mutation found in the patient.

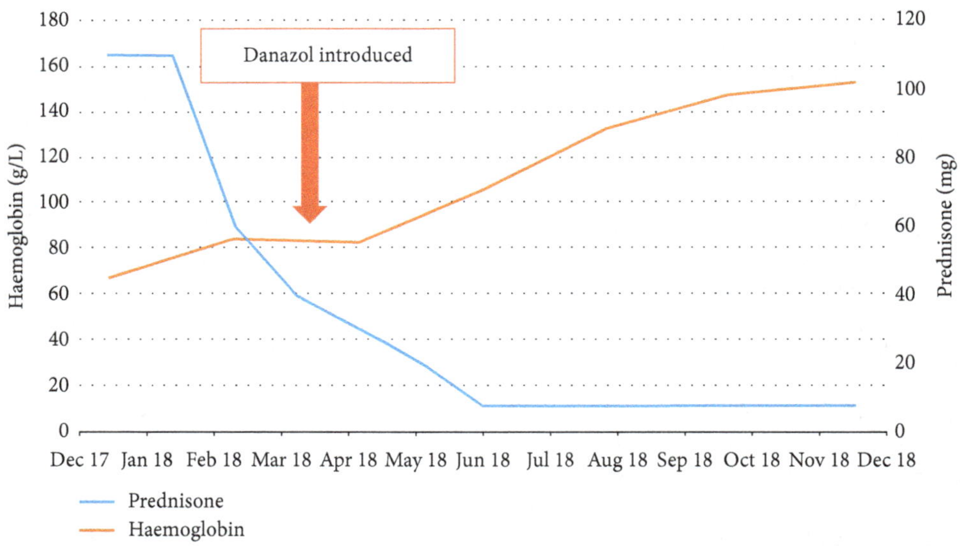

FIGURE 1: Line graph depicting improvement in haemoglobin despite decreasing prednisone dose following the introduction of danazol.

TABLE 1: Depicting figures of haemoglobin and prednisone as shown in Figure 1. Haemoglobin figures stated in November 2017 are pre- and posttransfusion.

Date	Nov 17	Nov 17	Dec 18	Feb 18	Apr 18	Jun 18	Aug 18	Oct 18	Dec 18
Haemoglobin (g/L)	47	77	67	84	83	105	133	148	153
Prednisone (mg)	7.5/5	110	110	60	30	7.5	7.5	7.5	7.5

3.3. Treatment. The mainstay treatment of DBA is with regular RBC transfusion and long-term corticosteroids [2, 3]. RBC transfusion intervals are typically every 4–6 weeks, and the cumulative iron loading can lead to significant endocrine, cardiac, hepatic, and joint dysfunction. The transfusional hemosiderosis can be minimised by chelation therapy but is usually poorly tolerated. Maintenance corticosteroids, whilst effective in about 80% of patients, have led to significant long-term toxicities causing a cessation in therapy in about half of patients [16].

Steroid refractory or intolerant patients may benefit from an AlloSCT [2, 7, 16]. Long-term registry data indicate 40% of patients are steroid dependent, 40% are transfusion dependent due to poor response or intolerance to steroids, and the remaining 20% are in haematologic remission (either spontaneous or post-AlloSCT) [17, 18]. Other treatments have been trialled in a small number of patients with minimal success. Immunosuppressive therapies including IVIG and cyclosporine have been used despite limited theoretical basis [1, 3, 7, 16]. Metoclopramide has been trialled on the basis of increasing prolactin levels to stimulate the erythroid precursor microenvironment, but with disappointing results [19]. Targeted therapy in the form of leucine remains experimental [2]. Clearly, there is a need for more effective and safer treatments that provide long-term control.

3.4. Danazol. Danazol is a synthetic androgen compound that inhibits pituitary gonadotrophins. It also has mild immunosuppressive properties via inhibition of TNF-alpha and IL-1 [20]. Its side effect profile is unsurprisingly related to hyperandrogenism but is also rarely associated with the development of hepatocellular carcinoma (HCC) and hepatocellular adenomas [21, 22].

Polycythaemia is a common side effect observed in testosterone-treated men, whereas haemoglobin levels in women with congenital adrenal hyperplasia also correlate with androgen levels [23]. More recently, testosterone has been shown to increase erythropoietin (EPO) levels while concurrently reducing hepcidin levels, therefore suggesting a molecular basis for androgen-induced erythropoiesis [24]. In addition, it has also been utilised to overcome EPO-resistance in renal-mediated anaemia [25, 26]. It stands to reason that danazol, a synthetic androgen, could also produce such effects in vivo leading to a targeted proliferation of erythroid precursors via the JAK/STAT signalling pathway [27].

Danazol has also shown activity in treating anaemia in other haematological conditions including aplastic anaemia, myelodysplasia, myelofibrosis, pure red cell aplasia, and other inherited bone marrow failure syndromes including Fanconi anaemia and dyskeratosis congenita [19, 28–33]. Jaime-Pérez et al. studied a cohort of 50 patients with aplastic anaemia of which 37 were treated with danazol. They found a response rate of 46% with a 41% five-year overall survival in the patients treated with danazol (compared with 92% in the remaining patients receiving allogeneic haematopoietic stem cell transplantation) [20]. Scheckenbach et al. collected data on eight patients with Fanconi anaemia who had been treated with danazol. They found that seven of the patients responded with marked improvement in both haemoglobin and platelets [31].

The patient had a haematological response to danazol, but a trial of oxymetholone earlier in life was found to be ineffective despite the fact that these medications are both androgens. We hypothesize that this may be due to the agonistic effects of danazol on glucocorticoid receptors, resulting in danazol having bimodal upregulating effects on erythropoiesis [34].

3.5. Relevance to Case. The patient developed steroid-resistant DBA after being on low-dose prednisone for 30 years, resulting in transfusion dependency. The addition of danazol led to a complete haematologic response sustained at 12 months (at time of writing) that was not seen even with salvage high-dose prednisone (2 mg/kg). The patient has significant toxicity from the chronic corticosteroid treatment including osteoporosis and central serous retinopathy in his 30s. In addition, he had life-threatening neutropenic sepsis from deferiprone, which was introduced when he became transfusion dependent after the prednisone response was lost. His prednisone is being tapered with the aim of transitioning to danazol monotherapy in the future. Whilst danazol is not completely benign (increased risk of HCC), it clearly has less risk and morbidity compared to long-term corticosteroids or an AlloSCT.

Other case reports highlighting the efficacy of danazol have been published. Flores Ballester et al. described a patient with a congenital hypoplastic left thumb who developed a hypoproliferative anaemia in his 30s [35]. He was diagnosed with adult-onset DBA after the identification of a pathogenic mutation in *RPL11*. He was unresponsive to steroids and became transfusion dependent. He was commenced on cyclosporine with minimal improvement until the addition of danazol (400 mg per day). The patient remains in haematologic remission for the last 16 months since starting danazol monotherapy.

4. Conclusions

Danazol is a relatively underutilised treatment in DBA with a plausible targeted molecular basis for overcoming erythroid hypoplasia. It is cheap and relatively nontoxic compared to long-term corticosteroids, immunosuppressive therapy, or AlloSCT. Whilst large prospective randomised controlled trials to confirm the efficacy of Danazol in DBA is not realistic due to the rarity of this condition, directed laboratory studies could be carried out as a surrogate to ascertain its utility in DBA patients.

References

[1] A. Vlachos and E. Muir, "How I treat Diamond-Blackfan anemia," *Blood*, vol. 116, no. 19, pp. 3715–3723, 2010.

[2] M. Bartels and M. Bierings, "How I manage children with Diamond—Blackfan anaemia," *British Journal of Haematology*, vol. 184, no. 2, pp. 123–133, 2018.

[3] S. E. Sjögren and J. Flygare, "Progress towards mechanism-based treatment for Diamond-Blackfan anemia," *Scientific World Journal*, vol. 2012, no. 2, Article ID 184362, 8 pages, 2012.

[4] H. Li, H. F. Lodish, and C. A. Sieff, "Critical issues in Diamond-Blackfan anemia and prospects for novel treatment," *Hematology/Oncology Clinics of North America*, vol. 32, no. 4, pp. 701–712, 2018.

[5] A. Vlachos, P. S. Rosenberg, E. Atsidaftos, B. P. Alter, and J. M. Lipton, "Incidence of neoplasia in Diamond Blackfan anemia: a report from the diamond blackfan anemia registry," *Blood*, vol. 119, no. 16, pp. 3815–3819, 2012.

[6] C. Muir, A. Dodds, and K. Samaras, "Mid-life extra-haematopoetic manifestations of Diamond–Blackfan anaemia," *Endocrinology, Diabetes & Metabolism Case Reports*, vol. 2017, Article ID 16-0141, 2017.

[7] A. Aspesi, C. Borsotti, and A. Follenzi, "Emerging therapeutic approaches for Diamond Blackfan anemia," *Current Gene Therapy*, vol. 18, no. 6, pp. 327–335, 2018.

[8] N. A. Paolini, A. W. MacInnes, and M. von Lindern, *Diamond-Blackfan Anaemia: From Genotype to Phenotype*, vol. 10, John Wiley & Sons, Ltd., Chichester, UK, 2001.

[9] R. Horos, H. IJspeert, D. Pospisilova et al., "Ribosomal deficiencies in Diamond-Blackfan anemia impair translation of transcripts essential for differentiation of murine and human erythroblasts," *Blood*, vol. 119, no. 1, pp. 262–272, 2012.

[10] S. Dutt, A. Narla, K. Lin et al., "Haploinsufficiency for ribosomal protein genes causes selective activation of p53 in human erythroid progenitor cells," *Blood*, vol. 117, no. 9, pp. 2567–2576, 2011.

[11] S. Mercurio, A. Aspesi, L. Silengo, F. Altruda, I. Dianzani, and D. Chiabrando, "Alteration of heme metabolism in a cellular model of Diamond-Blackfan anemia," *European Journal of Haematology*, vol. 96, no. 4, pp. 367–374, 2015.

[12] M. T. Elghetany, "Diamond-Blackfan anemia: death by heme toxicity?," *European Journal of Haematology*, vol. 96, no. 4, pp. 333-334, 2016.

[13] P. Jaako, S. Debnath, K. Olsson et al., "Disruption of the 5S RNP-Mdm2 interaction significantly improves the erythroid defect in a mouse model for Diamond-Blackfan anemia," *Leukemia*, vol. 29, no. 11, pp. 2221–2229, 2015.

[14] P. Jaako, J. Flygare, K. Olsson et al., "Mice with ribosomal protein S19 deficiency develop bone marrow failure and symptoms like patients with Diamond-Blackfan anemia," *Blood*, vol. 118, no. 23, pp. 6087–6096, 2011.

[15] A. Proust, L. Da Costa, P. Rince et al., "Ten novel Diamond-Blackfan anemia mutations and three polymorphisms within the rps19 gene," *Hematology Journal*, vol. 4, no. 2, pp. 132–136, 2003.

[16] R. T. Calado and D. V. Clé, "Treatment of inherited bone marrow failure syndromes beyond transplantation," *Hematology*, vol. 2017, no. 1, pp. 96–101, 2017.

[17] J. M. Lipton, E. Atsidaftos, I. Zyskind, and A. Vlachos, "Improving clinical care and elucidating the pathophysiology of Diamond Blackfan anemia: an update from the diamond Blackfan Anemia registry," *Pediatric Blood & Cancer*, vol. 46, no. 5, pp. 558–564, 2006.

[18] T. N. Willig, C. M. Niemeyer, T. Leblanc et al., "Identification of new prognosis factors from the clinical and epidemiologic analysis of a registry of 229 Diamond-Blackfan anemia patients. DBA group of Société d'Hématologie etd'Immunologie Pédiatrique (SHIP), Gesellshaft für Pädiatrische Onkologie und Hämatologie (GPOH), and the European Society for

Pediatric Hematology and Immunology (ESPHI)," *Pediatric research*, vol. 46, no. 5, pp. 553–561, 1999.

[19] T. M. Leblanc, L. Da Costa, I. Marie, P. Demolis, and G. Tchernia, "Metoclopramide treatment in DBA patients: no complete response in a French prospective study," *Blood*, vol. 109, no. 5, pp. 2266-2267, 2007.

[20] J. C. Jaime-Pérez, P. R. Colunga-Pedraza, C. D. Gómez-Ramírez et al., "Danazol as first-line therapy for aplastic anemia," *Annals of Hematology*, vol. 90, no. 5, pp. 523–527, 2011.

[21] K. Kobayashi, T. Shimokawa Miyama, K. Itamoto et al., "Development of hepatocellular carcinoma after long-term immunosuppressive therapy including danazol in a dog," *Journal of Veterinary Medical Science*, vol. 78, no. 10, pp. 1611–1614, 2016.

[22] J. Bartley, C. Loddenkemper, J. Lange et al., "Hepatocellular adenoma and focal nodular hyperplasia after long-term use of danazol for endometriosis: a case report," *Archives of Gynecology and Obstetrics*, vol. 269, no. 4, pp. 290–293, 2004.

[23] N. Karunasena, T. S. Han, A. Mallappa et al., "Androgens correlate with increased erythropoiesis in women with congenital adrenal hyperplasia," *Clinical Endocrinology*, vol. 86, no. 1, pp. 19–25, 2016.

[24] E. Bachman, T. G. Travison, S. Basaria et al., "Testosterone induces erythrocytosis via increased erythropoietin and suppressed hepcidin: evidence for a new erythropoietin/hemoglobin set point," *Journals of Gerontology Series A: Biological Sciences and Medical Sciences*, vol. 69, no. 6, pp. 725–735, 2014.

[25] D. Silverberg, D. Wexler, M. Blum, D. Schwartz, and A. Iaina, "The use of androgens in anaemia resistant to erythropoietin and i.v. iron in patients with heart and renal failure," *Nephrology Dialysis Transplantation*, vol. 19, no. 4, p. 1021, 2004.

[26] J. J. Carrero, P. Barany, M. I. Yilmaz et al., "Testosterone deficiency is a cause of anaemia and reduced responsiveness to erythropoiesis-stimulating agents in men with chronic kidney disease," *Nephrology Dialysis Transplantation*, vol. 27, no. 2, pp. 709–715, 2012.

[27] S. McGee, A. M. Havens, Y. Shiozawa, Y. Jung, and R. S. Taichman, "Effects of erythropoietin on the bone microenvironment," *Growth Factors*, vol. 30, no. 1, pp. 22–28, 2012.

[28] F. Cervantes, I. M. Isola, A. Alvarez-Larrán, J.-C. Hernández-Boluda, J.-G. Correa, and A. Pereira, "Danazol therapy for the anemia of myelofibrosis: assessment of efficacy with current criteria of response and long-term results," *Annals of Hematology*, vol. 94, no. 11, pp. 1791–1796, 2015.

[29] S. M. Lippman, B. G. M. Durie, H. S. Garewal, G. Giordano, and B. R. Greenberg, "Efficacy of danazol in pure red cell aplasia," *American Journal of Hematology*, vol. 23, no. 4, pp. 373–379, 1986.

[30] P. R. Colunga-Pedraza, J. E. Colunga-Pedraza, M. A. Garza-Ledezma et al., "Danazol as first-line therapy for myelodysplastic syndrome," *Clinical Lymphoma Myeloma and Leukemia*, vol. 18, no. 2, pp. e109–e113, 2018.

[31] T. Chuhjo, H. Yamazaki, M. Omine, and S. Nakao, "Danazol therapy for aplastic anemia refractory to immunosuppressive therapy," *American Journal of Hematology*, vol. 83, no. 5, pp. 387–389, 2008.

[32] K. Scheckenbach, M. Morgan, J. Filger-Brillinger et al., "Treatment of the bone marrow failure in Fanconi anemia patients with danazol," *Blood Cells, Molecules, and Diseases*, vol. 48, no. 2, pp. 128–131, 2012.

[33] A. Islam, S. Rafiq, M. Kirwan et al., "Haematological recovery in dyskeratosis congenita patients treated with danazol," *British Journal of Haematology*, vol. 162, no. 6, pp. 854–856, 2013.

[34] R. L. Barbieri and K. J. Ryan, "Danazol: endocrine pharmacology and therapeutic applications," *American Journal of Obstetrics and Gynecology*, vol. 141, no. 4, pp. 453–463, 1981.

[35] E. Flores Ballester, J. J. Gil-Fernández, M. Vázquez Blanco et al., "Adult-onset Diamond-Blackfan anemia with a novel mutation in the exon 5 of *RPL11*: too late and too rare," *Clinical Case Reports*, vol. 3, no. 6, pp. 392–395, 2015.

16

Oxford-AstraZeneca Coronavirus Disease-2019 Vaccine-Induced Immune Thrombocytopenia on Day Two

Azhar Kareem Razzaq [1] **and Ameer Al-Jasim** [2]

[1] *College of Medicine-University of Basrah, Department of Haematology, Baghdad, Iraq*
[2] *College of Medicine-University of Baghdad, Baghdad, Iraq*

Correspondence should be addressed to Azhar Kareem Razzaq; dr.azharalasady@gmail.com

Academic Editor: Pier Paolo Piccaluga

Introduction. Vaccines have been one of the most impactful human discoveries that have significantly changed life expectancy. Immune thrombocytopenic purpura (ITP) is an autoimmune disease characterized by platelet damage, life-threatening thrombocytopenia, and haemorrhage when the platelet count reaches below 20×10^9/mcL. Its pathogenesis involves viral mimicry or T-cell-induced immune destruction in antibody-negative cases. The clinical manifestations of thrombocytopenia vary according to the severity (level of platelets) and range from being asymptomatic to severe haemorrhage. ITP is treated with immunosuppression. *Case Presentation*. A 26-year-old Iraqi male laboratory analyst with an unremarkable medical history presented with severe thrombocytopenia 2 days after receiving the Oxford-AstraZeneca coronavirus disease-2019 vaccine. The patient was asymptomatic with unremarkable examination findings. However, his low platelet count was discovered accidentally, and the patient did not exhibit the resistance pattern of ITP and recovered successfully with regular immunosuppressant treatment. *Conclusion*. Patients with a history of thrombocytopenia can develop vaccine-induced thrombocytopenia earlier than the expected onset. Close monitoring, through regular complete blood counts, is highly recommended for patients with previous thrombocytopenia because the immune modulation process of the vaccine can worsen preexisting thrombocytopenia.

1. Introduction

Vaccines have become an impactful human discovery that has significantly changed life expectancy and disease incidence. However, adverse events and autoimmune phenomena, including immune thrombocytopenic purpura (ITP), have been reported in vaccination [1].

ITP is an autoimmune disease characterized by platelet damage that causes life-threatening thrombocytopenia through haemorrhage, when the platelet count drops below 20×10^9/mcL. The pathogenesis of vaccine-associated autoimmunity most likely involves virally induced molecular mimicry or a T-cell immune-mediated mechanism [2, 3].

The clinical manifestations of ITP range from asymptomatic to light purpuric rash all over the body to severe intracranial haemorrhage [4]. The usual treatments for such conditions are immunosuppressants, such as steroids and intravenous immunoglobulin (IVIG) [2].

Different vaccines have reportedly caused ITP through various mechanisms, eventually leading to thrombocytopenia. Thus, it is not unusual for a vaccine to cause ITP [1]. On the 8th of June 2021, Welsh et al. reported the occurrence of immune thrombocytopenia with the Pfizer and Moderna vaccines in their manuscript regarding the COVID-19 Vaccine Adverse Event Reporting System. We report the first case of immune thrombocytopenia induced by the Oxford-AstraZeneca coronavirus disease-2019 (COVID-19) vaccine [5].

In this case, we present an Oxford-AstraZeneca COVID-19 vaccine-induced immune thrombocytopenia that occurred on the second day in a 26-year-old man with a medical history of undiagnosed thrombocytopenia.

2. Case Presentation

A 26-year-old Iraqi male laboratory analyst presented with severe thrombocytopenia two days after receiving the Oxford-AstraZeneca COVID-19 vaccine. He had an unremarkable medical history, except for mild thrombocytopenia, ranging from 100 to 130×10^9. He had not sought consult for a provisional diagnosis. In addition to experiencing mild headaches, the patient had generally been asymptomatic. His low platelet counts were discovered incidentally through a routine complete blood count.

On examination, the patient was well, conscious, oriented, not in distress, and vitally stable. There was no gum or conjunctival bleeding, epistaxis, petechiae, purpura, or ecchymosis. Jaundice, organomegaly, and lymphadenopathy were also not noted.

Further laboratory testing revealed a platelet count of 64×10^9/L on day 2, which dropped to 35×10^9/L on day 3. The rest of his complete blood count results were unremarkable. His fibrinogen level was 145 mg/mL, and his prothrombin time, partial thromboplastin time, D-dimer, brain magnetic resonance imaging, and magnetic resonance venography were all normal.

The management plan consisted of hospital admission, methylprednisolone (pulse dose at 1 g/kg for 3 days), and IVIG (1 g/kg for 2 days).

The patient responded well to treatment and had a favourable outcome. On the fifth day, he had a platelet count of 90×10^9 L with a normal coagulation profile. His platelet count normalized in the second week. The patient was then discharged based on his improved blood count and was recommended for periodic follow-up.

3. Discussion

There have been at least 25 reports of ITP related to the COVID-19 vaccine. Reportedly, only the Pfizer and Moderna vaccines caused this adverse event. However, this side effect is not exclusively attributable to these vaccines [5–8].

Thrombocytopenia is not an unusual outcome of an immune modulation process, such as vaccination. It is expected to develop 4–30 days after vaccine administration [9]. In the present case, severe asymptomatic thrombocytopenia was noted 2 days after the Oxford-AstraZeneca COVID-19 vaccine had been administered. This contradicted the known onset and symptomatology of vaccine-induced thrombocytopenia. This deviation was attributed to the patient's undiagnosed thrombocytopenia.

The patient's good clinical response to the standard ITP regimen confirmed the immune-induced process of thrombocytopenia. This was most likely associated with the corresponding vaccine. The clinical scenario was similar to that of patients who received the Moderna and Pfizer vaccines [5, 8].

The deleterious effects of aggressive immunosuppression on vaccine-induced thrombocytopenia should not be overlooked. In prior studies, postvaccination immunosuppressive therapy attenuated the immune response to the administered vaccine [10].

4. Conclusion

In conclusion, patients with a history of thrombocytopenia can develop vaccine-induced thrombocytopenia earlier than the expected onset. Further studies are warranted to investigate this phenomenon.

Close monitoring of patients with previous thrombocytopenia is highly recommended because the immune modulation process of the vaccine can worsen the preexisting thrombocytopenia. Thus, regular complete blood count is indicated after COVID-19 vaccination.

Consent

Written informed consent was obtained from the patient to publish his details.

References

[1] C. Perricone, F. Ceccarelli, G. Nesher et al., "Immune thrombocytopenic purpura (ITP) associated with vaccinations: a review of reported cases," *Immunologic Research*, vol. 60, no. 2-3, pp. 226–235, 2014.

[2] D. B. Cines and V. S. Blanchette, "Immune thrombocytopenic purpura," *New England Journal of Medicine*, vol. 346, no. 13, pp. 995–1008, 2002.

[3] M. Rinaldi, C. Perricone, O.-D. Ortega-Hernandez, R. Perricone, and Y. Shoenfeld, "Immune thrombocytopaenic purpura: an autoimmune cross-link between infections and vaccines," *Lupus*, vol. 23, no. 6, pp. 554–567, 2014.

[4] V. Saudagar, S. Patil, S. Goh, and S. Pothiawala, "Vigilance regarding immune thrombocytopenic purpura after COVID-19 vaccine," *Irish Journal of Medical Science*, vol. 1971, pp. 1-2, 2021.

[5] K. J. Welsh, J. Baumblatt, W. Chege, R. Goud, and N. Nair, "Thrombocytopenia including immune thrombocytopenia after receipt of mRNA COVID-19 vaccines reported to the vaccine adverse event reporting system (VAERS)," *Vaccine*, vol. 39, no. 25, pp. 3329–3332, 2021.

[6] J. M. Helms, K. T. Ansteatt, J. C. Roberts et al., "Severe, refractory immune thrombocytopenia occurring after SARS-CoV-2 vaccine," *Journal of Blood Medicine*, vol. 12, pp. 221–224, 2021.

[7] E. J. Lee, D. B. Cines, T. Gernsheimer et al., "Thrombocytopenia following Pfizer and Moderna SARS-CoV-2 vaccination," *American Journal of Hematology*, vol. 96, no. 5, pp. 534–537, 2021.

[8] T. Shimabukuro, *COVID-19 Vaccine Safety Update*, Advisory Committee on Immunization Practices (ACIP), Atlanta, GA, USA, 2021.

[9] J. B. Bussel, J. M. Connors, and D. B. Cines, "Thrombosis with thrombocytopenia syndrome (also termed vaccine-induced thrombotic thrombocytopenia)," *American Society of Hematology*, vol. 25, 2021.

[10] K. A. Papp, B. Haraoui, D. Kumar et al., "Vaccination guidelines for patients with immune-mediated disorders on immunosuppressive therapies," *Journal of Cutaneous Medicine and Surgery*, vol. 23, no. 1, pp. 50–74, 2019.

17

Autoimmune Hemolytic Anemia in a Renal Transplant Patient Following Seasonal Influenza Vaccination

Imran Gani,[1] George Hinnant,[1] Rajan Kapoor,[1] and Natasha Savage[2]

[1]*Department of Nephrology, Hypertension and Transplant Medicine, Augusta University Health, Augusta, Georgia*
[2]*Department of Pathology, Augusta University Health, Augusta, Georgia*

Correspondence should be addressed to Imran Gani; igani@augusta.edu

Academic Editor: S Aref

Vaccines aim to prevent disease occurrence, its severity, and resultant complications. Our patient, a 58-year-old male, received seasonal influenza vaccination as part of routine health maintenance. Three days later, he presented with malaise, fever, and yellowish discoloration of eyes. His labs showed hyperbilirubinemia, anemia, elevated lactate dehydrogenase, and low haptoglobin, consistent with hemolytic anemia. Autoimmune hemolytic anemia has been associated with vaccine use and may result from phenomena of molecular mimicry and cross-reactivity with the possible role of vaccine adjuvants as well. An underlying structural defect of the red blood cell membrane may make them prone to hemolysis. The differential diagnosis and work-up of hemolytic anemia is extensive, as performed in our case. Management strategies for vaccine-induced hemolysis may involve supportive care, red blood cell transfusion, steroids, and intravenous immunoglobulin.

1. Introduction

Seasonal influenza vaccine aims to protect against infection by influenza virus and resultant complications. Vaccines have been associated with autoimmune phenomena including triggering of autoimmune hemolytic anemias. Hemolytic anemia can present as chronic anemia secondary to chronic low-grade hemolysis or as brisk hemolysis leading to frank anemia that requires prompt medical treatment. Herein, we present a unique case of acute on chronic hemolytic anemia after a routine influenza vaccine in a kidney transplant patient.

2. Case Presentation

A 58-year-old Caucasian male with a past medical history of end-stage renal disease secondary to hypertension, hyperlipidemia, and diabetes mellitus type 2, received a living related kidney transplant in 1994. He was in his routine state of health with stable allograft function and was seen in internal medicine clinic for health maintenance visit where he received a seasonal influenza vaccine (0.5 ml intramuscular in the deltoid in October 2018—Quadrivalent Inactivated Influenza Vaccine IIV4). Three days later, he presented with malaise, chills, fever (up to 101.6 F), and yellowish discoloration of eyes. Physical examination confirmed icteric sclerae. His labs were significant for hemoglobin of 12.5 g/dl (baseline hemoglobin of approximately 14.4 g/dl), total bilirubin of 5.1 mg/dl, and mildly elevated AST, ALT, and ALP. Platelet count and serum creatinine were normal. LDH was elevated and haptoglobin was very low with an elevated reticulocyte percentage of 4.2%. He denied any new medications, history of allergy, or any autoimmune disease. Rapid flu test was negative for both influenza A and B. The clinical picture and labs were suggestive of hemolytic anemia post routine influenza vaccine.

On further work-up, blood culture, urine culture, and acute viral hepatitis panel for HBV, HCV, and HAV were negative. The conventional tube technique direct antiglobulin test (DAT)/Coombs test was negative. The Coombs test was performed by using a polyspecific antihuman globulin reagent and monospecific antibodies to IgG and C3d. Parvovirus B19, Epstein–Barr virus, and cytomegalovirus PCR were also negative. Iron studies and ferritin levels were normal. G6PD levels and pyruvate kinase levels were within normal range. Hemoglobin high-performance liquid chromatography (HPLC) was unremarkable. A right upper quadrant ultrasound demonstrated borderline hepatomegaly along with gallstones with no acute pathology.

On review of the patient's labs and clinical records, the patient had been having low degree hyperbilirubinemia since 2003 (Bilirubin 1.3–1.8). He had elliptocytes on red cell morphologic review in 2004 and 2007 that had been overlooked. He did not carry a formal diagnosis of any structural erythrocyte abnormality. A peripheral blood smear was ordered during his acute hemolytic event. It demonstrated normochromic and normocytic red blood cells. However, there was significant anisopoikilocytosis with a predominance of elliptocytes suggestive of hereditary elliptocytosis (Figure 1).

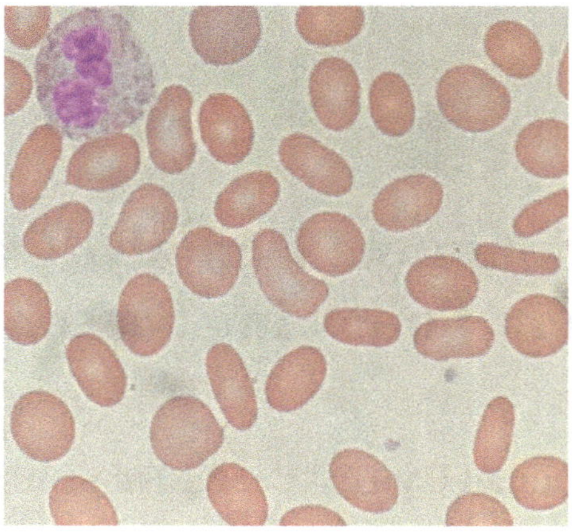

FIGURE 1: Morphologic review of the Wright–Giemsa stained peripheral blood smear revealed normochromic, normocytic red blood cells with anisopoikilocytosis. Many red blood cells (>25%) were elliptocytes. Elliptocytes are shaped like a pencil or thin cigar, with blunt ends and parallel sides.

3. Outcome and Follow-Up

The patient was managed conservatively with supportive care. As he was in a compensated hemolytic state, he did not require any blood transfusion. No steroids or intravenous immunoglobulin were used. Folic acid supplementation was started. Avoidance of hemolysis causing drugs in the future was suggested.

On follow-up, the patient had mild persistent anemia (hemoglobin 13.1–13.5 mg/dl) and resolving hyperbilirubinemia which stabilized close to his baseline bilirubin (1.9 mg/dl). His transaminitis resolved completely.

4. Discussion

Influenza vaccination can lower the risk of influenza and its complications. Kidney transplant patients, because of their iatrogenic immunosuppression, are at a higher risk of such infectious complications. Our patient received a quadrivalent, egg-grown, inactivated influenza vaccine and presented with hemolytic anemia 3 days later. Hemolytic anemia can occur after preventive vaccination. Influenza vaccine has been infrequently associated with autoimmune hemolytic anemia (AIHA). The exact mechanism of AIHA induced by vaccines is unknown. Molecular mimicry of host antigens by viral peptides inducing cross-reactivity by T-cells and B-cells has been proposed. Possible role of vaccine adjuvants has also been proposed [1].

There have been case reports of AIHA occurring a few days after influenza vaccination [2]. Other autoimmune manifestations after influenza vaccination reported include thrombocytopenia, vasculitis, and Guillain–Barré syndrome. Montagnani et al. reported two cases of AIHA after influenza vaccination. In the first case, an 83-year-old woman developed Coombs-positive AIHA two days after she received an influenza vaccine. The patient was treated with steroids and immunoglobulin. The second case describes a 74-year-old woman with underlying aortic valve disease who developed Coombs-positive AIHA approximately three days after she received an influenza vaccine. The patient died two days later after being hospitalized despite treatment with corticosteroids and blood transfusion [1]. In a case report by Shlamovitz and Johar a 50-year-old man with no past medical history developed Coombs-positive Evans syndrome (i.e., AIHA with autoimmune thrombocytopenia) four days after receiving influenza vaccine that responded to treatment with steroids and immunoglobulin [3]. A nine-year-old boy developed Coombs- negative autoimmune hemolytic anemia five days after receiving influenza vaccination twice. The anemia was severe and necessitated blood transfusion, but the patient eventually recovered without additional treatment [4].

Hemolytic anemias are broadly characterized as intrinsic and extrinsic (i.e., due to intrinsic disorders within the red blood cells or extrinsic to the red cell) or divided as intravascular or extravascular. Intrinsic hemolytic anemias include membrane disorders, enzyme deficiencies, hemoglobinopathies/thalassemias, and the only acquired intrinsic form, paroxysmal nocturnal hemoglobinuria. Extrinsic hemolytic anemias can be broadly divided into immune or nonimmune-mediated destruction of red blood cells.

Classic laboratory findings suggesting hemolysis are low haptoglobin level, elevated LDH, elevated bilirubin, and reticulocytosis [5]. Our patient had all these findings on laboratory work. When hemolytic anemia is suspected, the DAT/Coombs test and review of the peripheral smear are vital to deriving the correct diagnosis. A positive DAT/Coombs test is classic for an autoimmune facilitated process resulting from either a primary disorder or secondary to drugs, infections, or malignancy. However, Coombs- negative autoimmune hemolytic anemia is a well-described entity; therefore, immune-mediated hemolysis cannot always be ruled out when the Coombs test is negative [6]. 5–10% of all autoimmune hemolytic anemias are direct antiglobulin test negative [7]. The negative Coombs test may result from a lower number of IgG molecules per RBC, non-IgG immunoglobulin on the RBC (IgA, rarely IgM), or low-affinity autoantibodies [8]. Moreover, a positive DAT/Coombs test is not always associated with AIHA [9]. In patients where there is a high index of suspicion for AIHA despite a negative Coombs test, "Super Coombs" test is available at reference laboratories. Patients with DAT/Coombs-negative AIHA may suffer milder anemia and hemolysis as compared to patients with DAT/Coombs-positive AIHA [10].

A negative DAT/Coombs in the presence of hemolysis may suggest an intrinsic erythrocyte defect of hemoglobin synthesis, enzymes, or membrane disorders. It may also suggest a nonimmune-mediated extrinsic hemolysis, which would include microangiopathic hemolytic anemia among other entities. The distinctive morphologic appearance of the red blood cells on a peripheral smear may be supportive of a specific diagnosis.

Initial work-up of anemia may include an iron profile as iron deficiency is a common cause of anemia, particularly when microcytic. To complete the work-up of anemia, hyperbilirubinemia, and hemolysis, exclusion of hepatitis with acute viral hepatitis panel may be appropriate as hemolysis can be seen in this setting. In our patient, hepatitis was excluded. Polymerase chain reaction for Parvovirus, Epstein–Barr virus, and cytomegalovirus was negative ruling out the other more common viral causes. Next, intrinsic causes of hemolysis such as hemoglobinopathies/thalassemias can be investigated via HPLC or hemoglobin electrophoresis. In our patient, hemoglobinopathy/thalassemia was ruled out by a normal HPLC. Also, the absence of microcytosis made thalassemia diagnosis unlikely. This is particularly important as cases of alpha thalassemia with only 1 or 2 gene deletions will have a normal HPLC. A common enzyme deficiency was ruled out by normal G6PD and pyruvate kinase levels. However, it is important to note that G6PD levels in a G6PD-deficient patient may be normal during acute hemolysis, necessitating repeat testing once hemolysis has subsided. A peripheral blood smear review by a pathologist is critical to further help diagnosis and subclassify hemolysis. This test should be utilized early on as it is potentially a cost-saving technique where the pathologist can suggest a possible cause and direct further testing. In our patient, this revealed prominent elliptocytosis.

Hereditary elliptocytosis, also called as ovalocytosis, is an inherited disorder in which the red blood cells are oval or elliptical rather than biconcave. It is caused by mutations in various genes eventually affecting the integrity of red blood cell membrane proteins and cytoskeleton. This leads to diminished mechanical stability of the RBC membrane making them prone to hemolysis. Most cases of hereditary elliptocytosis are due to mutations in the *alpha-spectrin, beta-spectrin*, or *EPB41* genes. Diagnosis is usually made by review of the peripheral blood smear. The majority of patients with elliptocytosis are diagnosed incidentally as the disease is largely asymptomatic, as seen in our patient [11, 12]. Decompensated hemolysis resulting in symptomatic anemia may occur during acute illness or other conditions that impact red cell survival. This can be more severe in patients with underlying chronic hemolysis. In our patient, the influenza vaccine was the most likely culprit.

Piecing this together, the patient had an underlying hereditary elliptocytosis/ovalocytosis and was prone to chronic hemolysis due to diminished mechanical stability of the red blood cell membrane. Chronic low-degree persistent hyperbilirubinemia supported this diagnosis. In addition, the patient potentially developed an acute hemolytic insult from recent influenza vaccination.

Our patient was diagnosed with acute on chronic hemolytic anemia secondary to influenza vaccine with underlying hereditary elliptocytosis. A right upper quadrant ultrasound showed gallstones, which can be seen in patients with chronic hemolytic disorders (pigment stones), further supporting this diagnosis. In addition, the previously elevated bilirubin levels as well as prior noted elliptocytosis support this entity. The concordant acute AIHA diagnosis was supported by the development of hemolysis within a short time (3 days) after administration of influenza vaccine, absence of any new drug intake, and an extensive and negative work-up as mentioned above. The Naranjo algorithm used for determining the likelihood of adverse drug reaction due to the suspected drug categorized the event as "probable" adverse drug event. Of course, the elevated LDH, reticulocytosis, and suppressed haptoglobin support hemolysis in general.

5. Conclusion

Influenza vaccination may infrequently set off an episode of AIHA. The exact etiopathogenesis of such an event is not clearly understood. Molecular mimicry and role of vaccine adjuvants and other constituents have been proposed. An underlying erythrocyte membrane defect may act as a risk factor. Patients who receive an influenza vaccine should be counseled and educated about reporting any unusual signs and symptoms experienced after the vaccination.

References

[1] S. Montagnani, M. Tuccori, G. Lombardo et al., "Autoimmune hemolytic anemia following MF59-adjuvanted influenza vaccine administration: a report of two cases," *Annals of Pharmacotherapy*, vol. 45, p. 128, 2011.

[2] T. Shizuma, "Autoimmune hemolytic anemia following influenza virus infection or administration of influenza vaccine," *Journal of Blood Disorders & Transfusion*, vol. 5, no. 3, 2014.

[3] G. Z. Shlamovitz and S. Johar, "A case of Evans' syndrome following influenza vaccine," *The Journal of Emergency Medicine*, vol. 44, no. 2, pp. e149–e151, 2013.

[4] H. Tsuchiya, T. Ishii, H. Fujiwara, and I. Matsuda, "A case of Coombs-negative autoimmune hemolytic anemia, possibly caused by influenza vaccination," *Pediatrics International*, vol. 28, no. 1, pp. 78–81, 1986.

[5] L. Luzzatto, "Hemolytic anemias," in *Harrison's Principles of Internal Medicine, 20e*, J. Jameson, A. S. Fauci, D. L. Kasper et al., Eds., McGraw-Hill, New York, NY, USA, 2019, http://accessmedicine.mhmedical.com/content.aspx?bookid=2129&sectionid=192017418.

[6] T. Takahashi, "Direct antiglobulin test-negative autoimmune hemolytic anemia," *Acta Haematologica*, vol. 140, no. 1, pp. 18-19, 2018.

[7] G. Garratty, "Immune hemolytic anemia associated with negative routine serology," *Seminars in Hematology*, vol. 42, no. 3, pp. 156–164, 2005.

[8] G. B. Segel and M. A. Lichtman, "Direct antiglobulin ("Coombs") test-negative autoimmune hemolyticanemia: a review," *Blood Cells, Molecules and Diseases*, vol. 52, no. 4, pp. 152–160, 2014.

[9] A. Salama, "Clinically and/or serologically misleading findings surrounding immune haemolytic anaemias," *Transfusion Medicine and Hemotherapy*, vol. 42, no. 5, pp. 311–315, 2015.

[10] T. Kamesaki, T. Toyotsuji, and E. Kajii, "Characterization of direct antiglobulin test-negative autoimmune hemolytic anemia: a study of 154 cases," *American Journal of Hematology*, vol. 88, no. 2, pp. 93–96, 2013.

[11] T. L. Coetzer, "Erythrocyte membrane disorders," in *Williams Hematology, 9e*, K. Kaushansky, M. A. Lichtman, J. T. Prchal et al., Eds., McGraw-Hill, New York, NY, USA, 2019, http://accessmedicine.mhmedical.com/content.aspx?bookid=1581&sectionid=94304557.

[12] H. Bunn and S. E. Lux, "Inherited hemolytic disorders of the red cell membrane and red cell metabolism," in *Pathophysiology of Blood Disorders, 2e*, J. C. Aster and H. Bunn, Eds., McGraw-Hill, New York, NY, USA, 2017.

18

Splenomegaly in a Patient with a History of Pernicious Anemia; the Potential Therapeutic Effects of B12 Therapy

Alexis Lordi,[1,2] **Nida Ansari**,[2,3] **Michael Maroules**,[1,4] **and Anusha Manjegowda**[1,4]

[1]*St. Joseph's University Medical Center, 703 Main St., Paterson, NJ 07503, USA*
[2]*St. George's University School of Medicine, True Blue, Grenada*
[3]*Rowan University School of Osteopathic Medicine, Stratford, New Jersey, NJ 08084, USA*
[4]*Department of Hematology and Oncology, St. Joseph's University Medical Center, 703 Main St., Paterson, NJ 07503, USA*

Correspondence should be addressed to Nida Ansari; ansari28@rowan.edu

Academic Editor: John Frater

Splenomegaly is manifested by a variety of etiologies, one of which is macrocytic anemia. Macrocytic anemia has multiple causes in itself that include; folate (Vitamin B9) and Cobalamin (vitamin B12) deficiencies. In this case report, we present a patient with a history of pancytopenia, macrocytic anemia and vitamin B12 deficiency, who underwent a splenectomy. The differential diagnoses for the cause of the patient's splenomegaly included: lymphoma, infiltrative disease, and idiopathic splenomegaly. The pathology report from the splenectomy did not reveal any evidence of lymphoma or infiltrative disease, however, it did mention vascular congestion of the spleen. In theory, vascular congestion, due to extramedullary hematopoiesis in the spleen or sequestration of blood cell lineages, could lead to pancytopenia. In prior visits to the hospital this patient was diagnosed with: splenomegaly, and macrocytic anemia due to pernicious anemia. A splenectomy puts one at increased risk for infection by encapsulated organisms, and is to be avoided if possible. There are few case reports and studies that show vitamin B12 therapy can potentially cause a reversal in the splenomegaly as well as a reversal in the pancytopenia and macrocytic anemia. We hope to show that the least invasive treatment for vitamin B12, vitamin therapy, can be of use and effective.

1. Introduction

Splenomegaly due to exacerbated forms of normal splenic function is common in conditions such as infection, autoimmune disease, liver disease, leukemia, and hemolytic anemia. The spleen has multiple functions; it is involved with hematopoiesis, immunity, and filtering old, malformed, or damaged red blood cells [1]. An increase in red blood cell surface area, as in the case of macrocytic anemia, causes congestion of the splenic vasculature, potentiating pancytopenia. As the spleen works to overcome the congestion, hypertrophy of the organ may ensue resulting in splenomegaly [2]. The patient described in this case report has a past medical history of vitamin B12 deficiency but was noncompliant with treatment, developed progressively worsening splenomegaly, as well as pancytopenia. Initially, it was thought that this patient could have splenomegaly due to infiltrative disease or lymphoma, however, the pathology report was not consistent with either of the differentials and the diagnosis came to a standstill. This case report would like to highlight splenomegaly as one of the manifestations of Vitamin B12 deficiency and that treatment of vitamin B12 deficiency could potentially lead to splenic size regression and reversal of pancytopenia. It has been noted in previous literature, that a patient who had marked splenomegaly and pernicious anemia responded well to vitamin B12 therapy and in three months of vitamin therapy. The spleen was reduced by 2 cm and the pernicious anemia resolved [3]. However, there have not been many presented cases that show the association of splenomegaly and pernicious anemia. We aim to show that with vitamin B12 supplementation, a decrease in the degree of splenomegaly could prevent further, more invasive interventions such as splenectomies in these patients.

2. Case

A 48-year-old male with a past medical history of small bowel obstruction followed by exploratory laparotomy, pancytopenia, hepatosplenomegaly, pernicious anemia presented to ED with a chief complaint of left upper quadrant abdominal pain. He reported left upper quadrant pain, decreased appetite, and shortness of breath for a duration of about five to six days. He reported that the pain was exacerbated by deep breaths and that he was unable to walk more than a few feet without feeling short of breath. He additionally reported that his urine had turned dark orange. A urinalysis was done to rule out hematuria or myoglobinuria, which resulted negative for both. The patient reported early satiety and decreased appetite, along with decreased water intake which could be the reasoning for the dark color change of the patient's urine. He stated that he was "play-fighting" with his son and got punched in the stomach 2 weeks prior, but felt fine afterwards. During a previous hospital admission for small bowel obstruction, he was noted to have splenomegaly. He denied any similar presentation in any family members. He denied any allergies to food, medications, latex, dyes. He was not taking any home medications, OTC medications or herbal supplements at the time of presentation. He denied recent alcohol use, although he stated that he used to drink a 6 pack of beer a month. He denied substance use or tobacco use.

Upon the initial presentation in the ED, he was in mild distress from the abdominal pain. His vitals were stable. Physical exam revealed mild scleral icterus and sublingual jaundice. His abdominal exam showed a soft, non-distended abdomen, tenderness to palpation in LUQ, dullness to percussion in LUQ, spleen was palpable up to 3-4 inches below the rib cage, no hepatomegaly, no rebound, rigidity or guarding was appreciated. The remainder of the physical exam was unremarkable. Abdominal CT (Figure 1) showed increased splenomegaly from 17 cm previously to 20 cm currently, with inferior peri-splenic hemorrhage and the linear plane of hypoattenuation consistent with grade 3 laceration.

On this current admission, his lab results showed macrocytic anemia with hemoglobin of 6.9 g/dL, hematocrit of 21.7% and MCV of 101.4 fL. Patient was found to have a WBC of 2.1×10^3/mm3 indicating neutropenia but denied fever or recent sick contacts and thrombocytopenia of PLT: 125 K/mm3. His anemia panel showed no evidence of iron deficiency, B12 level was 137 pg/mL, folate level was 4.9 ng/mL. Patient also had lab findings of coombs negative hemolytic anemia with LDH of 560 unit/L, reticulocytosis of 17%, haptoglobin of <10, total bilirubin of 5 mg/dL secondary to vitamin B12 deficiency. The initial MMA was elevated at 385 and homocysteine was 11.8 about 2 years prior to this presentation. Patient had elevated levels of intrinsic factor antibodies and was diagnosed with pernicious anemia. He had been non-compliant with taking B12 supplements. On further investigation, it was found that in previous admissions he had an extensive hematologic workup including JAK testing, BCR-ABL testing, peripheral blood flow cytometry, and bone marrow aspirate and biopsy which was normal. On this admission, hemolytic workup resulted as a urobilinogen within normal limits, normal ALT, but an elevated LDH and positive reticulocytosis. A blood smear was not done at the time of hemolytic workup, but the splenic laceration could be the cause of a mixed acute hemolytic picture. Previous lab work would suggest that his hemoglobin count is consistently low; ranging from 9.4 to 11.7 since 2019.

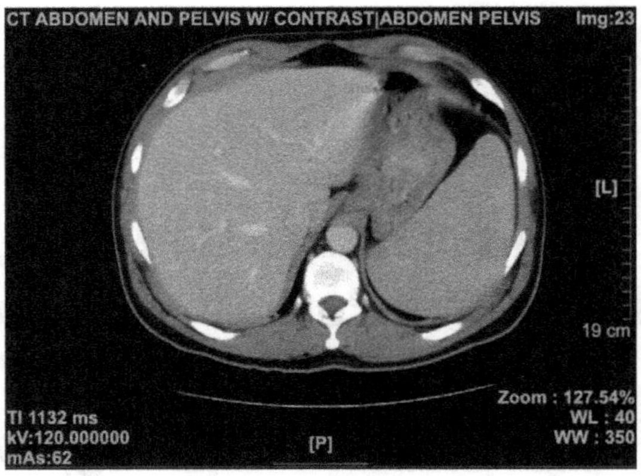

Figure 1: CT scan of abdomen and pelvis with contrast. Diagnosis of splenomegaly, 20 cm. Inferior peri-splenic hemorrhage, three grade laceration.

Patient underwent a splenectomy for the grade three splenic laceration. Pathology showed markedly enlarged spleen weighing 1260 grams with marked vascular congestion and measuring $22 \times 16 \times 7.5$ cm. There was no evidence of myeloid or lymphoid proliferative disease. It was concluded that the case of splenomegaly was caused by B12 deficiency secondary to pernicious anemia and non-compliance with vitamin supplementation. The patient was restarted on vitamin B12 intramuscular injections.

3. Discussion

Vitamin B12, also known as Cobalamin, deficiency classically causes macrocytic anemia. It has been hypothesized that the increase in size in red blood cells from macrocytosis can lead to congestion of the red pulp in the spleen and sequestration of other blood cell lineages [2]. Sequestration of the oversized red blood cells in the spleen over time in this patient leads to splenomegaly [2].

Vitamin B12 deficiency can be secondary to dietary restrictions such as a strict vegetarian diet, or autoimmune pernicious anemia. Once cobalamin is released from parietal cells, Intrinsic Factor forms a complex with vitamin B_{12} in the duodenum for absorption in the ileum to occur [4]. In a patient with pernicious anemia, autoantibodies are formed to prevent the release of Intrinsic Factor, therefore decreasing the amount of absorbed cobalamin [4]. When there is a decrease in the amount of available vitamin B12 there is a decrease in DNA synthesis, multilinear blood cell proliferation, and cellular metabolism. This results in ineffective erythropoiesis, leading to extramedullary hematopoiesis as a compensatory mechanism, manifesting as hepatosplenomegaly. [5] Extramedullary hematopoiesis typically occurs in the red pulp of the spleen. Clinical Manifestations of vitamin B12 deficiency include; shortness of breath, fatigue, pallor, loss of memory, poor balance, reduced sensation of touch, and tingling feet. [2]

Gedik et al. claim that out of 137 participants with pancytopenia, vitamin B12 deficiency was found to be the etiology in 24 of the participants [6]. It was the most frequent cause of pancytopenia. Halfdanarson et al. stated that severe megaloblastic anemia can be mistaken for leukemia which was also part of the workup for this patient but no significant pathology was found [3]. The initial presentation of vitamin B12 deficiency including pancytopenia, splenomegaly and leukoerythroblastosis is a common concern when considering a diagnosis of leukemia [3]. Our patient also had a blood smear that demonstrated leukoerythroblastosis, which is also described in the setting of infiltrative disease. In the Halfdanarson et al. article, a bone marrow examination of Cobalamin deficiency showed marked hypercellularity, with an increase in erythroid precursors, megaloblastic maturation, and a decreased amount of granulocytes. The megakaryocytes were normal in number but contained large nuclei. [3]. This case report reminds us to look into nutritional aspects when coming across a patient with splenomegaly and the pathology report does not show the clinical finding that was expected.

Pruthi, Rajiv K. et al. describe a patient who had marked splenomegaly, similar to this patient, and after three months of vitamin B12 therapy the spleen had decreased in size and the anemia had resolved [7]. A case report by Behera, Vineet, et al., describes a patient with megaloblastic anemia and a spleen palpable 13 cm below the left costal margin was treated with parenteral vitamin B12 1,000 mcg twice a week intramuscularly. Follow up at 1, 3 and 6 months showed sizeable improvement in his condition. As well as, serial abdominal ultrasounds showed gradual decreases in splenic size. A regression of 2 cm after 6 months was reported [1]. Our patient began to show signs of recovery of his blood counts within 3-4 weeks of parenteral vitamin B12 supplementation. He also had progressively worsening splenomegaly and pancytopenia in the setting of non-compliance with vitamin B12 therapy indicating the role of vitamin B12 deficiency in the development of splenomegaly. It is important to rule out B12 deficiency in the right clinical setting in all cases of splenomegaly to make sure that the patient is getting adequate B12 supplementation as it is the least invasive tool to reduce the size of the organ and in some cases, as seen above has been proven efficacious [7].

4. Conclusion

Splenomegaly is a rare manifestation of pernicious anemia. One of the major mechanisms is believed to be due to congestion in the red pulp of the spleen with macrocytic red blood cells which was seen in our patient. There have been few cases reported of pernicious anemia with concurrent splenomegaly reported as of 2014. It can be hypothesized that this patient's untreated B12 deficiency allowed for pancytopenia to persist secondarily from the vascular congestion causing splenomegaly. Hypothetically if this patient did not have a splenic laceration leading to a splenectomy, and had he been more adherent with B12 injections, the splenomegaly could have been reduced or at least controlled. Three months later, it was found that his pancytopenia had resolved. Previous literature demonstrates that it is possible to reverse splenomegaly secondary to B12 deficiency. This is something to consider in the management of those who present with B12 deficiency and splenomegaly.

References

[1] V. Behera, M. Randive, P. Sharma, and V. Nair, "Megaloblastic anemia presenting with massive reversible splenomegaly," *Indian Journal of Hematology and Blood Transfusion*, vol. 31, no. 2, pp. 297–299, 2014.

[2] S. Aubrey, B. Crooks, and M. Rashid, "Pancytopenia from severe cobalamin (vitamin B12) deficiency in johanson-blizzard syndrome," *European Journal of Clinical Nutrition*, vol. 67, no. 10, p. 1118, 2013.

[3] T. R. Halfdanarson, J. A. Walker, M. R. Litzow, and C. A. Hanson, "Severe vitamin B12 deficiency resulting in pancytopenia, splenomegaly and leukoerythroblastosis," *European Journal of Haematology*, vol. 80, no. 5, pp. 448–451, 2008.

[4] H. M. Al-Awami, A. Raja, and M. P. Soos, *Physiology, Gastric Intrinsic Factor*, StatPearls Publishing, Treasure Island, FL, USA, 2021, https://www.ncbi.nlm.nih.gov/books/NBK546655/.

[5] E. Keskin and M. Keskin, *Severe Vitamin* B_{12} *Deficiency in a 15-Year-Old Boy: Presentation with Haemolysis and Pancytopenia*, BMJ Publishing Group, London, UK, 2015, https://ncbi.nlm.nih.gov/pmc/articles/PMC4434362/.

[6] O. Yokus and H. Gedik, "Etiological causes of pancytopenia: a report of 137 cases," *Avicenna Journal of Medicine*, vol. 06, no. 04, pp. 109–112, 2016.

[7] R. K. Pruthi, "Reversible marked splenomegaly in pernicious anemia," *Annals of Internal Medicine*, vol. 119, no. 10, p. 1053, 1993.

19

HHV-8-Associated Lymphoproliferative Disorders and Pathogenesis in an HIV-Positive Patient

Carlo Guerrero,[1] Tania Jain,[2] and Katalin Kelemen[3]

[1]*Department of Medicine, Houston Methodist Hospital, Houston, TX, USA*
[2]*Adult Bone Marrow Transplantation Service, Memorial Sloan Kettering Cancer Center, New York, NY, USA*
[3]*Department of Laboratory Medicine and Pathology, Mayo Clinic, Phoenix, AZ, USA*

Correspondence should be addressed to Carlo Guerrero; carlo.a.guerrero@gmail.com

Academic Editor: Håkon Reikvam

Human herpesvirus 8 (HHV-8), also known as Kaposi's sarcoma-associated herpesvirus, is a DNA oncovirus known for its role in the development of Kaposi's sarcoma (KS) and several lymphoproliferative disorders (LPDs). HHV-8 promotes lymphoproliferation via the activation of the interleukin-6 receptor signaling pathway, as well as a host of other regulatory mechanisms. The spectrum of HHV-8-associated LPDs is increasing. The World Health Organization has recently updated the classification of HHV-8-associated LPDs by introducing HHV-8-positive germinotropic LPD (GLPD) in addition to the previously recognized entities of HHV-8-positive diffuse large B-cell lymphoma, not otherwise specified (DLBCL, NOS), primary effusion lymphoma (PEL), and HHV-8-positive multicentric Castleman's disease (MCD). We present here a case of an HIV-positive woman with a history of KS, who later developed three HHV-8-associated LPDs, including HHV-8-positive MCD, PEL, and GLPD. To the best of our knowledge, this is the first reported case of a patient with this combination of individually rare HHV-8-associated LPDs. This case illustrates the spectrum and the sequential development of the different clinical manifestations of HHV-8-associated diseases. Detection of HHV-8 can have clinical significance in the diagnosis and management of certain HHV-8-associated conditions. Recently discovered variants of HHV-8-associated LPDs indicate that this group represents a diverse spectrum of disorders, whose classification may require further refinement beyond the currently recognized entities.

1. Introduction

The first description of Kaposi's sarcoma (KS) was made in 1872 by the eponymous dermatologist Moritz Kaposi [1]. He documented what we now characterize as the "classic" form of KS, slow-growing skin tumours seen predominantly in elderly men of Mediterranean or Jewish ancestry [2]. More than a century later, the epidemic of human immunodeficiency virus (HIV) in North America unleashed a more aggressive form of KS associated with the acquired immunodeficiency syndrome (AIDS). This led to the discovery of human herpesvirus 8 (HHV-8), also known as Kaposi's sarcoma-associated herpesvirus, as the causative infectious agent of KS [3].

Since the discovery of its link to KS, HHV-8 has been recognized to be associated with several lymphoproliferative disorders (LPDs), including HHV-8-positive multicentric Castleman's disease (MCD), primary effusion lymphoma (PEL), HHV-8-positive germinotropic lymphoproliferative disorder (GLPD), and HHV-8-positive diffuse large B-cell lymphoma, not otherwise specified (DLBCL, NOS). The 2016 update of the WHO Classification of Tumours of Haematopoietic and Lymphoid Tissues included HHV-8-positive GLPD as a newly classified entity within the category of HHV-8-associated LPDs [4]. These HHV-8-associated LPDs constitute a spectrum of disorders which can be distinguished from one another based on their clinical manifestations, microscopic appearance, localization, immunophenotype, genetic profile, and the presence of an Epstein–Barr virus (EBV) coinfection. However, there have been reported cases that have overlapping features of several of these HHV-8-associated LPDs, and which may also manifest clinically in ways distinct from these WHO-classified disorders [5–7].

We present a case of an HIV-positive woman who developed KS, HHV-8-positive MCD, PEL, and GLPD. Through this case report, we aim to illustrate the pathologic spectrum of three HHV-8-associated LPDs and highlight the role that HHV-8 plays in the development of its associated LPDs, including a discussion of key mechanisms by which it promotes cellular proliferation. We emphasize the long-term effects of HHV-8 infection in the immunocompromised host, resulting in sequential development of several different LPDs in the same patient over time. Finally, we discuss several fundamental questions that arise from this case regarding the spectrum of HHV-8-associated LPDs.

2. Case

The patient is an African-American woman originally from Zimbabwe, who moved to the United States in 2007 at the age of 41. She was diagnosed with HIV/AIDS and KS in 2001 and was treated at that time with combination antiretroviral therapy (ART). Her medical records from Zimbabwe were not available for review. She established medical care in the United States in 2007. In late 2007, she was diagnosed with new KS lesions and HHV-8-positive MCD. Her CD4 count was 162 cells/μL, and her HIV viral load was 256 copies/mL. She had associated anemia, hypoalbuminemia, and elevated sedimentation rate. She was treated with rituximab and vincristine from 2008 to 2013, with intermittent interruptions in treatment due to cytopenias.

In January 2014, she presented to our institution for a sepsis-like illness and worsening diffuse lymphadenopathy. Her infectious workup was unrevealing. Her CD4 count was 307 cells/μL, and her HIV viral load was undetectable (i.e., <20 copies/mL). A core biopsy of an enlarged right inguinal lymph node was performed. The morphologic findings were consistent with the patient's known diagnosis of MCD, plasmacytic type. The lymph node architecture was preserved, and there was dense polyclonal plasma cell proliferation filling the paracortex. HHV-8 latency-associated nuclear antigen (LANA) immunostain was positive, with virus-infected cells localized primarily within germinal centers. Occasional germinal centers stood out due to the replacement of the germinal centers by large plasmacytoid cells (i.e., plasmablasts). Some of these atypical germinal centers showed lambda-light chain restriction of the plasmablasts, meeting the criteria of HHV-8-positive GLPD (Figure 1). EBV-encoded small RNA (EBER) in situ hybridization was positive for EBV. Her presenting signs and symptoms were ultimately attributed to progression of MCD, especially since she had not received vincristine treatment for six weeks prior to presentation due to severe cytopenias. She was treated with cyclophosphamide, vincristine, and valganciclovir during that admission and was continued on this regimen along with rituximab as an outpatient.

Over the next several months, she developed worsening left upper quadrant abdominal pain, anemia, and thrombocytopenia, which were attributed to progressive splenomegaly. She had hepatosplenomegaly seen on imaging since at least 2010, but she was asymptomatic from this until 2014. She underwent a laparoscopic splenectomy in May 2014, with subsequent improvement in her pain and cytopenias. The histology of the spleen showed extended red pulp due to congestion, fibrosis, and focal extramedullary hematopoiesis. There was no evidence of MCD, KS, or infectious mononucleosis (i.e., EBV) noted in the specimen.

In June 2014, she was readmitted to our hospital, this time for progressive dyspnea. She was diagnosed with nonischemic heart failure with reduced ejection fraction. Her CD4 count was 746 cells/μL, and her HIV viral load was undetectable (i.e., <20 copies/mL). She had a large right pleural effusion, which was drained via thoracentesis. Analysis showed this to be a malignant pleural effusion, which contained abundant large plasmablasts, positive with CD138, MUM1, CD30, HHV-8 LANA immunostaining, and lambda-light chain restricted by in situ hybridization, but negative for CD45, CD20, PAX5, CD79a, and CD3, consistent with PEL (see Figure 2). She was treated with a dose-adjusted regimen of etoposide, prednisolone, vincristine, and cyclophosphamide (EPOCH minus doxorubicin due to history of heart failure) for eight cycles, leading to a complete response.

As of most recent follow-up in March 2019, the patient is alive and remains in complete remission based on positive emission tomography (PET) results, resolution of her symptoms, and normalization of her laboratory testing. To the best of our knowledge, the patient has been maintained on ART since her HIV diagnosis without significant interruptions in treatment or the development of opportunistic infections. There was no apparent testing performed to assess for HHV-8 viremia, although there was a positive serum HHV-8 antibody (IgG) result in April 2014.

3. Discussion

Along with EBV, HHV-8 is classified into the gamma subfamily of Herpesviridae. Both DNA human oncoviruses utilize gene products which promote unregulated cell proliferation, particularly in immunosuppressed hosts. One of the key factors in the development of HHV-8-associated LPDs is the activation of the interleukin-6 receptor (IL-6R) signaling pathway, which, among other functions, promotes lymphoproliferation and angiogenesis [8, 9]. HHV-8-infected plasmablasts can be identified by their expression of the HHV-8 gene product known as LANA, a protein which may also function to increase the expression of human IL-6 (hIL-6) [10]. HHV-8 also encodes a functional homolog of hIL-6 called viral interleukin-6 (vIL-6), which can also activate the IL-6R but without the need for its coreceptor, gp80 [11].

Like other virally mediated lymphomas, HHV-8 potentiates an antiapoptotic effect via its constitutive activation of the family of transcription factors known as nuclear factor-kappa B (NF-κB) [12]. In latently infected tumour cells, HHV-8 activates NF-κB through its gene product known as viral FLICE inhibitory protein (vFLIP) [13]. Inhibition of NF-κB has been shown to induce apoptosis in

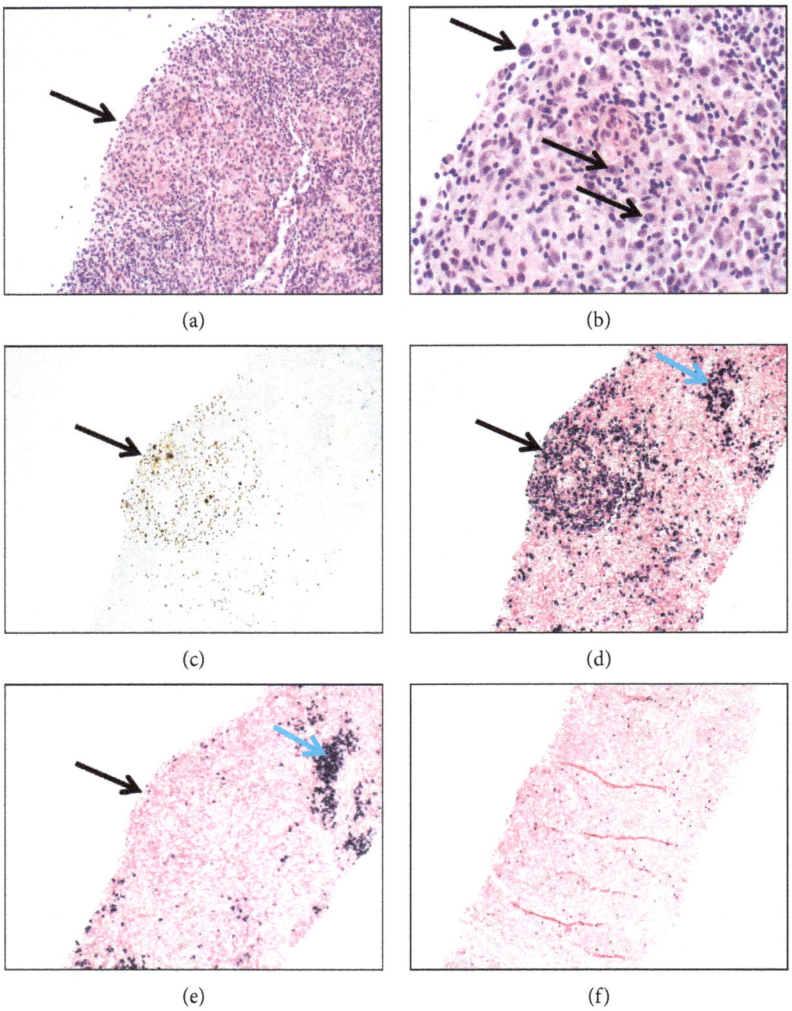

FIGURE 1: Pathologic findings in an inguinal lymph node core biopsy. (a) Germinal center showing large atypical plasmablasts. The arrow indicates the germinal center (H&E, 200x). (b) Germinal center, arrows point to plasmablasts (H&E, 500x). (c) The plasmablasts (arrow) are positive for HHV-8 (immunostaining, anti-HHV-8 (13b10) mouse monoclonal antibody by Cell Marque, 200x). (d, e) The germinal center (black arrows) contains lambda-light chain-restricted plasmablasts (in situ hybridization, DNA probes by Ventana that react with lambda mRNA and Kappa mRNA, respectively, 200x). The paracortex adjacent to the germinal center contains polyclonal plasma cells (blue arrows). (f) EBV-positive cells throughout the lymph node core biopsy (EBER in situ hybridization, DNA probe to EBV-encoded RNA-1 by Ventana, 100x).

PEL [14]. A full review of the known or proposed mechanisms through which HHV-8 exerts its oncogenic effects is beyond the scope of this article and is covered in detail elsewhere [15].

HHV-8-associated LPDs show key features that distinguish one from another in most cases (see Table 1). Our patient met the typical features seen with HHV-8-positive MCD, PEL, and GLPD, with the exception that GLPD is usually seen in HIV-negative patients. However, cases of HHV-8-positive GLPD have previously been described in patients with HIV [6].

The identification of HHV-8 via staining for the nuclear antigen LANA is crucial for making the correct diagnosis. It helps to distinguish the HHV-8-associated LPDs from similar-appearing HHV-8-negative malignancies such as plasmablastic lymphoma and HHV-8-negative MCD. Assessing for the presence of EBER can also be helpful; it tends to be positive in GLPD and PEL and negative in MCD and DLBCL. It is uncertain what role, if any, that EBV has in the pathogenesis of GLPD and PEL, as cases of each condition have been described in EBV-negative patients [6, 16].

Diagnostic challenges can arise when observed cases do not neatly fit into one of the WHO-defined conditions on the HHV-8-associated LPD spectrum. Examples include a case of HHV-8^+/EBV$^+$ DLBCL, NOS, and another of HHV-8^+/EBV$^+$ MCD [17, 18]. The rarity of the HHV-8-associated LPDs likely contributes to the fact that the currently recognized entities fail to capture the full spectrum of reported cases. This leaves room for more detailed characterization of these disorders in future classification systems.

Many unanswered questions remain regarding our understanding of the spectrum of HHV-8-associated LPDs.

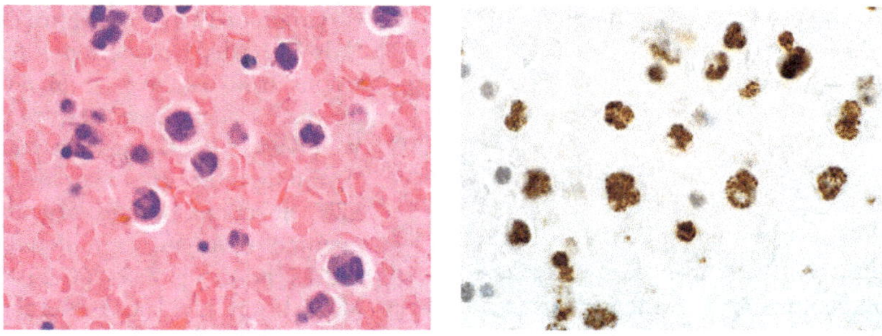

(a) (b)

FIGURE 2: Primary effusion lymphoma, cell block preparation. (a) Large atypical cells with irregular nuclei and visible nucleoli (H&E, 1000x). (b) The large cells in the pleural effusion are positive for HHV-8 (immunostaining, anti-HHV-8 (13B10) mouse monoclonal antibody by Cell Marque, 1000x).

TABLE 1: Typical features of the HHV-8-associated lymphoproliferative diseases.

Feature	DLBCL, NOS	GLPD	MCD	PEL
Clinical presentation	Diffuse LAN, constitutional symptoms, splenomegaly HHV-8 MCD usually present	Localized LAN	Diffuse LAN, constitutional symptoms, splenomegaly	Serous effusions, no LAN
Immunosuppression	+/–	–	+/–	+/–
Microscopy	Sheets of PB/IB, effacement of nodal architecture	PB/IB in germinal centers, nodal architecture intact	PB/IB in mantle zones Interfollicular plasmacytosis	PB/IB in serous effusions (esp. pleural, pericardial, peritoneal)
Phenotype	CD20 +/–, CD138 –	CD20 –, CD138 –	CD20 +/–, CD138 –	CD20 –, CD138 +/–
Clonality	Monoclonal	Poly- or oligoclonal	Polyclonal	Monoclonal
Ig	IgM λ +	Monotypic κ or λ, any heavy chain	IgM λ +	–
HHV-8 (LANA)	+	+	+	+
EBV (EBER)	–	+	–	+
Prognosis	Poor	Good	Poor, but improving	Poor
Treatment	EPOCH or CHOP plus rituximab if CD20+, ART if HIV+	Chemotherapy (e.g., CHOP) or surgical resection +/–RT, ART if HIV+	No organ failure: rituximab Organ failure: chemotherapy and/or rituximab ART if HIV+	EPOCH or CHOP plus rituximab if CD20+, ART if HIV+

CD: cluster of differentiation; CHOP: cyclophosphamide, doxorubicin, vincristine, prednisone; EPOCH: etoposide, prednisolone, vincristine, cyclophosphamide, doxorubicin; IB: immunoblast; Ig: immunoglobulin; LAN: lymphadenopathy; PB: plasmablast; RT: radiation therapy.

For example, what causes an HHV-8-infected patient to develop one disease entity on this spectrum and not another? Why do some patients, such as the one we report here, develop multiple HHV-8-associated LPDs? The sequential development in our patient of a lambda-restricted MCD followed by a lambda-restricted PEL leads one to question whether there is a clonal relationship between these two entities or if they developed independently under the influence of HHV-8. Given their rarity, the creation of a biobank for HHV-8-associated LPDs would be a reasonable step to facilitate research in this area and to help answer these lingering questions.

Our patient has maintained a complete response from her three HHV-8-associated LPDs for five years now, since she was diagnosed with PEL. Her treatment regimen for PEL followed current guidelines of the National Comprehensive Cancer Network, which includes treatment recommendations for HHV-8-positive MCD, PEL, and DLBCL, NOS [19]. However, in its current iteration, it does not cover treatment for HHV-8-positive GLPD, which generally has a favorable prognosis when treated with chemotherapy or surgical resection with or without radiotherapy [20]. Clinical experience with GLPD is extremely limited as only about 20 cases have been published in the literature to date.

As previously noted, immunocompromise (often but not exclusively due to HIV infection) is a significant risk factor that enhances the virulence of HHV-8 in susceptible hosts. Antiretroviral therapy is a critical component of treatment for HIV-positive patients diagnosed with HHV-8-associated LPDs, as it has been shown to improve survival in this cohort [21]. ART is generally not given as sole treatment of HHV-8-associated LPDs, although this may occur when patients are otherwise not good candidates for chemotherapy. Rituximab therapy should be considered in any HHV-8-associated LPD with CD20 positivity.

4. Conclusion

The HHV-8-associated LPDs represent a spectrum of disorders which can range from reactive lymphoid hyperplasia to aggressive lymphomas. Except for GLPD, they are usually seen in immunosuppressed patients, who appear to be more susceptible to the host of oncogenic factors employed by HHV-8. Identification of HHV-8 and other key features are critical to establishing the correct diagnosis, with the understanding that a minority of cases may not be easily characterized due to our evolving understanding of these disorders.

Abbreviations

AIDS: Acquired immunodeficiency syndrome
ART: Antiretroviral therapy
CHOP: Cyclophosphamide, doxorubicin, vincristine, prednisone
DLBCL, NOS: Diffuse large B-cell lymphoma, not otherwise specified
EBV: Epstein–Barr virus
EPOCH: Etoposide, prednisolone, vincristine, cyclophosphamide, doxorubicin
GLPD: Germinotropic lymphoproliferative disorder
HHV-8: Human herpesvirus 8
hIL-6: Human interleukin-6
HIV: Human immunodeficiency virus
KS: Kaposi's sarcoma
LANA: Latency-associated nuclear antigen
LPD: Lymphoproliferative disorder
MCD: Multicentric Castleman's disease
PEL: Primary effusion lymphoma
WHO: World Health Organization.

References

[1] M. Braun, "Moriz kaposi, m.d," *CA: A Cancer Journal for Clinicians*, vol. 32, no. 6, pp. 340-341, 1982.

[2] J. Iscovich, P. Boffetta, R. Winkelmann, P. Brennan, and E. Azizi, "Classic Kaposi's sarcoma in jews living in Israel, 1961–1989," *AIDS*, vol. 12, no. 15, pp. 2067–2072, 1998.

[3] Y. Chang, E. Cesarman, M. Pessin et al., "Identification of herpesvirus-like DNA sequences in AIDS-associated Kaposi's sarcoma," *Science*, vol. 266, no. 5192, pp. 1865–1869, 1994.

[4] S. H. Swerdlow, E. Campo, N. L. Harris et al., *WHO Classification of Tumours of Haematopoietic and Lymphoid Tissues*, IARC, Lyon, France, 4th edition, 2017.

[5] E. L. Courville, A. R. Sohani, R. P. Hasserjian, L. R. Zukerberg, N. L. Harris, and J. A. Ferry, "Diverse clinicopathologic features in human herpesvirus 8-associated lymphomas lead to diagnostic problems," *American Journal of Clinical Pathology*, vol. 142, no. 6, pp. 816–829, 2014.

[6] B. Gonzalez-Farre, D. Martinez, M. Lopez-Guerra et al., "HHV8-related lymphoid proliferations: a broad spectrum of lesions from reactive lymphoid hyperplasia to overt lymphoma," *Modern Pathology*, vol. 30, no. 5, pp. 745–760, 2017.

[7] W. Wang, R. Kanagal-Shamanna, and L. J. Medeiros, "Lymphoproliferative disorders with concurrent HHV8 and EBV infection: beyond primary effusion lymphoma and germinotropic lymphoproliferative disorder," *Histopathology*, vol. 72, no. 5, pp. 855–861, 2018.

[8] M.-Q. Du, H. Liu, T. C. Diss et al., "Kaposi sarcoma-associated herpesvirus infects monotypic (IgMlambda) but polyclonal naive B cells in Castleman disease and associated lymphoproliferative disorders," *Blood*, vol. 97, no. 7, pp. 2130–2136, 2001.

[9] Y. Aoki, E. S. Jaffe, Y. Chang et al., "Angiogenesis and hematopoiesis induced by Kaposi's sarcoma-associated herpesvirus-encoded interleukin-6," *Blood*, vol. 93, no. 12, pp. 4034–4043, 1999.

[10] J. An, A. K. Lichtenstein, G. Brent, and M. B. Rettig, "The Kaposi sarcoma-associated herpesvirus (KSHV) induces cellular interleukin 6 expression: role of the KSHV latency-associated nuclear antigen and the AP1 response element," *Blood*, vol. 99, no. 2, pp. 649–654, 2002.

[11] M. Chatterjee, J. Osborne, G. Bestetti, Y. Chang, and P. S. Moore, "Viral IL-6-induced cell proliferation and immune evasion of interferon activity," *Science*, vol. 298, no. 5597, pp. 1432–1435, 2002.

[12] S. A. Keller, D. Hernandez-Hopkins, and J. Vider, "NF- B is essential for the progression of KSHV- and EBV-infected lymphomas in vivo," *Blood*, vol. 107, no. 8, pp. 3295–3302, 2006.

[13] H. Matta and P. M. Chaudhary, "Activation of alternative NF-B pathway by human herpes virus 8-encoded Fas-associated death domain-like IL-1 -converting enzyme inhibitory protein (vFLIP)," *Proceedings of the National Academy of Sciences*, vol. 101, no. 25, pp. 9399–9404, 2004.

[14] S. A. Keller, E. J. Schattner, and E. Cesarman, "Inhibition of NF-kappaB induces apoptosis of KSHV-infected primary effusion lymphoma cells," *Blood*, vol. 96, no. 7, pp. 2537–2542, 2000.

[15] S. Li, L. Bai, J. Dong, R. Sun, and K. Lan, "Kaposi's sarcoma-associated herpesvirus: epidemiology and molecular biology," in *Infectious Agents Associated Cancers: Epidemiology and Molecular Biology. Advances in Experimental Medicine and Biology*, Q. Cai, Z. Yuan, and K. Lan, Eds., pp. 91–127, Springer, Singapore, 2017.

[16] L. Arvanitakis, E. A. Mesri, R. G. Nador et al., "Establishment and characterization of a primary effusion (body cavity-based) lymphoma cell line (BC-3) harboring kaposi's sarcoma-associated herpesvirus (KSHV/HHV-8) in the absence of Epstein-Barr virus," *Blood*, vol. 88, no. 7, pp. 2648–2654, 1996.

[17] A. Papoudou-Bai, E. Hatzimichael, L. Kyriazopoulou, E. Briasoulis, and P. Kanavaros, "Rare variants in the spectrum of human herpesvirus 8/Epstein-Barr virus-copositive lymphoproliferations," *Human Pathology*, vol. 46, no. 10, pp. 1566–1571, 2015.

[18] A. Shivane, A. Pearce, N. Khatib, and M. E. F. Smith, "EBV+ HHV-8+ multicentric castleman disease with plasmablastic aggregates in an HIV+ man: an evolving clinicopathologic entity," *International Journal of Surgical Pathology*, vol. 26, no. 4, pp. 338–341, 2018.

[19] National Comprehensive Cancer Network, *B-cell Lymphomas*, National Comprehensive Cancer Network, Fort Washington,

PA, USA, 2019, https://www.nccn.org/professionals/physician_gls/pdf/b-cell.pdf.

[20] M.-Q. Du, T. C. Diss, H. Liu, H. Ye, R. A. Hamoudi et al., "KSHV- and EBV-associated germinotropic lymphoproliferative disorder," *Blood*, vol. 100, no. 9, pp. 3415–3418, 2002.

[21] E. Boulanger, L. Gérard, J. Gabarre et al., "Prognostic factors and outcome of human herpesvirus 8-associated primary effusion lymphoma in patients with AIDS," *Journal of Clinical Oncology*, vol. 23, no. 19, pp. 4372–4380, 2005.

Autosplenectomy in a Patient with Paroxysmal Nocturnal Hemoglobinuria (PNH)

Ethan Burns,[1] Kartik Anand,[1] Gonzalo Acosta,[1] Malcolm Irani,[1] Betty Chung,[2] Abhishek Maiti,[3] Ibrahim Ibrahim,[4] and Lawrence Rice[1]

[1]*Houston Methodist Hospital, Department of Medicine, 6550 Fannin St, Houston, TX 77030, USA*
[2]*Houston Methodist Hospital, Department of Pathology and Genomic Medicine, 6550 Fannin St, Houston, TX 77030, USA*
[3]*The University of Texas MD Anderson Cancer Center, Division of Cancer Medicine, 1515 Holcombe Blvd, Houston, Texas 77030, USA*
[4]*University of Texas Southwestern, Department of Internal Medicine, Division of Hematology/Oncology, 5323 Harry Hines Blvd, Dallas, TX 75390, USA*

Correspondence should be addressed to Ethan Burns; eaburns312@gmail.com

Academic Editor: Håkon Reikvam

Autosplenectomy (AS) is a known complication of diseases such as sickle cell anemia, celiac disease, and inflammatory bowel disease. We report the first known case of AS due to paroxysmal nocturnal hemoglobinuria (PNH). A 24-year-old Caucasian male had evidence of hemolytic anemia at the age of 14 and was diagnosed with PNH at the age of 16. He had recurrent episodes of sepsis due to dialysis line infections from poor hygiene, and blood cultures had been positive for multiple organisms including *Staphylococcus aureus*, *Enterococcus faecalis*, and *Streptococcus pneumoniae*. The patient's peripheral blood smears since the age of 14 years demonstrated Howell–Jolly bodies in conjunction with thrombocytopenia and hemolytic anemia, but abdominal ultrasonography reported a normal appearing spleen. The patient presented with septicemia two years after starting eculizumab, and his peripheral blood smear showed extensive Howell–Jolly bodies, Pappenheimer bodies, acanthocytes, and target cells. Splenic ultrasonography demonstrated an atrophic spleen with multifocal scarring, and absent splenic uptake of liver-spleen scintigraphy, consistent with AS. Clinicians should remain vigilant of the potential sequelae of PNH and consider the possibility of the development of AS.

1. Introduction

PNH is an acquired hemolytic disease involving the hematopoietic progenitor cells of the bone marrow. The incidence and prevalence of PNH is 0.13/100,000 and 1.59/100,000 person/year, respectively [1]. Symptoms vary and arise secondarily to ongoing hemolytic anemia and thrombophilia and may include fatigue, urine discoloration, and pain. The only FDA approved therapy is eculizumab, a humanized monoclonal antibody that prevents the cytolytic and proinflammatory effects of the terminal complement system by acting against the C5 component of the complement cascade [2].

Hemolytic diseases can lead to repeated splenic infarcts, resulting in splenic atrophy and eventual loss of function. This can be histopathologically correlated with the presence of basophilic nuclear remnants in circulating erythrocytes known as Howell–Jolly bodies. In general, infiltrative hematologic diseases and thromboembolic diseases may predispose the spleen to infarction [3]. The following case illustrates the first known report of AS attributed to PNH.

2. Case

A 24-year-old Caucasian male with a history that includes Addison's disease, developmental delay, hypogammaglobulinemia, PNH complicated by lower extremity thrombosis, minimal change disease (MCD), and end-stage renal disease (ESRD) presented with headaches, fevers, and neck stiffness for several days after a tunneled dialysis catheter was placed for hemodialysis.

The patient was diagnosed with Addison's disease at the age of 14 years following a workup for ongoing fatigue. At that time, he was also found to have macrocytic anemia (hemoglobin 9.3 G/dL, hematocrit 26.9 G/dL, and mean cell volume 114 FL), thrombocytopenia (platelets 16,000 U/L), elevated lactate dehydrogenase (1261 U/L), and reticulocytosis (3.6%). His direct antiglobulin test, platelet antibodies, and HIV antibodies were negative, and the ADAMTS13 activity level was normal. Hemoglobin electrophoresis was not suggestive of hemoglobinopathy. His peripheral blood smear reported anisopoikilocytosis, mild to moderate schistocytes, and Howell–Jolly bodies. Splenic ultrasound with Doppler studies were normal. Slightly increased osmotic fragility was present, and bone marrow biopsy reported a hypercellular marrow with predominance of erythroid precursors. Further evaluation including bone marrow biopsies, cytogenetic analysis, and autoimmune panels failed to confirm a cause for this patient's hemolytic anemia. After returning to the clinic with progressive fatigue and hematuria, the diagnosis of PNH was made when flow cytometry indicated PNH clonal populations in 38% of red blood cells (RBCs), 68% granulocytes, and 71% monocytes. Since the patient's anemia was transfusion independent and without evidence of thromboembolic disease, treatment with eculizumab was not offered until two years after the confirmed diagnosis which the patient refused. His renal function declined over time, and initial renal biopsies reported hemosiderosis due to PNH. His renal function continued to worsen over the next three years, and he eventually developed significant proteinuria (20 g/24 h) prompting repeat kidney biopsy. The results indicated significant hemosiderosis due to PNH as well as effacement of podocyte foot processes consistent with MCD. He was treated with prednisone and later rituximab for MCD. Rituximab was later discontinued after the patient developed new onset hypogammaglobulinemia after starting rituximab. His proteinuria resolved with continued steroid therapy, but his renal function did not improve, requiring initiation of hemodialysis. After the diagnosis of ESRD, the patient was agreeable to eculizumab and started therapy. The patient's clinical course was further complicated by recurrent catheter-associated infection.

Over the past two years, the patient has been treated for frequent episodes of sepsis due to coagulase-negative *Staphylococcus aureus* bacteremia, methicillin-sensitive and resistant *Staphylococcus aureus* bacteremia, *Enterococcus faecalis* meningitis, and *Streptococcus pneumoniae* bacteremia and pneumonia. It was thought that the patient's recurrent infections were from poor tunneled dialysis catheter hygiene and maintenance.

On the current admission, peripheral blood smear demonstrated the presence of numerous Howell–Jolly bodies (Figure 1), Pappenheimer bodies, acanthocytes, and target cells. Splenic sonogram now showed multifocal scarring and splenic atrophy, measuring 7.9 × 3.9 × 3.3 cm, suggestive of recurrent infarctions (Figure 2). Liver-splenic scintigraphy with ^{99m}Tc-labelled colloid did not show splenic uptake, consistent with AS (Figure 3). The patient continued to have recurrent episodes of staphylococcus bacteremia, leading to tunneled dialysis catheter removal and transition to peritoneal dialysis.

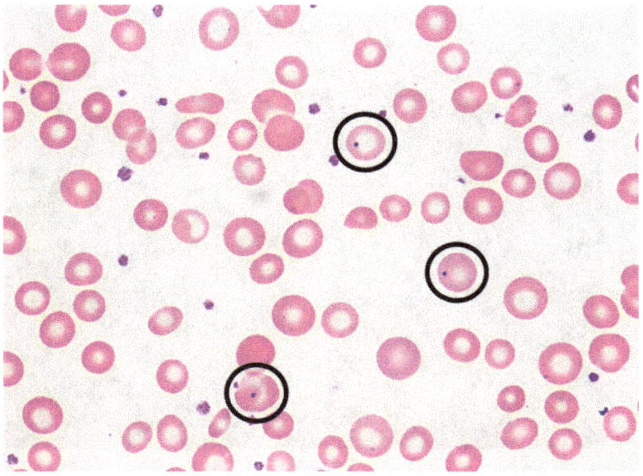

FIGURE 1: Peripheral blood smear (1000x oil, magnification): normocytic normochromic anemia with mild anisopoikilocytosis and three erythrocytes (black circles) with Howell–Jolly bodies (nuclear remnants) and adequate numbers of appropriately granulated platelets.

3. Discussion

PNH is caused by an acquired somatic mutation in the X-linked phosphatidylinositol glycan complementation class-A (*PIG-A*) gene that results in an absence of glycosylphosphatidylinositol linked surface anchored proteins on hematopoietic stem cells [4]. This leads to an absence of the decay accelerating factor (CD55) and membrane attack complex-inhibitory protein (CD59) on the surface of hematopoietic cells. Most human cells, including platelets and white blood cells, express surface CD55, CD59, and membrane cofactor protein (CD46), another inhibitor of complement-mediated effects [4]. Erythrocytes lack CD46 [4], and in the presence of a *PIG-A* mutation, circulating CD55 and CD59 deficient red blood cells cannot prevent complement binding, leading to complement-mediated intravascular destruction. Chronic hemolysis is due to unregulated activation of the alternative pathway of the complement system [5]. The alternative, lectin, and classical complement pathways converge at C3 activation. C3 spontaneously hydrolyzes and leads to the formation of C3 convertase, which in turn activates C3, C5, and the membrane attack complex (MAC) [5]. The presence of CD59 interrupts the formation of a fully functional MAC via inhibition of C9 polymerization; in the absence of CD59, unregulated formation of MAC leads to chronic intravascular hemolysis [5]. Transient decreases in pH or stress imposed on the body by surgery, infection, or inflammation may enhance complement-mediated effects, which may perpetuate brisk intravascular hemolysis and precipitate recurrent hypercoagulable events [5].

In sickle cell anemia (SCA), the spleen is one of the first organs injured as the disease manifests [6]. Though it may be

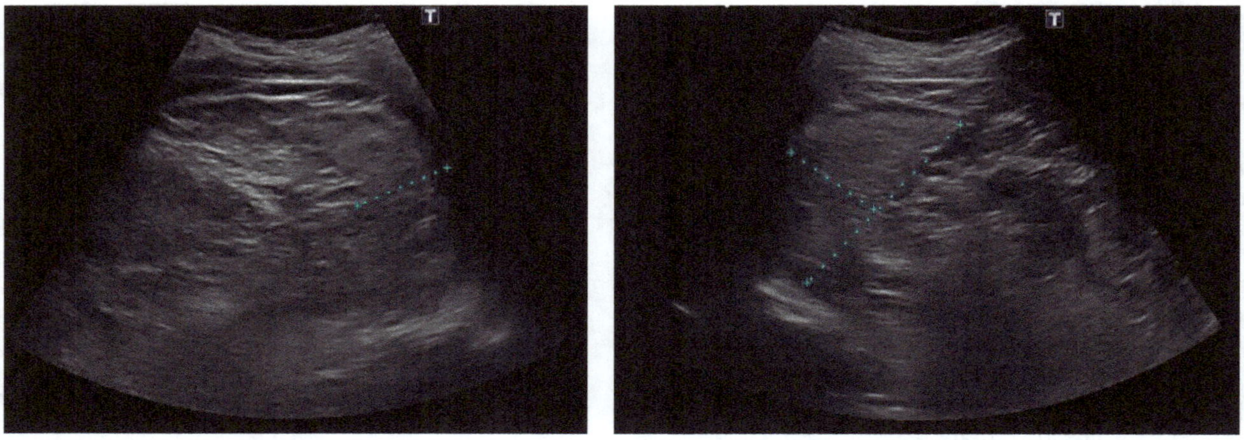

(a) (b)

Figure 2: Splenic ultrasound. (a) Transverse dimension: 3.3 centimeters. (b) Long axis: 7.9 centimeters and anteroposterior: 3.9 centimeters. Atrophic spleen suggestive of multiple repeated episodes of infarction.

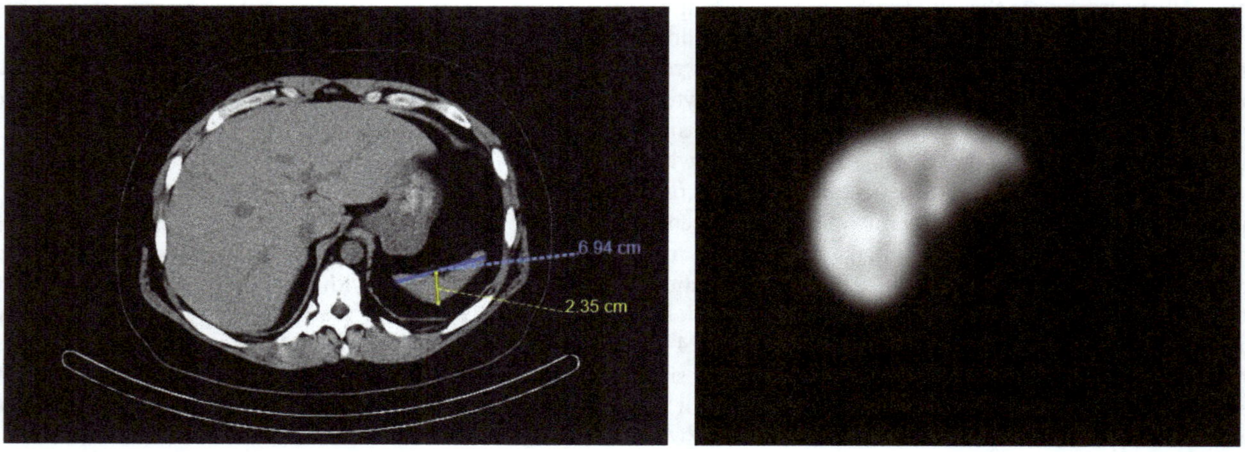

(a) (b)

Figure 3: (a) CT showing atrophic spleen without the presence of calcification. (b) Liver-splenic scintigraphy demonstrating hepatic uptake of radioactive ^{99m}Tc-labelled colloid but absent splenic uptake.

clinically silent, evidence of AS with Howell–Jolly bodies is often present within the first 12 months of life, with complete loss of splenic function by 5 years [6]. The mechanism of splenic destruction is related to a combination of upregulation of RBC adhesion molecules, diminished RBC deformability causing occlusion of splenic microcirculation, and recurrent vaso-occlusive episodes leading to progressive fibrosis, atrophy, and eventual AS [6]. This case demonstrated evidence of splenic damage on peripheral blood smear during the patient's initial presentation of hemolytic anemia, indicating that splenic damage may have started to occur early in PNH onset and suggesting a relationship between this patient's PNH and AS. Over time, it is possible that treatment delay and recurrent septicemia-induced PNH exacerbations led to repeated splenic ischemic infarcts, eventually resulting in AS.

The mechanism of PNH-induced AS is unknown, but hypercoagulability may be involved. In PNH, thromboembolism can occur at any site including the intra-abdominal vasculature and is attributable to 40–67% of deaths [7]. Approximately 29–44% of patients will have thromboembolic disease over the course of PNH [7], and patients with a granulocyte colony factor count of >50% have a 34.5% 10-year incidence of thrombosis [8]. Although less common, arterial thrombosis may also occur, usually in the cerebral or coronary circulation [9, 10]. Arterial complications including ischemic strokes and myocardial infarction have occasionally been described as the initial manifestations of PNH [9, 10].

PNH-induced hypercoagulability occurs via a myriad of proposed mechanisms. During hemolysis, a decrease in nitric oxide (NO) production and an increase in circulating cell-free hemoglobin-mediated NO scavenging results in enhanced endothelial molecule expression and cGMP mediated platelet activation [11–15]. In addition, the tissue factor (CD142) is abnormally expressed in hemolytic anemias including PNH and is thought to contribute to hypercoagulability [16, 17]. Furthermore, procoagulant phospholipid microparticles released during episodes of hemolysis may also contain elements of tissue factor, predisposing patients to hypercoagulable events [18], and tissue ischemia. The complement and coagulation cascades are closely interlinked, substantially increasing patient risk for thrombus formation. Thrombin has been demonstrated to play a role in PNH via activation of the C3 and C5 components of the complement system. This increases the risk of thrombosis via a positive feedback loop where thrombin increases complement-mediated hemolysis leading to a cycle of hypercoagulability [7]. In this case, recurrent PNH flares due to sepsis likely led to recurrent hypercoagulability, recurrent splenic vascular ischemia, and eventual AS. Treatment with eculizumab significantly reduces the risk of thrombosis and improves survival in patients with PNH [19]. The delay in treatment initiation despite a large PNH clone population, progressive symptoms, and significant anemia secondary to patient refusal likely contributed to this patient's resultant AS, progressive decline in renal function, and development of deep venous thrombosis.

Eculizumab inhibits terminal complement activity by binding to C5 which is an important mechanism of defense against *Neisseria species*, thus vaccination is recommended [20–22]. Infections with other encapsulated organisms including *Haemophilus influenza* type B and *Streptococcus pneumoniae* are typically not associated with C5 or the alternative complement pathway but rather with C3 deficiency and deficiencies of components in the classical pathway [20, 21]. The spleen plays a crucial role in macrophage-mediated destruction of opsonized encapsulated bacteria, so splenic damage can also predispose patients to overwhelming infections by encapsulated organisms [21]. It also has roles in both the adaptive and innate arms of the immune system and serves as a filter for other hematogenous pathogens and antigens [23]. Due to the possibility of AS arising from PNH, the predisposition to infection by encapsulated organisms must be considered. This case indicates the possibility of splenic damage early in the presentation of PNH, so the presence of Howell–Jolly bodies on peripheral blood smear or recurrent infections may indicate the need for a workup to assess splenic size and function.

4. Conclusion

This is the first known case of autosplenectomy in a patient with PNH. This was probably due to a recurrent hypercoagulable environment from untreated PNH leading to repeated episodes of splenic ischemia, infarction, and eventual atrophy with autosplenectomy. This case demonstrates that splenic damage may present early in PNH onset, and presence of Howell–Jolly bodies or recurrent infections should prompt consideration of splenic imaging, especially given the propensity of PNH to manifest with thrombi in unusual locations.

Abbreviations

AS: Autosplenectomy
PNH: Paroxysmal nocturnal hemoglobinuria
MCD: Minimal change disease
ESRD: End-stage renal disease
SCA: Sickle cell anemia.

References

[1] A. Hill, P. Platts, S. Richards et al., "The incidence and prevalence of paroxysmal nocturnal hemoglobinuria (PNH) and survival of patients in yorkshire," *Blood*, vol. 108, no. 11, p. 985, 2006.

[2] R. P. Rother, S. A. Rollins, C. F. Mojcik, R. A. Brodsky, and L. Bell, "Discovery and development of the complement inhibitor eculizumab for the treatment of paroxysmal nocturnal hemoglobinuria," *Nature Biotechnology*, vol. 25, no. 11, pp. 1256–1264, 2007.

[3] M. Nores, E. H. Phillips, L. Morgenstern, and J. R Hiatt, "The clinical spectrum of splenic infarction," *American Surgeon*, vol. 64, no. 2, pp. 182–188, 1998.

[4] M. Bessler and J. Hiken, "The Pathophysiology of disease in patients with paroxysmal nocturnal hemoglobinuria," *Hematology*, vol. 2008, no. 1, pp. 104–110, 2008.

[5] R. A. Brodsky, "Paroxysmal nocturnal hemoglobinuria," *Blood*, vol. 124, no. 18, pp. 2804–2811, 2014.

[6] V. Brousse, P. Buffet, and D. Rees, "The spleen and sickle cell disease: the sick(Led) spleen," *British Journal of Haematology*, vol. 166, no. 2, pp. 165–176, 2014.

[7] A. Hill, R. J. Kelly, and P. Hillmen, "Thrombosis in paroxysmal nocturnal hemoglobinuria," *Blood*, vol. 121, no. 25, pp. 4985–4996, 2013.

[8] C. Hall, S. Richards, and P. Hillmen, "Primary prophylaxis with warfarin prevents thrombosis in paroxysmal nocturnal hemoglobinuria (PNH)," *Blood*, vol. 102, no. 10, pp. 3587–3591, 2003.

[9] H. Audebert, J. Planck, M. Eisenburg, H. Schrezenmeier, and R. L. Haberl, "Cerebral ischemic infarction in paroxysmal nocturnal hemoglobinuria," *Journal of Neurology*, vol. 252, no. 11, pp. 1379–1386, 2005.

[10] S. I. Iñigo, C. N. McDonell, A. G. Valls et al., "Patients with paroxysmal nocturnal hemoglobinuria (PNH)-data from the Spanish PNH registry," *Blood*, vol. 128, no. 22, p. 4811, 2016.

[11] M. T. Gladwin, J. R. Lancaster, B. A. Freeman, and A. N. Schechter, "Nitric oxide's reactions with hemoglobin: a view through the SNO-storm," *Nature Medicine*, vol. 9, no. 5, pp. 496–500, 2003.

[12] K. I. Ataga, "Hypercoagulability and thrombotic complications in hemolytic anemias," *Haematologica*, vol. 94, no. 11, pp. 1481–1484, 2009.

[13] J. Villagra, S. Shiva, L. A. Hunter, R. F. Machado, M. T. Gladwin, and G. J. Kato, "Platelet activation in patients with sickle disease, hemolysis-associated pulmonary hypertension, and nitric oxide scavenging by cell-free hemoglobin," *Blood*, vol. 110, no. 6, pp. 2166–2172, 2007.

[14] M. W. Radomski, R. M. J. Palmer, and S. Moncada, "Endogenous nitric oxide inhibits human platelet adhesion to vascular endothelium," *The Lancet*, vol. 330, no. 8567, pp. 1057-1058, 1987.

[15] C. R. Morris, S. M. Morris, W. Hagar et al., "Arginine therapy," *American Journal of Respiratory and Critical Care Medicine*, vol. 168, no. 1, pp. 63–69, 2003.

[16] P. Ziakas, L. Poulou, and A. Pomoni, "Thrombosis in paroxysmal nocturnal hemoglobinuria at a glance: a clinical review," *Current Vascular Pharmacology*, vol. 6, no. 4, pp. 347–353, 2008.

[17] H. A. Liebman and D. I. Feinstein, "Thrombosis in patients with paroxysmal noctural hemoglobinuria is associated with markedly elevated plasma levels of leukocyte-derived tissue factor," *Thrombosis Research*, vol. 111, no. 4-5, pp. 235–238, 2003.

[18] B. Hugel, G. Socié, T. Vu et al., "Elevated levels of circulating procoagulant microparticles in patients with paroxysmal nocturnal hemoglobinuria and aplastic anemia," *Blood Journal*, vol. 93, no. 10, pp. 3451–3456, 2018.

[19] A. Hill, R. J. Kelly, A. G. Kulasekararaj et al., "Eculizumab in paroxysmal nocturnal hemoglobinuria (PNH): a report of all 153 patients treated in the UK," *Blood*, vol. 120, no. 21, p. 3472, 2012.

[20] E. Benamu and J. G. Montoya, "Infections associated with the use of eculizumab," *Current Opinion in Infectious Diseases*, vol. 29, no. 4, pp. 319–329, 2016.

[21] S. Ram, L. A. Lewis, and P. A. Rice, "Infections of People with complement deficiencies and patients who have undergone splenectomy," *Clinical Microbiology Reviews*, vol. 23, no. 4, pp. 740–780, 2010.

[22] P. Bonanni, M. Grazzini, G. Niccolai et al., "Recommended vaccinations for asplenic and hyposplenic adult patients," *Human Vaccines & Immunotherapeutics*, vol. 13, no. 2, pp. 359–368, 2016.

[23] B. Styrt, "Infection associated with asplenia: risks, mechanisms, and prevention," *American Journal of Medicine*, vol. 88, no. 5, pp. 33N–42N, 1990.

21

Intrauterine Growth Retardation Complicated by Biermer's Disease: An Observation in Togo

Essohana Padaro,[1] Baguilane Douaguibe,[2] Kossi Agbétiafa,[1] Irénée Kueviakoe,[3] and Ahoefa Vovor[3]

[1]*Hematology Department, Campus Teaching Hospital, University of Lome, Lome, Togo*
[2]*Gynecology Department, Campus Teaching Hospital, University of Lome, Lome, Togo*
[3]*Hematology Department, Tokoin Teaching Hospital, University of Lome, Lome, Togo*

Correspondence should be addressed to Essohana Padaro; essohanapadaro@gmail.com

Academic Editor: Gergely Feher

Objective. To report the first case in Togo of Biermer's disease associated with intrauterine growth retardation (IUGR) in a 39-year-old pregnant woman. *Observation.* The patient with phenotype AA, born on 20/02/1978, G_2P_0 (a spontaneous abortion at 3 months), was referred to hematology on 17th March 2017 for anemia at 26 weeks of amenorrhea (WA). She had received martial treatment with ferrous fumarate 66 milligrams daily. At 26 weeks, the uterine height was 16 centimeters, and there was good fetal vitality. During ultrasound, there was a harmonious development of the fetus, but it was lower than that for the gestational age at 10th percentile based on fetal biometry, and anemia was at 65 g/l. She was then referred to hematology where she was found to have pancytopenia with macrocytic aregenerative anemia at 47 g/l (MCV at 109 fl), neutropenia at 1.02 g/l, and thrombocytopenia at 58 g/l. The myelogram found megaloblastosis at 53%, collapsed serum B12 vitamin at 61.7 pg/ml, normal serum folate at 9.9 ng/ml, increased serum homocysteine to 51.44 μmol/l, and elevated LDH. The search for intrinsic anti-factor antibodies was positive. Digestive endoscopy noted fundal atrophy. The patient was given vitamin B12 injection; at the 7th day, hemoglobin was observed at 94 g/l, then a normalization of the blood count after 3 weeks, and a good evolution of the pregnancy with delivery at 38 WA of a newborn, female, weighing 1960 g with 500 grams of placenta, with a size of 40 cm, and a cranial perimeter of 29 cm. The child had stunted weight growth (at 16 months; weight = 7 kg; height = 69 cm). *Conclusion.* Biermer's disease as a maternal cause of IUGR and infantile hypotonia is a reality in Togo. It requires management in patients and especially during pregnancy to avoid neurological complications in children born from mothers with this disease.

1. Introduction

Biermer's disease (BD) also called pernicious anemia is an autoimmune atrophic gastritis with dryness of Castle's intrinsic factor (IF) responsible for vitamin B12 deficiency. It is usually diagnosed in the presence of megaloblastic anemia, neurologic symptoms, or atrophic gastritis [1]. This entity accounts for more than 25% of the etiologies of vitamin B12 deficiency in adults and results from malabsorption caused by autoimmune gastritis [2]. It is manifested by anemic and/or digestive and/or neurological signs. The diagnosis is based on the demonstration of chronic atrophic gastritis, the positivity of anti-FI (anti-intrinsic factor) and/or anti-GPC (antigastric parietal cell) autoantibodies in the serum, and/or the decrease of selective vitamin B12 [1]. The association of Biermer's disease with autoimmune diseases such as type 1 diabetes (insulin-dependent), autoimmune thyroiditis (especially Hashimoto's), or vitiligo is common [3]. Through an increase of homocysteine induced by vitamin B12 deficiency, several studies have reported venous thrombosis during Biermer's disease [1, 4]. During pregnancy, the causes or factors associated with an increased risk of intrauterine growth retardation (IUGR) are extremely numerous and can be grouped into maternal, placental, and fetal anemia [5].

Maternal anemia, irrespective of its origin, is one of the causes of IUGR and neonatal hypotrophy. Anemia in pregnant women is detrimental to fetal growth and pregnancy outcomes [6]. Low birth weight and preterm delivery have been persistently linked to anemia in pregnancy [7]. Chronic maternal diseases include heart disease and chronic hypertension, SLE, diabetes with vascular complications, chronic nephropathies, proven thrombophilias, chronic respiratory diseases, and also chronic gastrointestinal and intestinal pathologies, including Biermer's disease [5].

In Togo, a recent study reported cases of Biermer's disease in its classic presentation [8]. In the literature, no reports of Biermer's disease associated with IUGR have already been reported in Togo. We report the first observation of Biermer's disease associated with IUGR in a 39-year-old pregnant woman.

2. Observation

The patient, born on 20/02/1978, was referred to hematology of the Campus Teaching Hospital by the gynecologist on 17th March 2017 for an exploration of severe chronic anemia. She was pregnant and at 26 WA. She was a second gesture, nulliparous, and antecedent of spontaneous abortion at 3 months. She was seen in gynecology at 13 weeks of amenorrhea (WA). She had a regular cycle, the date of the last menstruation well known confirmed by the ultrasound of the first trimester. Physical examination revealed conjunctival paleness and moderate asthenia. The prenatal checkup blood count showed anemia at 7 g/l, the deep drop the parasitological examination of the stools were without abnormalities; and the electrophoresis of hemoglobin (Hb) showed a normal Hb AA. She was not an alcoholic; she had received martial treatment with ferrous fumarate 66 milligrams per day. At 26 WA, clinical examination showed the persistence of mucous pallor and asthenia, a weight of 57 kg, a height of 163 cm, a blood pressure (BP) of 120/60 mm·Hg in both arms, and negative proteinuria. Obstetrically, the uterine height was 16 cm, and there was good fetal vitality. During ultrasound, there was a harmonious development of the fetus, but it was lower than that for the gestational age at 10th percentile based on fetal biometry. The amniotic fluid amount was normal. The uterine artery Doppler and the fetal brain Doppler were normal. The control hemogram had objectified anemia at 65 g/l. In view of etiological research of anemia, this patient was referred to hematology before the signs of IUGR complication.

The clinical examination in hematology had found the relatively compensated anemic syndrome. The general condition was good. There were no digestive or neurological signs. After hematological examination, pancytopenia with macrocytic aregenerative anemia 47 g/l (MCV at 109 fl) (reticulocytes at 23 g/l), leukopenia at 3.4 g/l, neutropenia at 1.02 g/l, and thrombocytopenia at 58 g/l were observed. The myelogram by sternal puncture found megaloblastosis at 53%. On a biochemical basis, the serum vitamin B12 assay showed a collapsed vitamin B12 at 61.7 pg/ml (208–963.5), normal serum folates at 9.9 ng/ml (7.2–15.4), increased serum homocysteine to 51.44 μmol/l (3.36–20.44 μmol/l), and elevated LDH (6044 IU/l) > 13 normal. Immunological marking of anti-intrinsic factors (IF) performed at the CERBA Laboratory in France was positive. Upper gastrointestinal endoscopy with biopsies noted fundal atrophy with erosive bulbitis. Anatomopathological examination showed chronic atrophic gastritis without *Helicobacter pylori*. The anti-IF antibody had not been researched on biopsy specimens. The diagnosis of BD had been posited with certainty. IUGR was secondary to this chronic anemia related to BD.

The patient was given vitamin B12 deep intramuscular injection (1000 μg daily during 10 days and then a monthly injection for lifetime). Under this treatment, reticulocyte crisis was noted at the 7th day (reticulocytes at 94.3 g/l) with a hemoglobin rate of 94 g/l and a gradual normalization of the blood count after 3 weeks. On the gyneco-obstetrical level, good evolution of the pregnancy was noted, which resulted in a delivery on 3rd June 2017 by caesarean section at 38 WA of a newborn, female, of 1960 grams with 500 grams of placenta. The size of the newborn was 40 cm with a cranial perimeter of 29 cm. In October 2018, the child had a stunted weight loss because at 16 months, the child weighed only 7 kg for a height of 69 cm. However, she had good neurological development.

3. Discussion

Biermer's disease (formerly called pernicious anemia) is an autoimmune atrophic gastritis, predominantly fundic, responsible for vitamin B12 deficiency (cobalamin) by malabsorption of the latter [1]. Vitamin B12 is the cofactor of methylmalonyl mutase and methionine synthetase. Vitamin B12 is a ubiquitous coenzyme involved in a large number of intracellular enzyme reactions [9]. These are essentially the reactions that lead to the synthesis of DNA and the synthesis of methionine from homocysteine. Vitamin B12 deficiency is responsible for elevated homocysteine, methylmalonic acid, and propionylcarnitine [10]. B12 hypovitaminosis is common in adults and the elderly, with prevalence ranging from 15 to 40%, depending on the studies and the definition used [10]. It is often not diagnosed early because of poor clinical manifestations. However, its potentially serious hematological and neuropsychiatric complications require the diagnostic investigation of any patient with vitamin B12 deficiency, irrespective of the cause. Biermer's disease accounts for 25% of the etiologies of vitamin B12 deficiencies in adults according to the series [2]. The prevalence of Biermer's disease is 0.1% in the general population and 1.9% in subjects over 60 years of age [10]. Alteration of DNA synthesis results in blockage of maturation affecting mainly fast-multiplying cells and gives rise to hematological and mucocutaneous syndromes. Hematologically, DNA synthesis blockade and conserved synthesis of RNA are at the origin of cytoplasmic nucleotide asynchrony. Intramedullary abortion linked to inefficient hematopoiesis and megaloblastosis is responsible for clinicobiological images that can simulate true hemolytic anemia [11]. The patient has biological signs of hemolysis including an increase in LDH.

On the obstetrical side, recent studies have shown the effects of homocysteine on the fetus. Indeed, homocysteine results from the transmethylation of methionine. Its metabolism depends primarily on three enzymes and several vitamin cofactors. Genetic abnormality in these enzymes or deficiency of these vitamins leads to hyperhomocysteinemia (HHCh). HHCh is usually biologically defined by a fasting value >15 μmol/l. HHCh is among the congenital hypercoagulable states and is a long-known vascular disease risk factor. The discovery that HHCh may also be responsible for several pregnancy complications has only recently been made [12]. Studies in this area are still scarce and report on limited numbers of patients. It nevertheless appears clear that HHCh is associated with the syndromes of repeated miscarriage, preeclampsia, placental abruption, thromboembolic events, neural tube defects, and perhaps fetal death in utero and intrauterine growth retardation [12].

Also, methyl donors (B12 and folates) regulate the monocarbon cycle, which plays a key role in epigenetic/epigenomic regulation by methylation [13]. Methyl donor deficiency produces intrauterine growth retardation and promotes developmental abnormalities, mainly of the central nervous system. In addition, high levels of homocysteine associated with such deficiency are a risk factor for various neurodegenerative pathologies. The authors studied the consequences of periconceptional and gestational deficiency on the embryonic brain development in Wistar rats [13]. Morphometric study showed retarded growth of deficient embryos that also affected the brain, with atrophy of structures such as the hippocampus, cortex, and subventricular zone. In addition, they demonstrated that methyl donor deficiency was associated with a posttranslational modification corresponding to an irreversible *N*-homocysteinylation of neuronal proteins, in particular, associated with the cytoskeleton. This modification induces the aggregation of proteins, a phenomenon involved in many neurodegenerative diseases. The combination of these different mechanisms sheds new light on the developmental defects and cognitive disorders associated with early methyl donor deficiency, highlighting the importance of "fetal programming" in the occurrence of certain neurological pathologies [1, 12]. The patient had an increase in homocysteine that allows us to understand the IUGR and then the hypotonia at birth and the secondary stunted weight loss. Indeed, hypotonia and/or psychomotor retardation of the infant may have a metabolic cause.

Very recently, Savall et al. in 2015 [14] presented a case of suspicion of methylmalonic aciduria in an infant that allowed us to revisit the diagnosis of neuro-Biermer in his mother in whom there was no hematological sign. However, she had a painful obstetric history (several miscarriages and a baby died of bilateral renal agenesis at birth) and gave birth to a girl of 2.88 kg and 46 cm in January 2015, at 39 WA, healthy outside with slight intrauterine growth retardation [14]. For the patient situation, it is rather the presence of Biermer's disease that allowed the follow-up and the diagnosis of this stunted weight growth retardation. The maternal vitamin B12 deficiency is not always responsible for hematological abnormalities, thus delaying the diagnosis. In our patient, we can discuss the role of hyperhomocysteinemia induced by vitamin B12 deficiency as the cause of the first miscarriage. Barro et al. [15] also reported three similar cases of complex obstetric history and IUGR related to Biermer's disease. Infants born to mothers who are vitamin B12 deficient and exclusively breastfed are at high risk for neurological complications. Neonatal screening for this deficiency through the determination of blood or urinary methylmalonic acid may help avoid these complications and quickly diagnose the maternal cause [14]. We started vitamin B12 supplementation in infants.

4. Conclusion

Biermer's disease as a very rare maternal cause of intrauterine growth retardation and infantile hypotonia is becoming a reality in Togo. Vitamin B12 therapy should be provided lifelong to prevent relapses of neurological conditions and fetal consequences that may be irreversible. We advocate special care from birth for children born to mothers with this disease.

References

[1] W. Ammouri, Z. Mezalek Tazi, H. Harmouche, M. Maamar, and M. Adnaoui, "Venous thromboembolism and hyperhomocysteinemia as first manifestation of pernicious anemia: a case series," *Journal of Medical Case Reports*, vol. 11, no. 1, p. 250, 2017.

[2] J. Zittoun, "Anémies macrocytaires carentielles," *Encycl Méd Chir Hématologie*, Elsevier SAS, Paris, France, 2002.

[3] E. AndrèsAndrès, S. Affenberger, S. Vinzio, E. Noel, G. Kaltenbach, and J.-L. Schlienger, "Carences en vitamine B12 chez l'adulte: étiologies, manifestations cliniques et traitement," *La Revue de Médecine Interne*, vol. 26, no. 12, pp. 938–946, 2005.

[4] P. Venkatesh, N. Shaikh, M. F. Malmstrom, V. R. Kumar, and B. Nour, "Portal, superior mesenteric and splenic vein thrombosis secondary to hyperhomocysteinemia with pernicious anemia: a case report," *Journal of Medical Case Reports*, vol. 8, no. 1, p. 286, 2014.

[5] L. J. Salomon and V. Malan, "Bilan étiologique du retard de croissance intra-utérin (RCIU)," *Journal de Gynécologie Obstétrique et Biologie de la Reproduction*, vol. 42, no. 8, pp. 929–940, 2013.

[6] Y. M. Al-Farsi, D. R. Brooks, M. M. Werler, H. J. Cabral, M. A. Al-Shafei, and H. C. Wallenburg, "Effect of high parity on occurrence of anemia in pregnancy: a cohort study," *BMC Pregnancy and Childbirth*, vol. 11, no. 1, p. 7, 2011.

[7] F. M. D. Moghaddam Tabrizi and S. M. S. Barjasteh, "Maternal hemoglobin levels during pregnancy and their association with birth weight of neonates," *Iranian Journal of Pediatric Hematology Oncology*, vol. 5, no. 4, pp. 211–217, 2015.

[8] E. Padaro, I. M. D. Kuéviakoé, Y. Layibo, K. Agbétiafa, M. Kolou, and A. Y. Sébgéna, "Biermer's disease in the hematology service of campus teaching hospital of Lomé: 13 cases from January 2013 to December 2014," *Mali Medical Tome*, vol. 32, no. 3, pp. 34–39, 2017.

[9] L. Federici, N. Henoun Loukili, J. Zimmer, S. Affenberger, F. Maloisel, and E. Andrès, "Manifestations hématologiques

de la carence en vitamine B12: données personnelles et revue de la littérature," *La Revue de Médecine Interne*, vol. 28, no. 4, pp. 225–231, 2007.

[10] K. Serraj, M. Mecili, and E. Andrès, "Signes et symptômes de la carence en vitamine B12," *Revue Critique de la Littérature mt*, vol. 16, no. 1, pp. 13–20, 2010.

[11] M. J. Koury and P. Ponka, "New insights into erythropoiesis: the roles of folate, vitamin B12, and iron," *Annual Review of Nutrition*, vol. 24, no. 1, pp. 105–131, 2004.

[12] Y. Aubard, N. Darodes, and M. Cantaloube, "Hyperhomocysteinemia and pregnancy—review of our present understanding and therapeutic implications," *European Journal of Obstetrics & Gynecology and Reproductive Biology*, vol. 93, no. 2, pp. 157–165, 2000.

[13] R. Kerek, *Conséquences d'une Carence en Donneurs de Méthyles sur le Développement Cérébral: Implication du Programme Neurogénique et Rôle de L'homocystéine .Auteur IdRef*, https://www.idref.fr/178157279visitéle27/12/2018.

[14] A. Savall, C. Durousset, C. Gay, and P. Cathébras, "Une cause pernicieuse d'hypotonie du nourrisson," *La Revue de Médecine Interne*, vol. 36, no. 2, p. A134, 2015.

[15] C. Barro, V. Ducros, B. Bonaz et al., "Homocystéine et fausses couches: à propos de trois cas cliniques," *Annales de Biologie Clinique*, vol. 60, no. 3, pp. 325-326, 2002.

22

A Sudden Onset of Severe Thrombocytopenia While using Evolocumab

Ikuo Inoue,[1] **Yasuhiro Takenaka**,[1,2] **Yoshitora Kin**,[3] **Satoshi Yamazaki**,[4] **Yuichi Ikegami**,[1] **Daigo Saito**,[1] **and Akira Shimada**[1]

[1]*Department of Endocrinology and Diabetes, Faculty of Medicine, Saitama Medical University, 38 Morohongo, Moroyama, Iruma, Saitama 350-0495, Japan*
[2]*Department of Physiology, Graduate School of Medicine, Nippon Medical School, 1-25-16 Nezu, Bunkyo, Tokyo 113-0031, Japan*
[3]*Department of Internal Medicine, Fukaya Red Cross Hospital, 5-8-1 Kamishibatyohnishi, Fukaya, Saitama 366-0052, Japan*
[4]*Kumagaya-geka Hospital, 3811-1 Sayata, Kumagaya, Saitama 360-0023, Japan*

Correspondence should be addressed to Ikuo Inoue; i1901018@saitama-med.ac.jp

Academic Editor: Tomás J. González-López

A 72-year-old man with a 10-year history of coronary heart disease started evolocumab treatment once a month after developing excess myalgia due to therapy with a 3-hydroxy-methylglutaryl CoA reductase inhibitor. No side effects such as myalgia symptoms had been reported during the first 14 months of evolocumab treatment; however, he suddenly presented with acute severe thrombocytopenia following the 14th treatment. His platelet count continued to decrease to a nadir of 1,000/μL. His platelet-associated immunoglobulin G level had elevated to 790 ng/10^7 cells. He started receiving a combination of steroid therapy, high-dose immunoglobulin therapy, and platelet transfusions, but the first-line therapy was ineffective. He was subsequently treated with a thrombopoietin receptor agonist, and his platelet count recovered to 250,000/μL.

1. Introduction

3-Hydroxy-methylglutaryl CoA (HMG-CoA) reductase inhibitor (statin) therapy reduces coronary heart disease (CHD) events through decreasing low-density lipoprotein-cholesterol (LDL-C) levels. However, between 5% and 10% of statin users develop statin intolerance. Statin intolerance refers to an inability to use statins because of myalgia symptoms or elevated serum creatine kinase levels. It has been reported that patients with statin intolerance may have an increased risk of CHD events [1]; therefore, new and efficient LDL-C-lowering drugs via a different mechanism from statins are necessary.

Recently, proprotein convertase subtilisin/kexin type 9 (PCSK9) inhibitors have safely been administered to patients worldwide. Evolocumab, a PCSK9 inhibitor, became available in Japan in 2016, and 3 months later, alirocumab was also made available. Evolocumab [2] and alirocumab [3] are human immunoglobulin G2 and G1 monoclonal antibodies, respectively, against PCSK9 expressed by hepatocytes. Evolocumab or alirocumab therapy reduces CHD events through decreasing LDL-C levels, as seen in statin therapy. Evolocumab and alirocumab have been reported to be effective for patients with CHD without severe side effects. Mild adverse effects, such as an allergic reaction at the injection site, have been observed with the use of evolocumab or alirocumab. There has been no reported incidence of serious systemic hypersensitivity reactions such as anaphylaxis [4]. Moreover, during the clinical use of evolocumab or alirocumab, significant hematologic changes such as thrombocytopenia have not been reported so far. Furthermore, even in large-scale intervention studies, the incidence of side effects secondary to evolocumab or alirocumab use during follow-up has been reported to be similar to that of the placebo [4]. Here, we describe a rare case of thrombocytopenia that developed during the use of evolocumab.

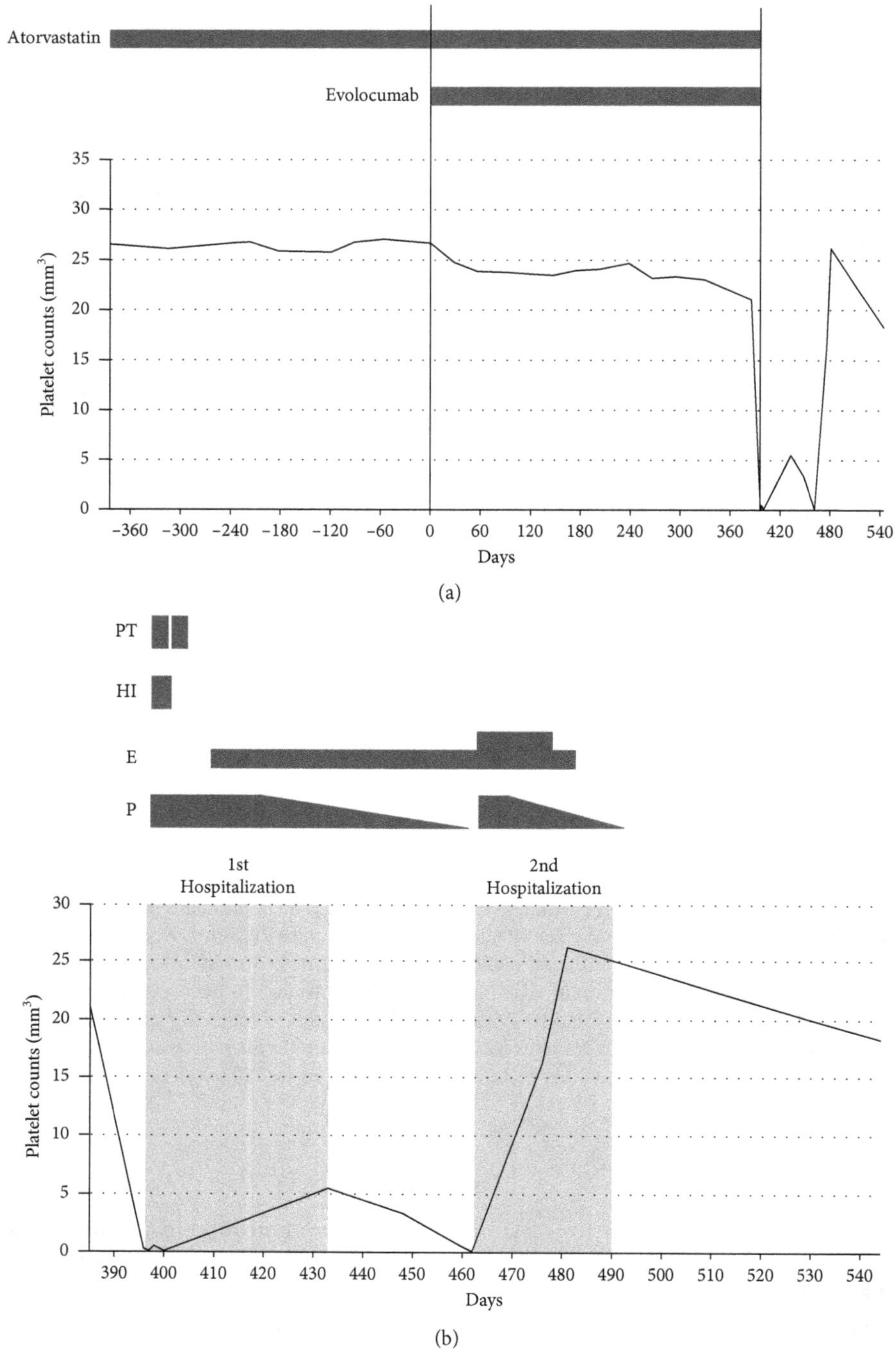

FIGURE 1: Patient's platelet counts relative to the time courses of his treatment before (a) and after (b) hospitalization. In (a) and (b), the Y-axis and the X-axis represent platelet counts and the number of days before and after the first treatment of evolocumab, respectively. Day 0 indicates the initial day of evolocumab therapy. The periods of atorvastatin and evolocumab treatment are indicated above the graph in (a). PT, platelet transfusions (two injections); HI, high-dose immunoglobulin (25 g per day for 5 consecutive days); E, eltrombopag (thin line, 12.5 mg; thick line, 25 mg per day, respectively); P, prednisone (starting with 1 mg/kg).

2. Case report

A 72-year-old man with a 10-year history of CHD and hyperlipidemia started evolocumab therapy once a month after he had developed excess myalgia due to statin treatment. His hematological laboratory data were normal. His CHD diagnosis had been supported by coronary computed tomographic angiography findings. He had complained of chest pain at various times between the age of 65 and 70 years. He had a family history of CHD.

The patient had no thrombocytopenia during his monthly combined treatment with evolocumab (140 mg) and low-dose atorvastatin (2.5 mg per day). His platelet count was largely unchanged (225,000–260,000/μL) for 14 months from the first evolocumab administration. On the 13th and just prior to the 14th treatment with evolocumab, his platelet count was 211,000 and 210,000/μL, respectively; however, it suddenly decreased to 1,000/μL on day 12 following his 14th treatment with evolocumab (Figure 1(a)), and he presented with symptoms of acute severe thrombocytopenia. A physical examination revealed nonpalpable petechial purpura over his face, extending to the neck, the front and back of the trunk, and both limbs. In addition, sudden-onset gingival bleeding and epistaxis were observed. He also presented with nasal bleeding, ocular hyperemia, and hemorrhages in the buccal mucosa. He was immediately admitted to a hospital.

The patient's platelet count at admission was 3,000/μL. His platelet count continued to decrease over 12 days following evolocumab discontinuation to a nadir of 1,000/μL, and he had slight anemia. The patient's reticulocyte count, serum iron level, and direct antiglobulin test results were normal (data not shown). Although his red blood cell count, hemoglobin, and hematocrit values slightly decreased from 3.39 to 3.27×10^4 cells/μL, from 11.5 to 11.1 g/dL, and from 34.8 to 33.8%, respectively, these changes were not significant. His white blood cell count slightly increased from 3,430 to 4,100/μL. A bone marrow aspiration examination revealed neither increase in the number of megakaryocytes nor any morphologic abnormalities. A cytogenetic study of megakaryocytes showed normal karyotype and absence of chromosomal rearrangements such as translocations and deletions. He tested negative for *Helicobacter pylori* infection. Inflammatory workup was performed for the negative erythrocyte sedimentation rate, anti-ribonucleoprotein antibody, anti-double-stranded DNA antibody, rheumatoid factor, and complement levels. Cytomegalovirus, human immunodeficiency virus, Epstein–Barr virus, immunoglobulin G (IgG), and IgM were not detected in the patient. Spleen size was measured using abdominal echo examination. His spleen was 9 cm long and 4 cm wide, which was in the normal range. His platelet-associated immunoglobulin G (PAIgG) level was elevated at 790 ng/10^7 cells. Therefore, the patient was newly diagnosed with immune thrombocytopenia.

The patient started a combination of steroid therapy, high-dose immunoglobulin therapy, and platelet transfusions (Figure 1(b)). After platelet transfusion therapy, his platelet count increased after 1 h, but was decreased again by 4 h. He was treated with prednisone (1 mg/kg/day for 3 weeks), but this resulted in no improvement of the thrombocytopenia and the initial therapy was ineffective. Owing to persistent thrombocytopenia, he was started on eltrombopag, which is a small molecule thrombopoietin receptor agonist, at a low starting dose of 12.5 mg. Thereafter, in addition to 25 mg eltrombopag, we administered a daily dose of 60 mg prednisone to achieve a >250,000/μl platelet count. Three months later, his platelet count had returned to normal and remained at approximately 200,000/μL during the 2-month follow-up period post-initiation of eltrombopag (Figure 1(b)). No bleeding complications were observed post-discharge. Currently, without steroid administration, his platelet count is stable at approximately 183,000/μL.

3. Discussion

Here, we describe a rare complication of severe thrombocytopenia that occurred while using evolocumab. There are two possible mechanisms of thrombocytopenia: decreased platelet production and increased platelet destruction. When a platelet count decreases, megakaryocytes usually increase in number as a compensatory action. However, in our case, a bone marrow aspiration examination revealed no increase in the number of megakaryocytes. Therefore, in the present case, we should consider both platelet destruction, as well as incomplete maturation of megakaryocytes, as the potential mechanism leading to thrombocytopenia.

The patient was diagnosed with acute ITP instead of drug-induced immune thrombocytopenia (DITP), although our assays were inconclusive. In general, DITP occurs 1 to 2 weeks after the initial administration of a particular drug with a sudden decrease in platelet counts to <100,000/μL [5, 6]. This causes clinically significant hemorrhage in patients, and deaths have been reported [7]. In our case, the patient's platelet counts were within the normal range from the first to the 14th evolocumab administration, but suddenly dropped 12 days after the 14th administration (Figure 1(a)). In some cases, DITP can occur following intermittent use of a drug such as quinine, the oldest reported cause of thrombocytopenia, for an extended period of time [5, 7, 8]. Thus, we were unable to exclude the possibility that evolocumab was relevant to the development of drug-induced and immune-mediated destruction of platelets in the patient. PAIgG level was elevated during thrombocytopenia, which may have largely bound to platelets and induced platelet aggregation or lysis, resulting in fewer platelets. Another possibility was that evolocumab impaired the maturation of megakaryocytes to produce platelets, although they were normal in number. Human megakaryocytes express PCSK9 transcripts at low level [9]. Thus, evolocumab potentially interacted with a part of the PCSK9 on the surface of megakaryocytes, which might have, in turn, caused disturbances in the signaling pathways of megakaryocyte differentiation.

To date, there have been no reported cases of severe thrombocytopenia involving patients receiving evolocumab. Barale et al. reported reduced platelet reactivity to agonists, such as adenosine diphosphate and collagen, in patients with familial hypercholesterolemia after 8-week treatment with evolocumab or alirocumab [10]. Although the presence of significant changes in the platelet count were not described in their report, senile or damaged platelets with decreased function may be quickly removed from the blood, resulting in fewer platelets.

Plasma PCSK9 levels have been shown to positively correlate with the platelet count in patients with stable coronary artery disease with unknown physiological mechanisms [11]. In our case, although the plasma PCSK9 level was not measured before or after the onset of thrombocytopenia, it is plausible that the administered evolocumab formed a drug-target complex with PCSK9 to block its function, thereby facilitating degradation and reducing the plasma PCSK9 levels. A prompt reduction in the plasma PCSK9 level via interaction with the drug may have led to a decreased platelet count. The relationship between the plasma PCSK9 level and the platelet count in patients with hypercholesterolemia needs to be investigated.

Significant hematologic changes, such as thrombocytopenia, have not been reported with the clinical use of evolocumab or alirocumab. However, hematologic parameters, especially changes in platelet count, should be carefully monitored during PCSK9 inhibitor therapy. We believe that our case report provides a new insight into the pharmacological aspects of lipid-lowering drugs in patients with coronary heart disease.

Supplementary Materials

Supplementary Figure 1: speculative schema of the mechanism of evolocumab-dependent platelet destruction through immune mechanisms. PCSK9-evolocumab complex containing IgG interacting with the platelet Fc receptors (a) and evolocumab-platelet membrane complex harboring neoantigenic determinants where excess evolocumab attaches onto the platelet membrane (b). In the former case, IgG directed against the PCSK9-evolocumab complex as the antigen was generated, and the complex bound to the platelet Fc receptor through the antibodies. PAIgG, platelet-associated immunoglobulin G. (*Supplementary Materials*)

References

[1] M.-C. Serban, L. D. Colantonio, A. D. Manthripragada et al., "Statin intolerance and risk of coronary heart events and all-cause mortality following myocardial infarction," *Journal of the American College of Cardiology*, vol. 69, no. 11, pp. 1386–1395, 2017.

[2] L. Fala, "Repatha (evolocumab): second PCSK9 inhibitor approved by the FDA for patients with familial hypercholesterolemia," *Am Health Drug Benefits*, Spec Feature, vol. 9, pp. 136–139, 2016.

[3] M. Manniello and M. Pisano, "Alirocumab (Praluent): First in the new class of PCSK9 inhibitors," *P T*, vol. 41, no. 1, pp. 28–53, 2016.

[4] A. Hirayama, S. Yamashita, H. Inomata et al., "One-year efficacy and safety of evolocumab in Japanese patients—A pooled analysis from the open-label extension OSLER studies —," *Circulation Journal*, vol. 81, no. 7, pp. 1029–1035, 2017.

[5] J. N. George and R. H. Aster, "Drug-induced Thrombocytopenia: Pathogenesis, Evaluation, and Management," *Hematology*, vol. 2009, no. 1, pp. 153–158, 2009.

[6] N. Ali and H. E. Auerbach, "New-onset acute thrombocytopenia in hospitalized patients: pathophysiology and diagnostic approach," *Journal of Community Hospital Internal Medicine Perspectives*, vol. 7, no. 3, pp. 157–167, 2017.

[7] R. H. Aster and D. W. Bougie, "Drug-induced immune thrombocytopenia," *New England Journal of Medicine*, vol. 357, no. 6, pp. 580–587, 2007.

[8] J. C. Reddy, M. A. Shuman, and R. H. Aster, "Quinine/quinidine-induced thrombocytopenia: a great imitator," *Archives of Internal Medicine*, vol. 164, no. 2, pp. 218–220, 2004.

[9] F. Paciullo, S. Momi, and P. Gresele, "PCSK9 in haemostasis and thrombosis: possible pleiotropic effects of PCSK9 inhibitors in cardiovascular prevention," *Thrombosis and Haemostasis*, vol. 119, no. 3, pp. 359–367, 2019.

[10] C. Barale, K. Bonomo, F. Noto et al., "Effects of PCSK9 inhibitors on platelet function in adults with hypercholesterolemia," *Atherosclerosis*, vol. 263, pp. e30–e31, 2017.

[11] S. Li, C.-G. Zhu, Y.-L. Guo et al., "The relationship between the plasma PCSK9 levels and platelet indices in patients with stable coronary artery disease," *Journal of Atherosclerosis and Thrombosis*, vol. 22, no. 1, pp. 76–84, 2015.

23

Ceftriaxone-Induced Immune Hemolytic Anemia: In Vitro Reversal with Peptide Inhibitor of Complement C1 (PIC1)

Kenji M. Cunnion,[1,2,3,4] Lisa M. Feagin,[5] Michael F. Chicella,[1,5] Cortney L. Kaszowski,[1] Pamela S. Hair,[1] Jessica Price,[1,5] and William C. Owen[1,2,3]

[1]*Department of Pediatrics, Eastern Virginia Medical School, 700 West Olney Road, Norfolk, VA 23507, USA*
[2]*Children's Specialty Group, 811 Redgate Avenue, Norfolk, VA 23507, USA*
[3]*Children's Hospital of the King's Daughters, 601 Children's Lane, Norfolk, VA 23507, USA*
[4]*Department of Microbiology and Molecular Cell Biology, Eastern Virginia Medical School, 700 West Olney Road, Norfolk, VA 23507-1696, USA*
[5]*Department of Pharmacy, Children's Hospital of the King's Daughters, 601 Children's Lane, Norfolk, VA 23507, USA*

Correspondence should be addressed to Kenji M. Cunnion; cunniokm@evms.edu

Academic Editor: Håkon Reikvam

We report a case of ceftriaxone-induced immune hemolytic anemia in a 10-year-old with chronic active Epstein–Barr virus disease and hemophagocytic lymphohistiocytosis. After chemotherapy, she became febrile and received ceftriaxone. She rapidly developed respiratory failure and anemia. Her direct antiglobulin test was positive for IgG and C3. To confirm this was ceftriaxone-induced complement-mediated hemolysis, we adapted the complement hemolysis using human erythrocytes (CHUHE) assay by adding exogenous ceftriaxone to the patient's serum which enhanced lysis of her erythrocytes. We confirmed that ceftriaxone initiated a classical complement pathway-mediated hemolysis by *in vitro* reversal with peptide inhibitor of complement C1 (PIC1).

1. Introduction

Ceftriaxone-induced immune hemolytic anemia (CIIHA) is a rare complication that can lead to shock, multiorgan dysfunction, and death. Ceftriaxone is the second most common agent to cause drug-induced hemolytic anemia [1]. The majority of documented cases of CIIHA have occurred in children [1]. Cases of CIIHA are primarily reported in patients with an underlying condition of sickle cell disease or HIV with fatalities in 30% of those published [2]. Because this is a type 2 hypersensitivity reaction, the disease process can progress rapidly after re-exposure [3]. Here, we report a case of CIIHA in a 10-year-old female with chronic active Epstein–Barr virus (EBV) disease and hemophagocytic lymphohistiocytosis (HLH).

CIIHA is mediated by anticeftriaxone antibodies that bind to circulating ceftriaxone creating immune complexes that initiate classical complement pathway activation, which lyses erythrocytes [4]. Anticeftriaxone antibodies develop in 12.5% of patients frequently exposed to ceftriaxone [5], but CIIAH is a very rare complication. Standard evaluation for suspected CIIAH includes a direct antiglobulin test (DAT) and evaluation for the presence of anticeftriaxone antibodies. CIIAH is inferred as the diagnosis if the DAT is positive for complement and the presence of anticeftriaxone antibodies is confirmed. However, those test results do not prove that the anticeftriaxone antibodies are interacting with ceftriaxone to initiate classical complement pathway-mediated hemolysis.

In order to prove the mechanism of action for this patient, we utilize new technologies including the complement hemolysis using human erythrocytes (CHUHE) assay and peptide inhibitor of complement C1 (PIC1). The CHUHE assay utilizes human serum and human erythrocytes to measure complement-mediated hemolysis for the specific serum and specific erythrocytes that are coincubated [6, 7]. PIC1 is a small peptide inhibitor of classical pathway complement activation which acts by inhibiting enzymatic activation of C1, the first component of the cascade [8–10].

2. Methods

2.1. Ethics Statement. This case report was reviewed by the Eastern Virginia Medical School IRB and determined to not constitute human subjects research.

2.2. Reagents. The patient's blood and sera were provided as discarded deidentified samples from residual specimens in the blood bank. PIC1 derivative PA-dPEG24 [8] was synthesized by the PolyPeptide Group (San Diego, CA). Standard veronal complement buffers were utilized [6].

2.3. Modified CHUHE Assay. The patient's sera (0.1 ml) were combined with ceftriaxone (10 μg/ml final concentration) in an ice-water bath for 30 minutes to enhance immune complex formation. This solution was then warmed to 24°C, and her erythrocytes (5×10^7) were added, with or without PIC1 (final concentration 0.75 mM). Samples were incubated at 37°C for 1 hour, and hemolysis was stopped by the addition of 2.0 ml of GVBS-EDTA buffer (veronal-buffered saline with 0.1% gelatin and 10 mM EDTA). Erythrocytes were sedimented, and free hemoglobin was measured by spectrophotometry at 412 nm. Due to the limited amount of serum and erythrocytes available, we could only perform n = 2 independent experiments performed in duplicate.

2.4. Statistical Methods. Quantitative data were analyzed determining means, standard error (SEM), and Student's t-test using Excel (Microsoft, Redmond, WA).

3. Case Presentation

A 10-year-old female with chronic active EBV disease and HLH was evaluated in the emergency department for fever and possible sepsis after recently receiving chemotherapy. In the emergency department, she received a dose of ceftriaxone (50 mg/kg). She had received ceftriaxone on three previous occasions with no history of adverse reaction. Within one hour, she developed back pain, tachycardia, and tachypnea. Over the next three hours, she developed worsening distress and failed continuous positive airway pressure support and required endotracheal intubation with mechanical ventilation. She also experienced hypotension requiring fluid resuscitation and a continuous epinephrine infusion.

Prior to receiving ceftriaxone, she had an erythrocyte hemoglobin concentration of 11.9 g/dL. Four hours later, her hemoglobin had decreased to 6.1 g/dL, followed by a point-of-care hemoglobin of 5.1 g/dL. There were spherocytes on her peripheral blood smear as well as red blood cell aggregation. A DAT report was sent after confirmation of the hemoglobin decrease and was positive for both IgG and C3. Urinalysis demonstrated hemoglobinuria and bilirubinuria. She required four packed red blood cell transfusions (each 10 mL/kg) over 72 hours, after which her hemoglobin stabilized at her initial baseline. High-dose methylprednisolone was begun during the first day of admission. On admission, one day later, and five days later, her total bilirubin levels were 1.5 mg/dL, 10.7 mg/dL, and 23.1 mg/dL, respectively, with 90% being unconjugated. On admission, her LDH was 514 U/L and increased to 42,093 U/L two days later. Her renal function declined 24 hours after ceftriaxone, with her BUN doubling from 12 mg/dL to 25 mg/dL and serum creatinine tripling from 0.3 mg/dL to 0.9 mg/dL. She continued to require inotropic blood pressure support for three days and required mechanical ventilation for sixteen days. Her presentation was highly suggestive of CIIHA and did not include red urine or severe anemia making the suspicion for cold agglutinin syndrome low.

The American Red Cross tested a blood sample from the day after admission and reported "Our testing was not definitive due to unexpected reactivity at the 37°C phase of testing with one set of controls. However, all controls were acceptable at the antihuman globulin phase of testing. The strong reactivity at 37°C and the reactivity at the antihuman globulin phase of testing indicate a strong likelihood that the patient has antibody to ceftriaxone." In order to evaluate whether this was ceftriaxone-initiated hemolysis, we adapted the complement hemolysis using human erythrocytes (CHUHE) hemolytic assay utilizing the patient's serum and erythrocytes and adding exogenous ceftriaxone. These experiments showed that adding ceftriaxone (10 μg/ml) to her serum increased complement-mediated hemolysis ($p = 0.02$) of her erythrocytes (Figure 1). We also evaluated whether the hemolysis was occurring via the classical complement pathway by adding peptide inhibitor of complement C1 (PIC1). Adding PIC1 (0.75 mM) in addition to ceftriaxone to her serum and erythrocytes decreased hemolysis compared with adding ceftriaxone alone ($p = 0.03$), returning hemolysis to the level of the no-ceftriaxone control. Together, these tests confirmed that the hemolysis was initiated by ceftriaxone and mediated via the classical complement pathway. These results raise the possibility that a classical pathway complement inhibitor could be employed therapeutically to moderate the disease process by blocking complement opsonization (e.g., C3b, iC3b, and C3d) of erythrocytes and inhibiting hemolysis. A terminal complement pathway inhibitor could also inhibit hemolysis, but would not stop complement opsonization of the erythrocytes.

4. Discussion

Here, we describe a case of CIIHA where we utilized new technologies to confirm the etiology and mechanisms of hemolysis. We modified the CHUHE assay [6, 7] by adding exogenous ceftriaxone and showed that hemolysis of the patient's erythrocytes was enhanced in the presence of ceftriaxone, confirming that ceftriaxone was the initiating stimulus. This result is consistent with a mechanism of

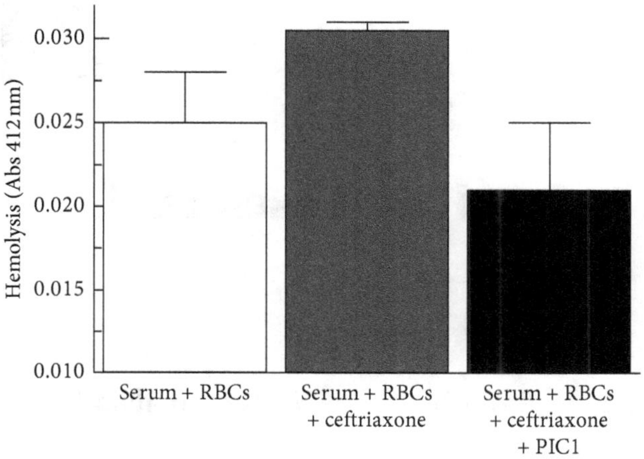

FIGURE 1: Modified CHUHE assay testing the patient's serum and erythrocytes. Addition of exogenous ceftriaxone increased hemolysis over baseline ($p = 0.02$). Addition of PIC1 (0.75 mM) to the patient's serum, to which ceftriaxone was added, resulted in decreased hemolysis compared with the addition of ceftriaxone alone ($p = 0.03$). Means ± SD are shown for 2 independent experiments.

"innocent bystander" complement-mediated hemolysis indicative of a drug-dependent IHA. We then added a classical complement pathway inhibitor, PIC1 [8], which inhibited ceftriaxone enhancement of hemolysis, demonstrating that the hemolysis was mediated by the classical complement pathway. These results also suggest the potential for complement inhibitors to be used clinically in treating CIIHA to prevent further hemolysis in the correct clinical setting with a C3-positive DAT. The long half-life of ceftriaxone of 8-9 hours [11] suggests that complement activation and hemolysis will continue to occur for a period of time as evident in this patient's course and can potentially be moderated.

Abbreviations

EBV: Epstein–Barr virus
HLH: Hemophagocytic lymphohistiocytosis
DAT: Direct antiglobulin test
CHUHE: Complement hemolysis using human erythrocytes
PIC1: Peptide inhibitor of complement C1
CIIHA: Ceftriaxone-induced immune hemolytic anemia
HIV: Human immunodeficiency virus
LDH: Lactate dehydrogenase
BUN: Blood urea nitrogen
pRBC: Packed red blood cells.

Acknowledgments

This work was funded in part by a grant from the Commonwealth Transfusion Foundation, Richmond, Virginia, USA.

References

[1] P. A. Arndt, R. M. Leger, and G. Garratty, "Serologic characteristics of ceftriaxone antibodies in 25 patients with drug-induced immune hemolytic anemia (CME)," *Transfusion*, vol. 52, no. 3, pp. 602–612, 2011.

[2] G. Neuman, S. Boodhan, and I. Wurman, "Ceftriaxone-induced immune hemolytic anemia," *Annals of Pharmacotherapy*, vol. 49, no. 5, p. 616, 2015.

[3] D. Renard and A. Rosselet, "Drug-induced hemolytic anemia: pharmacological aspects," *Transfusion Clinique et Biologique*, vol. 24, no. 3, pp. 110–114, 2017.

[4] R. Kakaiya, J. Cseri, S. Smith, S. Silberman, T. C. Rubinas, and A Hoffstadter, "A case of acute hemolysis after ceftriaxone: immune complex mechanism demonstrated by flow cytometry," *Archives of Pathology & Laboratory Medicine*, vol. 128, no. 8, pp. 905–907, 2004.

[5] K. Quillen, C. Lane, E. Hu, S. Pelton, and S. Bateman, "Prevalence of ceftriaxone-induced red blood cell antibodies in pediatric patients with sickle cell disease and human immunodeficiency virus infection," *Pediatric Infectious Disease Journal*, vol. 27, no. 4, pp. 357-358, 2008.

[6] K. M. Cunnion, P. S. Hair, N. K. Krishna et al., "Discriminating complement-mediated acute transfusion reaction for type O+ red blood cells transfused into a B+ recipient with the complement hemolysis using human erythrocytes (CHUHE) assay," *Transfusion*, vol. 56, no. 7, pp. 1845–1848, 2016.

[7] K. M. Cunnion, P. S. Hair, N. K. Krishna et al., "Discriminating the hemolytic risk of blood type A plasmas using the complement hemolysis using human erythrocytes (CHUHE) assay," *Transfusion*, vol. 57, no. 3, pp. 517–524, 2016.

[8] J. A. Sharp, P. S. Hair, H. K. Pallera et al., "Peptide inhibitor of complement C1 (PIC1) rapidly inhibits complement activation after intravascular injection in rats," *PLoS One*, vol. 10, no. 7, Article ID e0132446, 2015.

[9] P. S. Kumar, H. K. Pallera, P. S. Hair et al., "Peptide inhibitor of complement C1 modulates acute intravascular hemolysis of mismatched red blood cells in rats," *Transfusion*, vol. 56, no. 8, pp. 2133–2145, 2016.

[10] J. A. Sharp, P. H. Whitley, K. M. Cunnion et al., "Peptide inhibitor of complement C1, a novel suppressor of classical pathway activation: mechanistic studies and clinical potential," *Frontiers in Immunology*, vol. 5, p. 406, 2014.

[11] Y. Zhao, M. E. Cudkowicz, J. M. Shefner et al., "Systemic pharmacokinetics and cerebrospinal fluid uptake of intravenous ceftriaxone in patients with amyotrophic lateral sclerosis," *Journal of Clinical Pharmacology*, vol. 54, no. 10, pp. 1180–1187, 2014.

24

Co-Amoxiclav Induced Immune Haemolytic Anaemia: A Case Report

H. G. C. S. Karunathilaka[1] **D. P. Chandrasiri,**[1] **P. Ranasinghe**[2] **V. Ratnamalala,**[1] **and A. H. N. Fernando**[1]

[1]*National Hospital of Sri Lanka, Colombo, Sri Lanka*
[2]*Department of Pharmacology, Faculty of Medicine, University of Colombo, Colombo, Sri Lanka*

Correspondence should be addressed to H. G. C. S. Karunathilaka; chathurikakarunathilaka@gmail.com

Academic Editor: Tatsuharu Ohno

Drug-induced immune haemolytic anaemia (DIIHA) is extremely rare. We herein report a case of DIIHA due to co-amoxiclav. A 53-year-old male being treated for left-sided pyelonephritis with intravenous co-amoxiclav developed symptoms and signs of anaemia on the third day of treatment. He was found to have evidence of haemolysis with a positive Coombs test and IgG antibodies and C3d. Co-amoxiclav was identified as the probable culprit, using the Naranjo adverse drug reaction probability scale. Upon discontinuation of the drug and blood transfusion, the patient's haematological parameters stabilised. Steroids were not required in the treatment. Diagnosis of DIIHA is made through a history of intake of co-amoxiclav, clinical and laboratory features of haemolysis, and a positive Coombs test. An autoantibody screen is most commonly negative. It is essential for clinicians to be aware about this rare complication caused by commonly prescribed drugs and be able to accurately diagnose and initiate treatment.

1. Introduction

Drug-induced immune haemolytic anaemia (DIIHA) is rare and occurs in about one per million per year [1]. The severity of DIIHA varies from acute severe intravascular haemolysis to subacute milder forms of extravascular haemolysis [2]. There are numerous drugs that have been incriminated in DIIHA. Common drugs causing DIIHA include antimicrobials (42%), nonsteroidal anti-inflammatory drugs (15%), and antineoplastic drugs (11%) [3]. Some of the common antibiotics causing DIIHA are cephalosporins, levofloxacin, nitrofurantoin, and piperacillin/tazobactam [4]. DIIHA is not commonly seen with co-amoxiclav, and we report a case of a DIIHA occurring in a 53-year-old male patient, prescribed this drug. Since DIIHA is generally under-reported, clinicians need to be aware about this rare but life-threatening adverse reaction to commonly prescribed drugs and its diagnosis and management.

2. Case Report

A 53-year-old male with a history of bronchial asthma (on inhaled salbutamol and corticosteroids) and diabetes mellitus (on gliclazide and metformin) presented to the National Hospital of Sri Lanka with fever, constitutional symptoms, dysuria, and left-sided loin pain for three days. Review of the other systems was normal. There were no known allergies to food or drugs. Patient informed about previous antibiotic usage as an outpatient; however, he was not sure which antibiotics were used and records were not traceable. However, he has not received intravenous antibiotics previously. On examination he was febrile, with significant left-sided renal angle tenderness, with normal vital signs, and no hepatosplenomegaly. The rest of the systemic examination was normal. He was empirically diagnosed with left-sided pyelonephritis and started on intravenous co-amoxiclav (1.2 g three times per day) on the day of presentation. Initial

TABLE 1: Changes in haemoglobin and red cell indices.

	Days				
	Baseline	3	7 (medication stopped)	10 (2 days after stopping)	14 (6 days after stopping)
Number of red cells (x10^9/L)	4.61	3.43	1.24	1.98	3.20
Haemoglobin (g/dL)	13.7	9.5	4	6	9.6
Haematocrit (HCT) (%)	39.4	30.8	13.2	19.7	29.7
Mean corpuscular volume (MCV) (fL)	85.4	89.8	106.4	99.5	92.8
Mean corpuscular haemoglobin (MCH) (pg)	29.7	27.7	32.2	30.3	30
Mean corpuscular haemoglobin concentration (MCHC) (g/dL)	34.7	30.8	30.3	30.4	32.3
Red cell distribution width (RDW) (%)	12.7	14.7	17.7	24.2	17.8
Reticulocyte count	1.5%	5.9%	15%	11.6%	5.4%
Reticulocyte index	1.3%	3.9%	4.4%	5.1%	3.6%

laboratory tests on admission showed a normal haemoglobin level of 13.7 g/dl (normal range 13–16.5 g/dL), a white blood cell count of 11,400/μL (normal range 7,000–11,000/μL), and a platelet count of 221,000/μL (normal range 150,000–450,000/μL). His urine microscopy showed a field full of pus cells, without any red cell or casts. Serum creatinine was normal (93 μmol/l) and remained in the normal range throughout admission. Inflammatory markers were markedly elevated on admission (C-reactive protein 400 mg/dl). The initial clinical diagnosis was confirmed by ultrasound scan of the kidneys, which did not reveal any other abnormalities, including hepatosplenomegaly.

On day 3 of the admission, apart from mild fatigue, fever and other symptoms, including loin tenderness, have improved. However, physical examination revealed a pale conjunctivae and mucous membranes, along with mild icterus, but the rest of the systemic examination was normal. He did not complain of any bleeding manifestations, including melena, and digital rectal examination was normal. Repeat blood counts on day three revealed a reduction in the haemoglobin (9.5 g/dl) and C-reactive protein (190 mg/dl) levels. He had a reticulocyte production index of 4.6 (reticulocyte count 15%; haematocrit 30.0%), with indirect hyperbilirubinaemia (total bilirubin 17.6 μmol/L; indirect bilirubin 11.4 μmol/L), with normal hepatic transaminase levels. Changes in haemoglobin and red cell indices are summarized in Table 1. A review of the peripheral blood smear revealed polychromasia, red cell agglutination, and numerous nucleated red blood cells (RBCs), without evidence of bite cells or blister cells to indicate G6PD deficiency. Direct Coombs test was positive with IgG and C3d. Antibody screening was negative. His haemoglobin dropped to 4 g/dl on post-admission day 7 (reticulocyte production index 4.4%, haematocrit 13.2%). The following investigations for other causes of acquired haemolytic anaemia were negative: hepatitis B and C serology, retroviral screening, mycoplasma antibody, Ham test, EBV/CMV IgM antibodies, and antinuclear antigen (ANA).

In view of a possible DIIHA co-amoxiclav was changed to intravenous ciprofloxacin (400 mg twice daily). Additionally, 2 units of cross matched blood were transfused (blood group A positive). He reported improvement after the blood transfusion and discontinuation of co-amoxiclav. His haemoglobin gradually increased, and at day 6 after discontinuation of co-amoxiclav, it was 9.5 g/dL. The drug review showed that the only new drug prescribed to him was co-amoxiclav for the empirical treatment of pyelonephritis. Other drugs were unchanged and could not have accounted for the onset and subsequent improvement after discontinuation of co-amoxiclav. The patient had no further haemolytic episodes. The patient was doing well at the follow-up one month later. Using the Naranjo adverse drug reaction probability scale (our patient scored 7, which makes the drug reaction "probable"), the patient's diagnosis was confirmed as haemolytic anaemia, possibly caused by co-amoxiclav [5].

3. Discussion

Immune haemolytic anaemia occurs when IgG and/or IgM antibodies bind to the surface of the red cells, initiating cell destruction via the complement and reticuloendothelial systems. The condition is classified into either autoimmune, alloimmune, or drug-induced, depending on the antigenic stimulus responsible for the immune response [3]. The patient presented in this case report satisfies the diagnostic criteria for immune haemolytic anaemia, as he met the clinical and serological criteria of haemolysis (indirect hyperbilirubinaemia, decreasing haemoglobin level, and peripheral blood smear consistent with haemolysis), along with a positive Coombs test [6]. Co-amoxiclav is an antibiotic used to treat a number of bacterial infections, and it is a combination consisting of amoxicillin and beta-lactamase inhibitor, clavulanic acid. To our knowledge, DIIHA due to co-amoxiclav is only rarely described in the literature, although other beta-lactam antibiotics, including amoxicillin, are known to cause DIIHA [7, 8].

Several mechanisms causing DIIHA are described in the literature. In general, DIIHA can be mediated through drug-induced antibodies or through a mechanism called non-immunologic protein adsorption [3]. Drug-induced antibodies can be either drug-dependent (DDA) or drug-independent antibodies (DIA) [3, 9]. DDAs need the presence of the drug to bind and lyse red cells, while DIAs can bind erythrocytes in absence of the causative drugs. However, DIIHA due to DIAs cannot be distinguished serologically from autoantibodies mediating warm autoimmune haemolytic anaemia, and hence, diagnosis depends upon clinical improvement on cessation of the causative drug [10]. The mechanism of co-amoxiclav-induced immune haemolysis resembles ceftriaxone induced haemolysis and is characterized by "immune complex-type" reactions [10]. Immune complex-type reactions occur with DDAs as a result of loose binding with red cells, while a covalent binding will result in a so-called "drug-adsorption mechanism" (penicillin-type) reaction [3, 9]. In cases of DDA-mediated DIIHA, the antibody screen is typically negative and only positive if tested in the presence of the drug or with RBC coated with the drug, respectively [10]. Although not performed in the current patient, this can be used as a test to confirm the diagnosis, where mixing washed group O RBCs, patient serum and the implicated drug will result in a strongly positive Coombs test. Subsequently, specificity can be demonstrated by showing that the Coombs test is negative when normal serum is used instead of patient serum and when drug is omitted from the reaction mixture.

Management of DIIHA includes the discontinuation of the suspected drug and red cell transfusion, resulting in a haemoglobin improvement over 7–10 days [3]. Our patient improved with these measures. There is no proven benefit and therefore no recommendation for steroid therapy in DIIHA, at least as far as drug-dependent antibodies are involved, and withdrawing the culprit drug is the most important step [10]. In cases of drug-independent antibodies, which are autoantibodies, steroid therapy can be tried, but also in these cases, the immediate withdrawal of the responsible drug is the most important therapeutic measure [10]. If glucocorticoids are required, they are recommended to be given for 1–3 weeks (1–2 mg/kg/day orally) [4, 5]. Intravenous steroids are reserved for those with severe haemolysis, requiring a rapid response, and other immunosuppressants such as cyclophosphamide and azathioprine can also be used in those who do not respond.

In conclusion, DIIHA is underestimated and underreported, as many cases may not lead to dramatic haemolysis, requiring interventions. However, with increasing antibiotic use and increased reliance on newer generations of antibiotics, such rare but life-threatening adverse reactions may be more frequent. Therefore, it is essential for clinicians to recognize this rare complication caused by commonly prescribed drugs and be aware of its accurate diagnosis and management.

References

[1] E. Garbe, F. Andersohn, E. Bronder et al., "Drug induced immune haemolytic anaemia in the Berlin case-control surveillance study," *British Journal of Haematology*, vol. 154, no. 5, pp. 644–653, 2011.

[2] Q. A. Salama, R. Stamps, E. Massey et al., "Guidelines on the management of drug-induced immune and secondary autoimmune, haemolytic anaemia," *British Journal of Haematology*, vol. 177, no. 2, pp. 208–220, 2017.

[3] G. Garratty, "Drug-induced immune hemolytic anemia," *Hematology*, vol. 2009, no. 1, pp. 73–79, 2009.

[4] G. Garratty, "Immune hemolytic anemia associated with drug therapy," *Blood Reviews*, vol. 24, no. 4-5, pp. 143–150, 2010.

[5] C. A. Naranjo, U. Busto, E. M. Sellers et al., "A method for estimating the probability of adverse drug reactions," *Clinical Pharmacology and Therapeutics*, vol. 30, no. 2, pp. 239–245, 1981.

[6] B. C. Gehrs and R. C. Friedberg, "Autoimmune hemolytic anemia," *American Journal of Hematology*, vol. 69, no. 4, pp. 258–271, 2002.

[7] G. Garratty and P. A. Arndt, "Positive direct antiglobulin tests and haemolytic anaemia following therapy with beta-lactamase inhibitor containing drugs may be associated with nonimmunologic adsorption of protein onto red blood cells," *British Journal of Haematology*, vol. 100, no. 4, pp. 777–783, 1998.

[8] J. Gmür, M. Wälti, and K. A. Neftel, "Amoxicillin-induced immune hemolysis," *Acta Haematologica*, vol. 74, no. 4, pp. 230–233, 1985.

[9] P. A. Arndt, "Drug-induced immune hemolytic anemia: the last 30 years of changes," *Immunohematology*, vol. 30, no. 30, pp. 44–54, 2014.

[10] H. B. Leicht, E. Weinig, B. Mayer, J. Viebahn, A. Geier, and M. Rau, "Ceftriaxone-induced hemolytic anemia with severe renal failure: a case report and review of literature," *BMC Pharmacology and Toxicology*, vol. 19, no. 1, p. 67, 2018.

25

Sevoflurane-Induced Thrombocytopenia in Post-Robotic-Assisted Paraesophageal Hernia Repair

Sara Alhaj ,[1] James Tran,[1] Muhammad Nazim,[2] Praveen Tumula,[3] and Hassan Ahmed [2]

[1]*Texas Tech University Health Sciences Center School of Medicine, Amarillo, TX, USA*
[2]*Department of Surgery, Texas Tech University Health Sciences Center School of Medicine, Amarillo, TX, USA*
[3]*Texas Oncology, Amarillo, TX, USA*

Correspondence should be addressed to Sara Alhaj; sara.alhaj@ttuhsc.edu

Academic Editor: Kostas Konstantopoulos

Background. Transient transaminitis is an expected outcome from liver retraction after foregut surgeries. However, severe thrombocytopenia is usually not a sequela of that. We present a case in which sevoflurane is suspected of inducing thrombocytopenia as it was the only newly introduced medication to the patient during the hospital course. Thrombocytopenia may present in a variety of settings in hospitalized patients. However, managing this occurrence requires deep exploration of pathophysiology that can cause decreased platelets, which may be a challenging task in certain circumstances. The liver plays an important role in thrombopoiesis by releasing megakaryocyte growth factors. Therefore, liver dysfunction can present as thrombocytopenia or other platelet dysfunctions. *Objective.* To describe a presentation of thrombocytopenia possibly associated with anesthesia-induced transaminitis after a robotic paraesophageal hernia repair with mesh and fundoplasty with intraoperative esophagogastroduodenoscopy (EGD). *Methods.* A 55-year-old presented to the ED with abdominal pain and was found to have a large type IV paraesophageal hernia that was surgically treated with a robotic paraesophageal hernia repair with mesh. However, on the first postoperative day (POD) (#1), the patient developed new onset thrombocytopenia with transaminitis. Workup for thrombocytopenia failed to determine an etiology. With platelet transfusion, platelet count showed an upward trend. The patient was then evaluated and cleared for discharge by POD#5. *Results.* The patient's POD#1 daily labs showed elevated values for liver function tests and a low platelet count of 10,000 platelets per microliter with an international normalized value (INR) of 1.3. She had received two doses of intravenous acetaminophen just prior to surgery. Her platelet count responded to two units of platelets but decreased again immediately after. She continued to have transaminitis with down-trending liver enzymes. Peripheral smear on review showed no evidence of schistocytes. A heparin-induced thrombocytopenia (HIT) screening was negative. The patient was regularly evaluated, and the platelets stabilized and slowly started to trend up. The patient recovered by the morning of her POD#5 and was cleared for discharge. *Conclusion.* We are reporting on a case of acute postoperative thrombocytopenia that was associated with transaminitis and elevated liver enzymes. We are linking the role of the liver dysfunction in noncirrhotic patients with surgical abdominal procedures. Although liver retraction transaminitis possibly played a role in the laboratory findings in the patient, the acute drop in her platelet count could be closely related to the use of sevoflurane anesthetic considering its potential hepatotoxic side effects. We also cannot rule out the sevoflurane directly affecting the platelet count.

1. Introduction

Thrombocytopenia is defined as a platelet count less than 150,000 platelets/microliter which may be asymptomatic but can place the patient at risk of bleeding or can manifest as thrombotic events as well [1]. Thrombocytopenia is a commonly encountered condition in hospitalized patients regardless of the nature, duration, or severity of their illness. It can present as a challenge to treat due to the variety of the pathophysiology that can cause it. Platelets are produced in response to thrombopoietin (TPO) that is produced by the liver that can stimulate TPO receptors on hematopoietic stem cells to differentiate to platelet cells [1]. Therefore, the liver plays a vital role in the formation of platelets in the body. Many pathologies can affect the liver, which can be detected by elevated liver enzymes, hence impairing the functions that the liver secondarily controls. Upper gastrointestinal laparoscopic surgeries and the use of certain anesthetics have been linked to transient transaminitis with liver function impairment both of which are yet to be fully explained.

2. Case Presentation

A 55-year-old female with no known past medical history presented with abdominal pain and was found to have a large type IV paraesophageal hernia with approximately 75% of her stomach in the chest as well as the transverse colon with the presence of obstruction. She was found to be a candidate for a robotic paraesophageal hernia repair with mesh and fundoplasty and intraoperative EGD. The patient was taken to the operating room (OR), recovered well afterwards, and tolerated full liquids without any issues. However, on POD#1, the patient was found to have new onset thrombocytopenia which was not present prior to surgery. This trend is presented in Figure 1. The patient's platelets had dropped to 10,000 platelets/microliter with an INR of 1.3 (with normal range around 0.89–1.07), and complete metabolic panel was also significant for an aspartate transaminase (AST) level of 4461 and alanine transaminase (ALT) level of 2796, as shown in Figure 2; a normal AST level ranges around 8 to 48 units per liter (U/L), and a normal ALT level around 7 to 55 U/L. Her platelet count continued to trend down to as low as 9,000 platelets/microliter. She later received transfusion of 2 units of platelets which increased her platelets to 65,000 platelets/microliter which then abruptly decreased back to 18,000 shortly after. Peripheral smear showed no evidence of schistocytes, and a HIT screen was negative. The patient still showed transaminitis with down-trending liver enzymes and laboratory values significant for lactate dehydrogenase (LDH) of 2001 U/L (with normal range around 45–90 U/L), folate of 18 nmol/L (with normal range around 4.5–45.3 nmol/L), vitamin B12 of >1500 mg/L (with normal > 200 mg/L), fibrinogen of 220 mg/dL (with normal range around 200–400 mg/dL), INR of 1.5, prothrombin time (PT) of 17.9 s (with normal range around 11–15 s), and partial thromboplastin time (PTT) of 34 s (with normal range around 25–40 s). Bilirubin levels ranged between 0.3 and 1.3 mg/dL (with normal range around 0.1–1.2 mg/dL) throughout the hospitalization. Hemoglobin was 15.1 g/dL on admission with a gradual decrease to 11.0 g/dL (with normal range around 12.2–15.0 g/dL) during the hospitalization. No imaging was performed postoperatively to exclude causal relationship of a liver hematoma or other bleeding complication. Hepatitis C antibody was negative, and hepatitis B surface antibody (immune), surface antigens, and core antibody were negative. No bone marrow biopsy was performed. The patient did not have fever or C-reactive protein elevation, and no blood cultures were drawn. Ferritin was elevated at 402 μg/mL on POD#2 (with normal range around 12–150 μg/mL), but otherwise was within normal limits. Her platelets stabilized and slowly started to trend up with platelet transfusions, and the patient was evaluated the morning of her POD#5 and cleared for discharge.

3. Discussion

Reasons for thrombocytopenia can be grouped into the following broad categories: pseudothrombocytopenia, hemodilution, increased platelet consumption, increased platelet destruction, decreased platelet production, and increased platelet sequestration. However, we are presenting a perplexing case of postsurgical transaminitis and thrombocytopenia without a clear cause or predisposition. Prior to and during the patient's surgery, the patient exhibited liver enzyme values and platelets well within normal ranges. Paradoxically, this patient's symptoms of transaminitis and thrombocytopenia appear to have begun on POD#1 without a clear indication. There is literature that describes postsurgical platelet counts below 15,000 platelets/microliter following surgical procedures [2]. The nadir of the platelet count typically occurred within POD#1–4 with the platelets reaching normal ranges around POD#5[2]. This pattern seems to appear in major trauma, vascular, and abdominal surgeries as well as within populations of ICU patients [2]. It is also previously described that TPO introduction takes approximately three days to begin significantly increasing platelet counts [2].

From literature review, we hypothesize that this transient thrombocytopenia and transaminitis were a result of a brief slowdown of TPO production by the liver after sevoflurane exposure. The elevated liver enzymes seen on POD#1 may signify an acute irritation or damaging process of the liver. Acute irritation or damage to the liver may have resulted in hepatocellular slowing or halting due to an inflammatory or damaging process related to anesthetic use. As such, this would manifest mainly as an insufficient stimulation of megakaryocytes and thus inadequate platelet production [3]. Consequently, this would present as the profound thrombocytopenia as observed in this patient on POD#1 until the return to normal on POD#5.

This introduces the question as to what exactly factored into interrupted TPO production and why the liver was affected. On the one hand, hepatotoxicity is a risk of commonly used anesthetic agents in the United States. Sevoflurane, a commonly used anesthetic agent, has been implicated in cases of hepatotoxicity and at least one case of postoperative transaminitis with thrombocytopenia [4]. On the other hand, transient transaminitis has been associated with upper GI surgeries especially antireflux surgery [5]. This sequela has been linked to liver retraction during the procedure which was reported to resolve spontaneously with no clinical consequences. Although liver retraction plays a role in the postoperative transaminitis, the extent of the retraction during an upper GI surgery is irritation of segments II and III of the liver which constitute about 20–25% of its function [6]. The liver can meet its bodily function with up to 75% of its volume damaged [6]. Therefore, an extensive damaging process developed to cause the liver dysfunction which manifested in the form of significant transaminitis

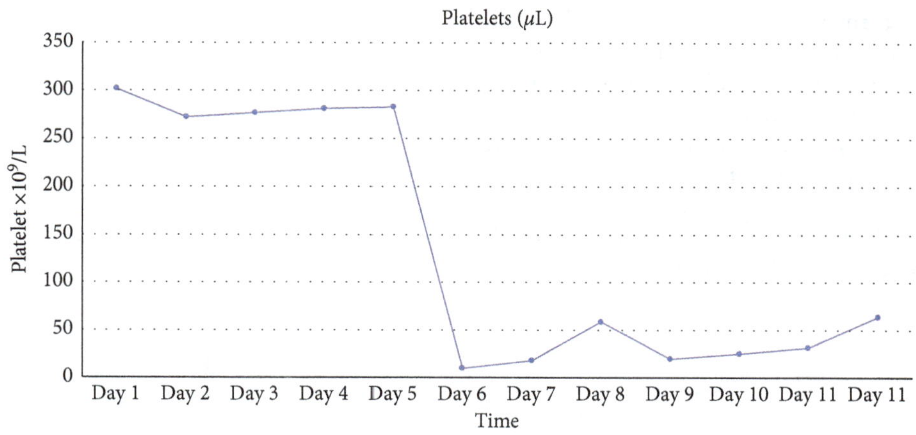

FIGURE 1: A graph depicting platelet count over time during this patient's hospital stay. The surgery was performed on hospital day 5.

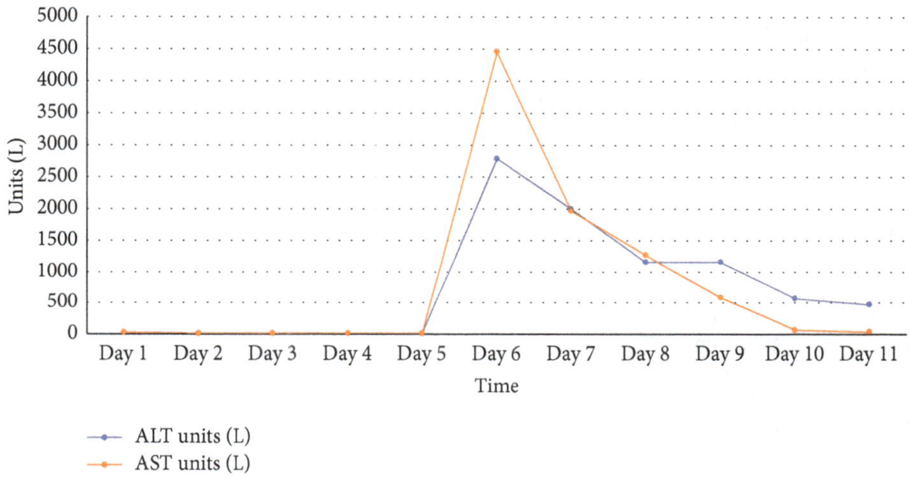

FIGURE 2: A graph depicting AST and ALT levels over time during this patient's hospital stay. Surgery was performed on hospital day 5.

and consequent thrombocytopenia. After literature review and patient workup, sevoflurane anesthetic is the agent to cause the apparent fulminant hepatitis and liver dysfunction.

Finally, the discussion that sevoflurane caused these symptoms raises suspicion whether it was a direct effect on platelet function and aggregation or whether it was through hepatic toxicity that manifested in reduced TPO production and consequent thrombocytopenia. The patient's elevated liver enzyme resolved earlier than her platelet counts—therefore, drug interactions with platelets must be considered. Notably, halothane, sevoflurane, and propofol appear to reversibly inhibit platelet function in a dose-dependent manner, and sevoflurane's suppression of thromboxane A2 is suspected [7]. Propofol and nitrous oxide both suppress calcium mobilization which may contribute to an effect on decreasing platelet function [7]. However, some literature suggests that isoflurane, enflurane, desflurane, barbiturates, etomidate, opioids, and muscle relaxants do not appear to significantly affect platelet number or function [7]. In another study, volatile anesthetics such as sevoflurane caused increased platelet aggregation [8]. The study showed sevoflurane to increase antithrombotic effect and platelet aggregation within 15 minutes after intubation and anesthesia [8]. Isoflurane and desflurane showed reversibility after 15 minutes of induction, whereas sevoflurane showed continued effect past 1 hour after intubation. The study did not show, however, significant change in platelet count, PTT, or PT immediately after anesthesia induction [8]. On the contrary, sevoflurane has previously demonstrated hepatotoxicity and reproducible hepatic dysfunction after anesthesia in patients with no prior history of liver disease [9]. Sevoflurane is a relatively safe drug in its class; however, its induction of compound A production may play a role in liver insults [9]. Additionally, repeated exposure to halogenated volatile anesthetics such as sevoflurane may cause drug sensitization further manifesting as hepatotoxicity [9].

4. Conclusion

We conclude that anesthesia-induced hepatotoxicity occurs after minimally invasive upper GI surgeries and can have effects on processes controlled by the liver. We demonstrate the impairment of thrombopoiesis led by the liver which caused this thrombocytopenia. Other liver functions can also be affected by this transient transaminitis that can be symptomatic in other patients. Further studies are required for exploring the different implications of minimally invasive surgery and sevoflurane use on liver functions and the body as a whole. Although transaminitis is possibly due to liver retraction, literature indicates that it is commonly short-lived and recovers spontaneously [5]. In addition, the liver has the capacity to function with as low as 25% of its capacity [6]. Therefore, there is more evidence to indicate that sevoflurane anesthetic played a larger role in the fulminant liver failure and loss of functionality in inducing thrombopoiesis.

References

[1] H. Schulze and R. A. Shivdasani, "Mechanisms of thrombopoiesis," *Journal of Thrombosis and Haemostasis*, vol. 3, no. 8, pp. 1717–1724, 2005.

[2] A. Greinacher and K. Selleng, "Thrombocytopenia in the intensive care unit patient," *Hematology*, vol. 2010, no. 1, pp. 135–143, 2010.

[3] D. J. Kuter, "The biology of thrombopoietin and thrombopoietin receptor agonists," *International Journal of Hematology*, vol. 98, no. 1, pp. 10–23, 2013.

[4] N. Shah and N. Ballone, "Hepatotoxicity after sevoflurane exposure in a patient with chronic hepatitis C," *Internal Medicine: Open Access*, vol. 5, no. 6, 2015.

[5] G. Morris-Stiff, R. Jones, S. Mitchell, K. Barton, and A. Hassn, "Retraction transaminitis: an inevitable but benign complication of laparoscopic fundoplication," *World Journal of Surgery*, vol. 32, no. 12, pp. 2650–2654, 2008.

[6] G. K. Michalopoulos, "Liver regeneration after partial hepatectomy," *The American Journal of Pathology*, vol. 176, no. 1, pp. 2–13, 2010.

[7] S. A. Kozek-Langenecker, "The effects of drugs used in anaesthesia on platelet membrane receptors and on platelet function," *Current Drug Targets*, vol. 3, no. 3, 2002.

[8] N. Bozdogan, H. Madenoglu, K. Dogru et al., "Effects of isoflurane, sevoflurane, and desflurane on platelet function: a prospective, randomized, single-blind, in vivo study," *Current Therapeutic Research*, vol. 66, no. 4, pp. 375–384, 2005.

[9] S. Rajan, D. Garg, K. C. Cummings, and A. A. Krishnaney, "Hepatotoxicity after sevoflurane anaesthesia: a new twist to an old story," *British Journal of Anaesthesia*, vol. 122, no. 4, pp. e63–e71, 2019.

26

Multiple Myeloma in a Patient with ANKRD26-Related Thrombocytopenia Successfully Treated with Combination Therapy and Autologous Stem Cell Transplant

Muhammad Husnain,[1] **Trent Wang**,[1,2] **Maikel Valdes**,[2] **James Hoffman**,[1,2] **and Lazaros Lekakis**[1,2]

[1]*Division of Hematology/Oncology, Department of Medicine, Miller School of Medicine, University of Miami, Miami, FL, USA*
[2]*Sylvester Comprehensive Cancer Center, University of Miami, Miami, FL, USA*

Correspondence should be addressed to Muhammad Husnain; muhammad.husnain@jhsmiami.org

Academic Editor: Yusuke Shiozawa

Ankyrin repeat domain-containing protein 26- (ANKRD26-) related thrombocytopenia is a rare, autosomal dominant condition caused by ANKRD26 gene mutation. ANKRD26-related thrombocytopenia is characterized by moderate thrombocytopenia with minimal bleeding, normal platelet size, and dysmegakaryopoiesis on bone marrow evaluation. ANKRD26 mutation has been previously associated with myeloid malignancies, including acute myeloid leukemia, myelodysplastic syndrome, and chronic myeloid leukemia. We report the first case of multiple myeloma in a patient with ANKRD26 related thrombocytopenia. The patient was successfully treated with contemporary combination therapy followed by melphalan-conditioned autologous stem cell transplant for his multiple myeloma despite preexisting thrombocytopenia.

1. Introduction

Ankyrin repeat domain-containing protein 26- (ANKRD26-) related thrombocytopenia is a rare, autosomal dominant condition caused by ANKRD26 gene mutation [1]. Its clinical hallmark includes moderate thrombocytopenia with minimal bleeding, normal platelet size, and dysmegakaryopoiesis on bone marrow evaluation. Mild polycythemia and leukocytosis have also been reported [2]. There is reported association between ANKRD26 mutation with myeloid malignancies, including acute myeloid leukemia, myelodysplastic syndrome, and chronic myeloid leukemia [2]. No known correlation with multiple myeloma has been previously identified. We report a case of multiple myeloma and ANKRD26-related thrombocytopenia (ANKRD26-RT) successfully treated with combination therapy and autologous stem cell transplant.

2. Case Presentation

A 64-year-old Caucasian man with a lifelong history of thrombocytopenia was found with elevated total protein of 10.3 g/dl, serum monoclonal spike of 3.5 g/dl, immunoglobulin G (IgG) of 5371 mg/dl, and free lambda light chains of 703 mg/dl with free kappa/lambda ratio of 0.08. Calcium and renal function were within normal limits. Hemoglobin was 16.6 g/dL, and platelet count was $33 \times 10^3/\mu L$. Skeletal survey was negative for any lytic lesions. Bone marrow examination showed adequate megakaryocytes with normal platelet morphology, and no dysmegakaryopoiesis or micromegakaryocytes were seen on the bone marrow. Erythrocytes and granulocytes were adequate in number without any significant abnormality.

The past medical history included essential hypertension and hypogonadism, but without neuropathy or dermatologic conditions. The diagnosis of thrombocytopenia stemmed from childhood and was accompanied by a penetrant family history of thrombocytopenia seen in his mother, maternal aunt, brother, and son. No genetic cause of the thrombocytopenia had been established, and questioning found no personal or family history of physical deformity, vision, hearing, or bleeding disorders. Laboratory review of his platelet count history ranged from 30 to $50 \times 10^3/\mu L$.

Repeat testing of hemoglobin was 17.9 g/dl with hematocrit of 55.6%. Peripheral blood examination showed normal appearing red and white blood cells, with erythrocytosis, and morphologically normal platelets that were decreased in number. Erythropoietin level was normal (12.2 mIU/mL), and molecular testing found no mutations in JAK2 V617F or BCR/ABL1 (p190 and p210). The erythrocytosis was attributed to use of testosterone supplementation for hypogonadism. A limited congenital thrombocytopenia testing panel was ordered and resulted negative for mutations in myeloproliferative leukemia protein (MPL), runt-related transcription factor 1 (RUNX1), myosin heavy chain 9 (MYH9), and Wiskott–Aldrich syndrome (WAS) gene mutations. Flow cytometry for platelet associated autoantibodies. Anti-glycoprotein IIb/IIIa antibodies, anti-glycoprotein Ib/Ix antibodies, and anti-glycoprotein CD36 antibodies were also negative.

After a period of monitoring, his serum IgG increased to 7063 mg/dl and monoclonal-spike to 5.4 g/dl. Albumin level was 2.7 g/dl, and beta-2 microglobulin level was 2.52 mg/dl. Repeat bone marrow biopsy showed 70% plasma cells with adequate megakaryocytes and normal platelet morphology, and he was diagnosed with International Staging System (ISS) stage II IgG lambda multiple myeloma. Treatment was now indicated, however complicated given his marked thrombocytopenia.

He started treatment with pulse doses of dexamethasone (40 mg daily for 4 days) with subsequent addition of bortezomib at $0.4\,mg/m^2$ with slow escalation to full dose ($1.3\,mg/m^2$) by week 3. Oral cyclophosphamide (600 mg/weekly) was added to this regimen during cycle 2. After 5 cycles of CyBorD (cyclophosphamide, bortezomib, and dexamethasone), the patient had normalization of IgG levels and decrease in M-spike to 0.62 g/dl consistent with a partial response. He was referred for consolidative melphalan-conditioned autologous stem cell transplant.

Stem cell mobilization with granulocyte colony-stimulating factor ($10\,mcg/kg \times 5$ doses and plerixafor $24\,mg \times 1$ dose) resulted in peak white blood cell count of $151 \times 10^3/\mu L$ and stem cell yield of 105.6×10^6 CD34+/kg in a single session (the highest recorded at our institution that year). The patient proceeded to high-dose melphalan ($200\,mg/m^2$) followed by infusion of 45×10^6 CD34+/kg autologous stem cells. Despite a robust and quick neutrophil engraftment on day +9, the patient encountered marked nausea and a severe pruritic skin rash that started after engraftment and lasted for 1-2 months, resembling a graft versus host reaction. After engraftment, his platelet count peaked as high as $84 \times 10^3/\mu L$ on $D + 21$ before slowly declining back to his baseline of about 30×10^3/cells 6 weeks after transplant. He continued to have stable disease after autologous transplant and started lenalidomide maintenance with aspirin prophylaxis.

At a subsequent follow-up visit after autologous transplant, a more comprehensive 21-gene-inherited thrombocytopenia panel was sent, and a heterogeneous mutation of ANKRD26 c.-128G>A in the 5′ untranslated region (5′ UTR) of chromosome 10 was identified. This was consistent with a diagnosis of ANKRD26-RT. The patient continues to have persistent thrombocytopenia in the range of $30–50 \times 10^3$ platelets. Given his significant family penetrance of thrombocytopenia, the patient and family were referred to genetic counseling for further evaluation.

3. Discussion

Point mutations in the 5′ UTR of ANKRD26 have now been reported in almost 60 unrelated families accounting for almost 200 cases of ANKRD26-RT [2, 3]. There are total of 17 different heterozygous mutations identified to date in the 5′ UTR of ANKRD26 with nucleotide substitutions at position c.-118C>T, c.-128G>T, and c.134G>A representing 75% of all mutant alleles [2, 3].

The mechanism by which ANKRD26 promotes thrombocytopenia is not clearly understood but the MAPK/ERK1/2 pathway has been implicated. ANKRD26 overexpression in megakaryocytes increases MAPK/ERK pathway activity in megakaryocytes and alters TPO/MPL function leading to thrombocytopenia [4]. CXCR4-SDF1 axis is also implicated in pathogenesis of ANRD26-RT as it directs megakaryocyte migration towards the vascular niche and permits terminal maturation and proplatelet formation [5]. Decreased expression of CXCR4 may lead to decreased terminal maturation of platelets and thus thrombocytopenia. Noris et al. have described 78 patients of ANKRD26-related thrombocytopenia from 21 families [1]. They have reported an increased number of megakaryocytes at all stages of maturation in bone marrows of these patients with dysmegakaryopoiesis, small megakaryocytes with hypolobulated nuclei, and typical micromegakarycytes. In our case, we did not see any dysmegakaryopoiesis, and the megakaryocytes in our patient were normal in number and morphology. Mild polycythemia and leukocytosis have also been reported in a small subset of patients with congenital thrombocytopenia, however without clear explanation [1]. In our case, the patient's polycythemia may have been attributed to preexistent testosterone supplementation use.

It is known that patients with ANKRD26 mutations are at increased risk of developing hematological malignancies including myelodysplastic syndrome, acute myeloid leukemia, and chronic myeloid leukemia. In the largest series of 118 patients with ANKRD26-RT, 10 (8%) ultimately developed myeloid malignancies [2]. Loss of RUNX1 and friend leukemia integration 1 transcription factor (FLI1) and increased signaling of MPL have been implicated in the pathogenesis of myeloid malignancies in the patients with ANKRD26 mutations [4]. ASXL1-mutated chronic myelomonocytic leukemia has also been reported in a patient with ANKRD26-RT [6]. Zhang et al. have previously described hereditary association between thrombocytopenia and hematological malignancies including one case of multiple myeloma in three families with germline ETV6 mutation [7], but there is no reported case of ANKRD26 RT and multiple myeloma. To our knowledge, this is the first case of multiple myeloma in a patient with ANKRD26-RT. While it is unclear whether this relationship was an incidental finding, ANKRD26 mutation was identified in 3.1% of African-American patients and 0.2% of Caucasian patients in a molecular profiling study of 718 multiple myeloma patients [8]. It is not known whether these mutations of ANKRD26, detected with a higher frequency in African American than in Caucasian multiple myeloma patients, were preferentially localized in the 5′ UTR part of this gene.

We demonstrated safe and successful treatment of multiple myeloma using contemporary combination therapy followed by melphalan-conditioned autologous stem cell transplant despite preexisting thrombocytopenia. Of interest, mobilization with filgrastim and plerixafor resulted in marked leukocytosis and extraordinary yield of CD34+ stem cells after only one session of apheresis. We postulate this may have been related to decreased surface CXCR4 expression which has been reported in association with ANKRD26-RT [5] along with CXCR4 antagonism by plerixafor, thus amplifying CXCR4 blockade.

The appearance of an autologous graft-versus-host skin eruption and the transient rise of platelets above pretransplant baseline remain unexplained. Perhaps, a rebound effect of increased CXCR4 after stem cell mobilization and posttransplant use of granulocyte colony stimulating factor contributed to the brisk yet temporary rise in platelets.

4. Conclusion

This to our knowledge is the first reported case of multiple myeloma in a patient with ANKRD-26RT. We demonstrate the safe and successful treatment of multiple myeloma using contemporary combination therapy followed by melphalan-conditioned autologous stem cell transplant despite preexisting thrombocytopenia.

Authors' Contributions

All authors contributed equally in concept, design, drafting, and final approval of the manuscript.

References

[1] P. Noris, S. Perrotta, M. Seri et al., "Mutations in ANKRD26 are responsible for a frequent form of inherited thrombocytopenia: analysis of 78 patients from 21 families," *Blood*, vol. 117, no. 24, pp. 6673–6680, 2011.

[2] P. Noris, R. Favier, M.-C. Alessi et al., "ANKRD26-related thrombocytopenia and myeloid malignancies," *Blood*, vol. 122, no. 11, pp. 1987–1989, 2013.

[3] H. Boutroux, A. Petit, A. Auvrignon et al., "Childhood diagnosis of genetic thrombocytopenia with mutation in the ankyrine repeat domain 26 gene," *European Journal of Pediatrics*, vol. 174, no. 10, pp. 1399–1403, 2015.

[4] D. Bluteau, A. Balduini, N. Balayn et al., "Thrombocytopenia-associated mutations in the ANKRD26 regulatory region induce MAPK hyperactivation," *Journal of Clinical Investigation*, vol. 124, no. 2, pp. 580–591, 2014.

[5] J. P. Salim, A. C. Glembotsky, P. R. Lev et al., "Differential expression of SDF-1 receptor CXCR4 in molecularly defined forms of inherited thrombocytopenias," *Platelets*, vol. 28, no. 6, pp. 602–606, 2017.

[6] J. Perez Botero, J. L. Oliveira, D. Chen et al., "ASXL1 mutated chronic myelomonocytic leukemia in a patient with familial thrombocytopenia secondary to germline mutation in ANKRD26," *Blood Cancer Journal*, vol. 5, no. 5, p. e315, 2015.

[7] M. Y. Zhang, J. E. Churpek, S. B. Keel et al., "Germline ETV6 mutations in familial thrombocytopenia and hematologic malignancy," *Nature Genetics*, vol. 47, no. 2, pp. 180–185, 2015.

[8] Z. Manojlovic, A. Christofferson, W. S. Liang et al., "Comprehensive molecular profiling of 718 multiple myelomas reveals significant differences in mutation frequencies between African and European descent cases," *PLoS Genetics*, vol. 13, no. 11, article e1007087, 2017.

27

A Case of Acquired Hemophilia A in a Patient with Exposure to COVID-19

Jorge D. Guerra,[1] **Jasmine Gowarty**,[2] **Jordan Buess**,[2] **James Mason**,[2] **and Kathleen Halka**[2]

[1]*Department of Internal Medicine, Baylor Scott & White Medical Center, Texas A&M University College of Medicine, Temple, TX, USA*
[2]*Department of Hematology and Medical Oncology, Baylor Scott & White Medical Center, Texas A&M University College of Medicine, Temple, TX, USA*

Correspondence should be addressed to Jorge D. Guerra; jorgedguerra@gmail.com

Academic Editor: Håkon Reikvam

Acquired Hemophilia A (AHA) is a very rare autoimmune condition involving immune-mediated depletion of Factor VIII, resulting in spontaneous hemorrhage. Failure to recognize AHA as a possible etiology of hemorrhage can result in delayed diagnosis and treatment. The COVID-19 pandemic has given rise to several hematologic conditions and complications, with a rare manifestation being Acquired Hemophilia A (AHA). An interesting case of AHA following SARS-CoV-2 infection is described, along with the treatment approach and a brief review of several cases describing AHA in association with COVID-19.

1. Introduction

Acquired Factor VIII deficiency, also referred to as Acquired Hemophilia A (AHA), is a rare condition that entails antibody-mediated depletion of Factor VIII, resulting in spontaneous hemorrhage in patients without a history of bleeding [1, 2]. Traditionally, AHA is found in elderly men or young women and is oftentimes associated with pregnancy or the postpartum period [1]. Data trends have suggested that approximately 50% of AHA cases are classified as idiopathic while the remaining half are associated with other autoimmune disorders, malignancies, infections, drugs, and certain dermatologic disorders [2]. Although hemarthrosis is classically associated with hemophilia A, there is a higher prevalence of hemorrhage from the soft tissues, abdomen, and retroperitoneum in acquired hemophilia as compared to congenital hemophilia [3]. Therefore, bleeding associated with AHA can be severe and life threatening as described in this case of *de novo* AHA occurring in the setting of recent infection with SARS-CoV-2, the virus causing COVID-19 in humans.

2. Case Report

A 74-year-old female with a history of recent infection with SARS-CoV-2, hypertension, and fibromyalgia presented as a transfer from an outlying facility with a history of gross hematuria beginning approximately four weeks after recovery from what was classified an NIH mild-grade COVID-19 illness [4]. Computed tomography (CT) scanning showed no findings concerning for malignancy. Prior to transfer, she underwent evaluation with urology to include cystoscopy, which identified bleeding from the right ureteral orifice, as well as retrograde pyelography and ureteroscopy, identifying a large clot in the right renal pelvis. She additionally required laser hemostasis treatment for renal calyceal bleeding and placement of ureteral stents. During her stay at the outside hospital, she received four units of blood for hemoglobin of less than 7.0 g/dL. Due to ongoing bleeding despite procedural interventions, she was transferred for higher level of care. Factor levels had been ordered prior to transfer but were send-out labs and thus not available for several days.

Her vitals were stable on arrival after transfer. Physical exam was significant for right costovertebral angle tenderness to palpation. Labs demonstrated normocytic anemia with hemoglobin of 10.1 g/dL (reference: 12–16 g/dL), elevated white blood cell count of 14.1×10^9/L (reference: $4.8–10.8 \times 10^9$/L), normal platelet count of 351×10^9/L (reference: $150–450 \times 10^9$/L), prolonged activated partial-thromboplastin time (aPTT) of 80.1 seconds (reference: 25.1–36.5 sec), and normal prothrombin time (PT) of 12.5 seconds (reference: 12.2–15.3 sec). Additional studies revealed creatinine of 1.73 (reference: 0.50–1.30 mg/dL) in this patient with previously normal renal function. Urinalysis and urine cultures did not reveal evidence of an infection. She was evaluated by the local urology service with additional procedures, including electrode fulguration of bleeding areas with placement of a right percutaneous nephrostomy drain. Interventional Radiology (IR) was subsequently consulted and performed renal angiography with embolization of an arteriovenous malformation in the right upper pole along with coiling of a nephrostomy tract pseudoaneurysm. Due to persistent bleeding after addressing these anatomical and procedure-related issues, Hematology/Oncology was consulted for suspicion of a bleeding disorder. Lab results from the outside facility became available at that time, demonstrating Factor VIII level of 3%. Based on this result and on mixing studies suggestive of inhibitor presence, the patient was empirically treated with factor eight inhibitor bypass agent (FEIBA) and prednisone. Repeat studies requested by the hematology service demonstrated Factor VIII activity of 0% with the presence of Factor VIII inhibitor measured at 48 Bethesda units (BU), confirming the diagnosis of AHA. The remaining factor levels were normal, without any other inhibitors identified. Other malignant, drug-induced, and infectious etiologies were investigated and results were ultimately unrevealing.

Due to ongoing bleeding, treatment escalations were required, including NovoSeven (a recombinant human coagulation Factor VIIa), cyclophosphamide, and ultimately a single dose of rituximab. Hematuria had nearly resolved by 48 hours after rituximab administration and had fully resolved by 72 hours, allowing discharge from the hospital with continued prednisone and cyclophosphamide use in the outpatient setting and planned rituximab treatments weekly to complete four infusions. Repeat labs one week after discharge revealed a Factor VIII activity of 18% with a reduced inhibitor level of 9.2 BU. Cyclophosphamide was stopped at this time due to neutropenia. Labs two weeks thereafter revealed no evidence of inhibitor, with a Factor VIII activity of 43%. After two additional weeks and completion of rituximab infusions, she achieved a normal Factor VIII activity level of 71%, with inhibitor no longer identified and with normal hemoglobin of 13.6 g/dL. She slowly weaned prednisone over the course of several weeks and has not had any recurrence of AHA.

3. Discussion

AHA is a rare etiology of life-threatening hemorrhage mediated by autoantibodies directed against Factor VIII [1, 2]. Although no predisposing disorder is identified in approximately half of cases, an awareness of associated conditions may lead to earlier diagnosis in patients presenting with hemorrhage and concomitant diagnoses associated with AHA [2]. Some of these established diagnoses associated with AHA include other viral illnesses, such as human immunodeficiency virus (HIV), Hepatitis B and C viruses, and Epstein-Barr virus (EBV), along with various autoimmune conditions, such as autoimmune hemolytic anemia (AIHA)—a better understood autoimmune hematologic disease [1, 5–7]. Several studies have demonstrated a close relationship between AIHA and T-helper type 2 (Th2) cell response—particularly T-helper 17 (Th17) cell and regulatory T-cell (Treg) immune dysregulation [6]. An increased number of Th17 cells in discordance are thought to be a contributing pathway of AIHA development and, with increasing levels, a predictive model correlating with AIHA disease activity [6]. Other studies of viral-induced immune dysregulation, specifically related to influenza and SARS-CoV-2, have demonstrated such imbalance in both Th cells and suppressor T-cell activity. Ongoing investigative efforts suggest that severe manifestations of COVID-19, as well as associated complications, could be related to these findings [8].

A review by Barcellini et al. discusses autoimmune complications in hematologic neoplasms, including development of AHA, AIHA, immune thrombocytopenia (ITP), systemic lupus erythematosus (SLE), rheumatoid arthritis (RA), and antiphospholipid syndrome (APS) [7]. Autoimmunity is described as complex, related to genetic and environmental factors, and primary immunodeficiencies leading to blunted, imbalanced immune response. Patients with this demographic have additional components of immunosuppression, further worsening immune dysregulation. Treg imbalance associated with miRNA dysregulation is one such component of immune dysregulation thought to be related to the development of various autoimmune conditions such as AHA [7]. Virus-derived miRNAs, as established in EBV, have also been implied in the pathogenesis of autoimmunity. Other noteworthy mechanisms that can induce autoimmunity include molecular mimicry, leading to T- and B-lymphocyte activation, clonality, and discordance. Such mechanisms are utilized by several viruses, bacteria, and parasites [7].

A search of the literature revealed three other cases of AHA attributed to COVID-19. The first case involved an 83-year-old female patient who presented with diffuse bruising a week after recovering from NIH mild-grade COVID-19. Treatment involved administration of both prednisone and rituximab [9]. The second case was of a 66-year-old male who had AHA *re-activation* causing hematoma in the trunk, which was identified in 2020 during admission for COVID-19 pneumonia. He had been previously diagnosed and treated for AHA in 2011, which was managed then with intravenous recombinant activated Factor VII, prednisone, and once-weekly cyclophosphamide for a total of 4 weeks. Remission was achieved at day 21. On relapse, he was managed with the same antihemorrhagic and immunosuppressive treatment with remission achieved at day 20. He additionally received lopinavir-ritonavir and supplemental oxygen for treatment of COVID-19 pneumonia [2]. The third case described a 65-year-old man who presented with symptoms of severe subcutaneous bleeding in his arm leading to fasciotomy and mass transfusion protocol. Work-up revealed elevated PTT, decreased Factor VIII, and elevated Factor VIII inhibitor levels. He had elevated SARS-CoV-2 antibody levels with a negative SARS-CoV-2 PCR test. It was concluded that the patient's new findings may have been linked to previous asymptomatic COVID-19. He was treated with a combination of NovoSeven, stress-dose steroids (with taper), a 4-week course of weekly rituximab, followed by a cyclophosphamide taper. Due to persistence of elevated inhibitor levels, the patient was also treated with two doses of FEIBA. Bleeding resolved and Factor VIII normalization was documented at 3-week follow-up [10].

While the pathophysiology of AHA remains unclear and the link with SARS-CoV-2 even more so, there is growing evidence associating COVID-19 with hematological and nonhematological autoimmune diseases including cold agglutinin autoimmune hemolytic anemia, thrombotic thrombocytopenic purpura, Guillain–Barré syndrome, and immune thrombocytopenic purpura [11–14]. Given these associations, as well as known associations of other viral infections with AHA, it is prudent to consider COVID-19-associated AHA in patients with hemorrhage occurring in the setting of recent or current SARS-CoV-2 infection.

4. Conclusion

To our knowledge, this is the third reported case in the literature of *de novo* AHA associated with SARS-CoV-2 infection and the first reported case of a spontaneous urological bleed due to AHA. This relationship was established given the absence of prior history of spontaneous bleeding, autoimmune disease, malignancy, or other offending agents or infections and the known dysregulation of the hemostatic system by SARS-CoV-2 [15]. Due to the severity and life-threatening nature of this disease, a high suspicion for AHA must be maintained in patients presenting with unexplained or worsening hemorrhage after exposure to SARS-CoV-2.

Consent

The patient described in this case was notified and formally consented on the nature of this publication.

Authors' Contributions

The manuscript has been read and approved by all authors.

References

[1] P. Knoebl, P. Marco, F. Baudo et al., "Demographic and clinical data in acquired hemophilia A: results from the European Acquired Haemophilia Registry (EACH2)," *Journal of Thrombosis and Haemostasis*, vol. 10, no. 4, pp. 622–631, 2012.

[2] M. Franchini, C. Glingani, G. De Donno et al., "The first case of acquired hemophilia A associated with SARS-CoV-2 infection," *American Journal of Hematology*, vol. 95, no. 8, 2020.

[3] R. Kruse-Jarres, C. L. Kempton, F. Baudo et al., "Acquired hemophilia A: updated review of evidence and treatment guidance," *American Journal of Hematology*, vol. 92, no. 7, pp. 695–705, 2017.

[4] Covid-19 Treatment Guidelines Panel, *Coronavirus Disease 2019 (COVID-19) Treatment Guidelines*, National Institutes of Health, 2021, https://www.covid19treatmentguidelines.nih.gov/.

[5] Y. Mizukawa and T. Shiohara, "Virus-induced immune dysregulation as a triggering factor for the development of drug rashes and autoimmune diseases: with emphasis on EB virus, human herpesvirus 6 and hepatitis C virus," *Journal of Dermatological Science*, vol. 22, no. 3, pp. 169–180, 2000.

[6] S. S. Michalak, A. Olewicz-Gawlik, J. Rupa-Matysek, E. Wolny-Rokicka, E. Nowakowska, and L. Gil, "Autoimmune hemolytic anemia: current knowledge and perspectives," *Immunity & Ageing*, vol. 17, no. 1, p. 38, 2020.

[7] W. Barcellini, J. A. Giannotta, and B. Fattizzo, "Autoimmune complications in hematologic neoplasms," *Cancers*, vol. 13, no. 7, Article ID 1532, 2021.

[8] S. Tahaghoghi-Hajghorbani, P. Zafari, E. Masoumi et al., "The role of dysregulated immune responses in COVID-19 pathogenesis," *Virus Research*, vol. 290, Article ID 198197, 2020.

[9] G. M. Olsen, H. M. Rinder, and C. A. Tormey, "De novo acquired hemophilia as an immune dysregulation phenomenon following SARS-CoV-2 infection," *Transfusion*, vol. 61, no. 3, pp. 989–991, 2021.

[10] K. Y. Wang, P. Shah, D. T. Roarke, and S. A. Shakil, "Severe acquired haemophilia associated with asymptomatic SARS-CoV-2 infection," *BMJ Case Reports*, vol. 14, no. 7, Article ID e242884, 2021.

[11] E. Zagorski, T. Pawar, S. Rahimian, and D. Forman, "Cold agglutinin autoimmune haemolytic anaemia associated with novel coronavirus (COVID-19)," *British Journal of Haematology*, vol. 190, no. 4, pp. e183–e184, 2020.

[12] N. Albiol, R. Awol, and R. Martino, "Autoimmune thrombotic thrombocytopenic purpura (TTP) associated with COVID-19," *Annals of Hematology*, vol. 99, no. 7, pp. 1673-1674, 2020.

[13] S. Abu-Rumeileh, A. Abdelhak, M. Foschi, H. Tumani, and M. Otto, "Guillain-Barré syndrome spectrum associated with COVID-19: an up-to-date systematic review of 73 cases," *Journal of Neurology*, vol. 268, no. 4, pp. 1133–1170, 2020.

[14] A.-A. Zulfiqar, N. Lorenzo-Villalba, P. Hassler, and E. Andrès, "Immune thrombocytopenic purpura in a patient with Covid-19," *New England Journal of Medicine*, vol. 382, no. 18, p. e43, 2020.

[15] E. Terpos, I. Ntanasis-Stathopoulos, I. Elalamy et al., "Hematological findings and complications of COVID-19," *American Journal of Hematology*, vol. 95, pp. 834–847, 2020.

28

Lenalidomide-Associated Immune Thrombocytopenia: A Case Report and Review of the Literature

William Forehand III[1], **Germame Ajebo**[1], **Michael Toscano**[2], **Anand Jillella**[1], **and Paul Dainer**[1]

[1]*Division of Hematology-Oncology, Medical College of Georgia, Augusta University, Georgia Cancer Center, Augusta, Georgia*
[2]*Department of Pathology and Laboratory Medicine, Augusta University, Augusta, Georgia*

Correspondence should be addressed to Paul Dainer; pdainer@augusta.edu

Academic Editor: Vincent Ribrag

Lenalidomide is indicated in the front-line management of multiple myeloma. More recently, it has been introduced for use in treating other hematologic malignancies. Although the drug is known to cause myelosuppression, there have been rare reports of lenalidomide-associated immune thrombocytopenia (ITP). Here, we review the literature on lenalidomide-associated ITP and report upon a 59-year-old man who was administered lenalidomide due to concern of progressive multiple myeloma more than a year following his having undergone an autologous hematopoietic stem cell transplant. His platelet count precipitously declined and lead to his hospitalization. Despite our withholding of the drug, he did not respond to platelet transfusions or administration of corticosteroids. He was successfully managed with intermittent immune globulin for several months before definitive treatment with splenectomy, which resulted in the complete resolution of his thrombocytopenia. A literature search identified a total of six additional cases of lenalidomide-associated ITP. Similarly, many of the reported cases were associated with persistent thrombocytopenia after discontinuation of the drug. Furthermore, these patients were generally managed successfully with standard ITP therapies, such as corticosteroids or intravenous immune globulin.

1. Introduction

Immune thrombocytopenia (ITP) is a disorder characterized by immune-mediated thrombocytopenia [1]. Idiopathic ITP is reportedly more common; however, ITP secondary to underlying conditions or drugs has been identified not infrequently and may be underdiagnosed [2–4]. Several subtypes of drug-induced ITP (DITP) have been described based on their proposed mechanisms: hapten-dependent, drug-dependent, fiban-induced, drug-specific, autoantibody, and immune complex.

In most circumstances, there must be ongoing exposure to the offending drug for the thrombocytopenia to persist [5]. Hence, the mainstay of managing DITP has been to discontinue the drug whenever possible. Furthermore, criteria have been proposed by George and others for assessing possible DITP cases [6]. Based on such criteria, a case of definitive DITP would require that the patient's thrombocytopenia recovers after the drug is discontinued; however, this definition would exclude cases of DITP of the autoantibody subtype from being considered definite DITP. In the autoantibody subtype of DITP, thrombocytopenia can persist following the removal of the offending drug. The mechanism of this subtype of DITP is thought to involve the production of autoantibodies to platelets that do not depend upon the presence of the drug for binding, such as in primary ITP. Autoantibody-type DITP has been reported with gold and sulfamethoxazole [5, 7].

There have been very few cases of lenalidomide-associated ITP reported in the literature [8–10]. Of these cases, several have been reported in which the thrombocytopenia persisted after stopping the lenalidomide [10]. Here, we report another distinct case of lenalidomide-associated ITP that persisted for months after stopping this agent, possibly placing it among the drugs which can cause the autoantibody subtype of DITP.

2. Case Presentation

The patient was a 59-year-old male who had been diagnosed with plasma cell myeloma in 2004 when he presented with pain and lytic lesions on a skeletal survey and an associated monoclonal IgG on a serum protein electrophoresis (SPEP) and immunofixation. A bone marrow biopsy demonstrated 30% lambda-restricted plasma cells at that time. He was treated with dexamethasone and thalidomide and achieved a very good partial response prior to receiving high-dose melphalan and underwent an autologous peripheral hematopoietic stem cell transplant (auto-HSCT) in July 2005. He achieved a complete response as a bone marrow aspirate, and biopsy in January 2006 revealed less than five percent polyclonal plasma cells. By the following month, his platelet count had recovered to 208,000/mm^3.

Following his recovery, the patient's care was transitioned back to his local hospital. In September 2006, he experienced increasing hip pain. Radiographic imaging revealed bilateral lesions in the femoral necks and pelvis. A bone marrow aspirate and biopsy at that time demonstrated maturing trilineage hematopoiesis and no monoclonal plasma cell population. An SPEP on September 25, 2006, demonstrated a rising M-spike of 0.65 g/dL. In October 2006, he underwent a right hip nail procedure to avoid an impending fracture. The pathologic specimen retrieved from that surgery showed fragments of bone with necrosis and interspersed poorly preserved crushed cells, which could not be definitively characterized.

By November 2006, his M-spike further increased to 0.77 g/dL. Based on the bone lesions and an increasing M-spike, a decision was made to initiate an attenuated course of lenalidomide and dexamethasone, along with a low dose of warfarin. The patient's transplant physician had recommended a 21-day 10 mg daily dose, which was initiated on December 30, 2006. He also received 40 mg dexamethasone every two weeks. No other new medications were initiated at that time. His chronic medications included metformin, glipizide, atenolol, pamidronate aspirin, fosinopril, gabapentin, lansoprazole, simvastatin, and ezetimibe. On January 26, 2007, the patient was admitted to the hospital for severe thrombocytopenia with a platelet count of 9,000/mm^3; his other blood counts at the time of admission included Hgb, 10.7 g/dL, which was similar to his Hgb level before initiating lenalidomide. His WBC count was normal at 5.8 k/mm^3. Further lenalidomide was withheld, and he was administered a 3-day course of 1 mg/kg prednisone along with a platelet transfusion; however, there was no increment in his platelet count. His HIV, hepatitis B, hepatitis C, and ANA screens were negative. On February 5, 2007, he underwent an abdominal ultrasound which demonstrated no evidence of portal hypertension or splenomegaly. Subsequently, he was transferred to the Augusta University Medical Center. At the time of transfer on February 6, 2007, his platelet count was 17,000/mm^3.

Following his transfer, he received transfusions of several more units of platelets on February 8th and 9th, but his platelets continued to decline and fell to a nadir of 5,000/mm^3 on February 9th. A bone marrow aspirate and biopsy were performed. The specimens obtained demonstrated maturing hematopoiesis with adequate megakaryopoiesis and no morphologic evidence of recurrent myeloma (Figure 1). His hepatic function tests and renal function remained normal throughout his clinical course. In the absence of abnormal bleeding, he was discharged and maintained under close observation as an outpatient.

Despite having had the lenalidomide withheld, his thrombocytopenia persisted, and he was readmitted to the hospital on February 18, 2007, after the onset of epistaxis, petechiae over his ankles, and melenic stools. He received intravenous gamma globulin (IVIG) on February 18th and achieved a rapid and robust platelet response. His platelets increased to 48,000/mm^3 on the following day and peaked at 110,000/mm^3 on February 22nd. The response was not sustained, and his platelets again decreased to 19,000/mm^3. He received an additional dose of IVIG, which again resulted in a transient response. A course of rituximab was added to the treatment regimen. He remained dependent on intermittent IVIG infusions until July 2, 2007, when he underwent a splenectomy, resulting in a sustained rise in his platelet count (Figure 2). His spleen had a normal weight of 244.5 gm, and microscopic examination demonstrated red pulp congestion and no abnormal cell populations (Figure 3). Within a few months, he developed new bone lesions with an associated hip fracture, and his serum paraprotein increased further. He was treated sequentially with thalidomide and prednisone and, later, bortezomib, liposomal doxorubicin, and dexamethasone with symptomatic improvement and no recurrence of significant thrombocytopenia. He was lost to follow-up after a year of treatment and reportedly expired of uncertain causes.

3. Methods

Using PubMed and Ovid, we searched the MEDLINE database using a date range from 1980–2020 for the keywords (lenalidomide) and (ITP) or (lenalidomide) and (immune thrombocytopenia). There were 24 search results. Only one result reported on a case of lenalidomide-associated ITP. A separate search using Google Scholar was conducted, using the keywords (lenalidomide) and (ITP). There were 569 search results. There were two additional articles or abstracts that reported on cases of lenalidomide-associated ITP. A summary of the search results is shown in Figure 4.

4. Discussion

Lenalidomide is a drug supported by national guidelines for the front-line management of plasma cell myeloma [11]. More recently, the U.S. Food and Drug Administration (FDA) approved the use of lenalidomide as maintenance therapy after auto-HSCT for patients with myeloma. The approval was based on evidence from two randomized, blinded trials of maintenance lenalidomide

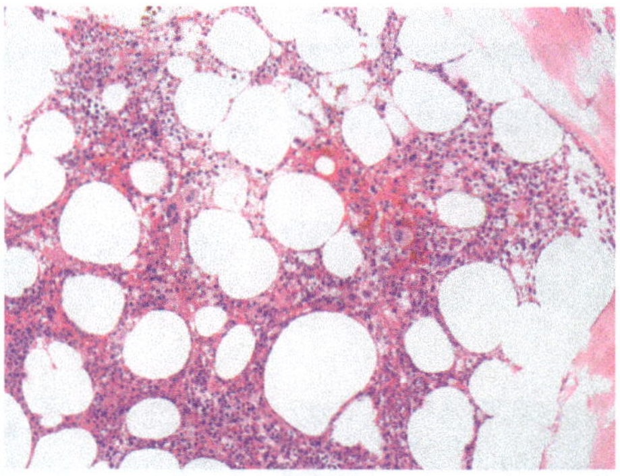

Figure 1: Bone marrow biopsy (200x). The bone marrow is normocellular with adequate trilineage hematopoiesis and normal maturation. Several megakaryocytes are present.

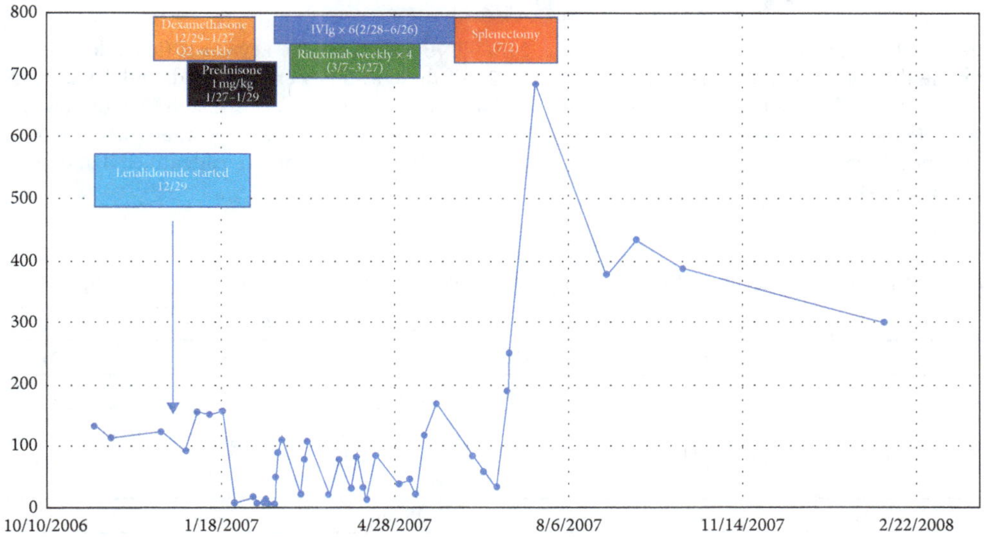

Figure 2: The platelet count and treatment history of the case.

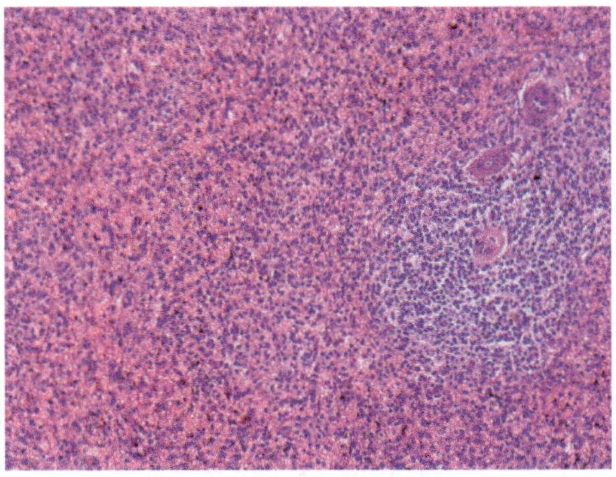

Figure 3: The spleen was 244.5 gm showing red pulp congestion, but no abnormal cell population. The perivascular white pulp is intact but attenuated.

versus placebo [12]. One of its well-known toxicities has been reversible myelosuppression; however, there have only been rare reports of DITP from lenalidomide [8–10]. Our MEDLINE and Google Scholar search only identified three reports with a total of six cases of lenalidomide-associated ITP (summarized in Table 1).

Most cases of DITP related to drugs other than lenalidomide have been associated with platelet recovery after stopping the drug. Improvement in platelet counts after removing exposure to the offending drug establishes drug dependence of the immune-mediated platelet destruction. Such cases, especially with recurrence of the

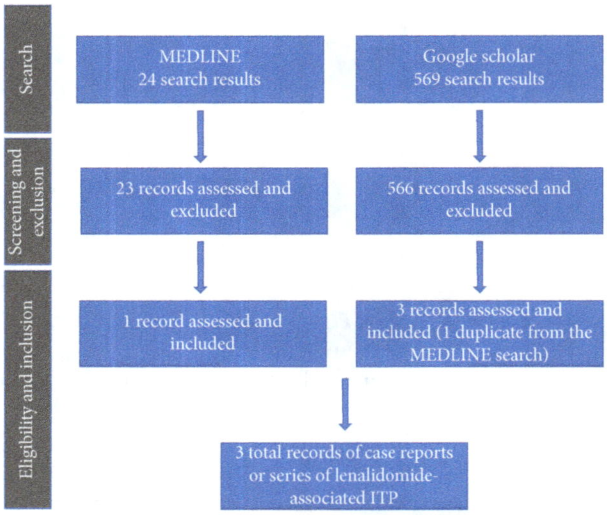

FIGURE 4: Literature search results, exclusion, and inclusion. A MEDLINE search for the keywords (lenalidomide) and (ITP) or (lenalidomide) and (immune thrombocytopenia) resulted in 24 results. 23 of these results were excluded, and 1 was assessed and included. Google Scholar was also searched using the keywords (lenalidomide) and (ITP). There were 569 results. 566 of these results were assessed and excluded as not related to lenalidomide and ITP. 3 of the 569 results were included in our report. Because one of the included Google Scholar results was a duplicate with the included MEDLINE, there were a total of 3 reports that were identified that those were case reports or case series of lenalidomide-associated ITP.

TABLE 1: A comparison of the cases of lenalidomide-associated ITP reported in the literature along with our case.

	Case 1[10]	Case 2 [10]	Case 3 [10]	Case 4 [10]	Case 5 [8]	Case 6 [9]	Our case
Age	66	76	78	66	27	74	59
Sex	F	F	F	F	M	F	M
Plasma cell dyscrasia subtype	IgGk MM	IgGλ MM	IgAλ amyloid	MM (subtype not reported)	MM (subtype not reported)	Light chain λ MM	IgGλ MM
Dose of len	15 mg	15 mg	15 mg	25 mg	25 mg	15 mg	10 mg
Previous autologous bone marrow transplant	No	No	No	No	Yes	No	Yes
Cycle of lenalidomide before developing thrombocytopenia	5	3	6	3	Received consolidation × 4 VRD and maintenance lenalidomide × 3 months	1	1
Treatment of ITP	Steroids, IVIg, rituximab	Steroids	Steroids	Steroids (prednisone)	Steroids and IVIG	Steroids	Steroids, IVIg, rituximab, splenectomy
Persistent thrombocytopenia after stopping lenalidomide	Yes	Yes, until steroids initiated. Responded to steroids at around 1 month after stopping lenalidomide	Yes, patient remained steroid-dependent	Yes	No, responded to steroid tapering	No, responded to steroid tapering	Yes, patient eventually obtained a long-term remission with splenectomy
Retreatment with lenalidomide was associated with recurrence of thrombocytopenia	Yes	Retreated, but no recurrent thrombocytopenia	Not retreated	Not retreated	Not retreated	Not retreated	Not retreated
Other manifestations	None reported	None reported	None reported	None reported	Alopecia, leukopenia	Rash, proteinuria	None

thrombocytopenia upon re-exposure to the drug, can be considered definitive DITP by criteria proposed by George and others [6]; however, such criteria do not capture those few cases characterized by autoantibodies able to destroy platelets without depending upon the presence of the inciting drug. Such cases of DITP can be associated with ongoing thrombocytopenia that resembles primary ITP. Here, we reported a case of secondary ITP associated with lenalidomide exposure that persisted after stopping lenalidomide for several months, long after its biotransformation and rapid renal clearance. Our case suggests that lenalidomide may be able to induce persistent immune-mediated platelet destruction. While cases of thrombocytopenia resolution after discontinuation of lenalidomide have been reported, our case is consistent with the report of Pompa and colleagues [10]. They describe four cases of lenalidomide-associated ITP (Table 1). These cases were also associated with persistent thrombocytopenia or ITP-therapy dependence after discontinuation of lenalidomide. In one case, thrombocytopenia was successfully treated with steroids, but immune thrombocytopenia recurred after the patient resumed lenalidomide. In a case reported by Meguri and colleagues, a patient with lenalidomide-associated ITP also developed a rash and proteinuria (Table 1). The authors implicated a broader immunologic dysregulation as the underlying mechanism of lenalidomide-associated ITP [9].

In conclusion, lenalidomide may be an underrecognized cause of the autoantibody subtype of DITP resulting from the induction of nondrug-dependent autoantibody-mediated platelet destruction. As in primary ITP, our patient was successfully managed with IVIG and splenectomy. To our knowledge, this is the first case to report the successful treatment of lenalidomide-associated ITP with splenectomy. Our case, along with the other cases reported in the literature, suggests that the management of lenalidomide-associated ITP may require both drug discontinuation and therapies traditionally used in primary ITP. Splenectomy may be a successful approach to attain a durable response in patients who otherwise remain steroid-refractory or IVIG-dependent; however, it should be noted that thrombopoietin receptor agonists were not clinically available during that time and should be considered in recalcitrant cases. Our report and those of others should alert the clinician to this unusual mechanism of lenalidomide toxicity as this drug is currently being utilized in the treatment of an increasing number of malignant hematologic neoplasms.

Authors' Contributions

P.D., W.F., and G.A. devised the study, collected data, and conducted the data analysis. W.F. drafted the manuscript. The manuscript was revised by P.D. and G.A. M.T. reviewed the pathology and provided pathology images. A.J. and P.D. provided the clinical care of the patient. All authors reviewed and approved the manuscript.

Acknowledgments

This work was supported by The Georgia Cancer Center of Augusta University.

References

[1] H. Kashiwagi and Y. Tomiyama, "Pathophysiology and management of primary immune thrombocytopenia," *International Journal of Hematology*, vol. 98, no. 1, pp. 24–33, 2013.

[2] W. M. Schoonen, G. Kucera, J. Coalson et al., "Epidemiology of immune thrombocytopenic purpura in the general practice research database," *British Journal of Haematology*, vol. 145, no. 2, pp. 235–244, 2009.

[3] G. Moulis, A. Palmaro, J.-L. Montastruc, B. Godeau, M. Lapeyre-Mestre, and L. Sailler, "Epidemiology of incident immune thrombocytopenia: a nationwide population-based study in France," *Blood*, vol. 124, no. 22, pp. 3308–3315, 2014.

[4] D. B. Cines, J. B. Bussel, H. A. Liebman, and E. T. Luning Prak, "The ITP syndrome: pathogenic and clinical diversity," *Blood*, vol. 113, no. 26, pp. 6511–6521, 2009.

[5] R. H. Aster, B. R. Curtis, J. G. McFarland, and D. W. Bougie, "Drug-induced immune thrombocytopenia: pathogenesis, diagnosis, and management," *Journal of Thrombosis and Haemostasis*, vol. 7, no. 6, pp. 911–918, 2009.

[6] J. N. George, G. E. Raskob, S. R. Shah et al., "Drug-induced thrombocytopenia," *Annals of Internal Medicine*, vol. 129, no. 11_Part_1, pp. 886–890, 1998.

[7] R. H. Aster, "Can drugs cause autoimmune thrombocytopenic purpura?," *Seminars in Hematology*, vol. 37, no. 3, pp. 229–238, 2000.

[8] C. I. Herold, C. Gasparetto, and G. M. Arepally, "Lenalidomide-associated ITP," *Case Reports in Hematology*, vol. 2011, Article ID 638020, 4 pages, 2011.

[9] Y. Meguri, Y. Kamara, A. Yamamoto, T. Masunari, N. Sezaki, and T. Kiguchi, "Development of unexpected severe thrombocytopenia just after initiating lenalidomide: possible involvement of an immunologic mechanism," *International Journal of Myeloma*, vol. 8, no. 1, pp. 1–3, 2018.

[10] A. Pompa, F. Guidotti, A. I. Gregorini et al., "Four cases of Lenalidomide-associated immune thrombocytopenia," *Blood*, vol. 128, no. 22, p. 4927, 2016.

[11] S. K. Kumar, "Management of multiple myeloma," *Journal of the National Comprehensive Cancer Network*, vol. 16, no. 5S, pp. 624–627, 2018.

[12] E. D. Pulte, A. Dmytrijuk, L. Nie et al., "FDA approval summary: lenalidomide as maintenance therapy after autologous stem cell transplant in newly diagnosed multiple myeloma," *The Oncologist*, vol. 23, no. 6, pp. 734–739, 2018.

29

Necrotizing Bacterial Myositis as the Initial Presentation of Severe Aplastic Anaemia

Synne Dragesund Rørvik[1] **Kristoffer Stange Larsen,**[2] **Lars Helgeland,**[3,4] **Håvard Dale,**[4,5] **Birgitta Ivarsen,**[6] **Øystein Bruserud,**[1] **and Tor Henrik Anderson Tvedt**[1,7]

[1]*Department of Medicine, Haukeland University Hospital, Bergen, Norway*
[2]*Department of Medicine, Haraldsplass Deaconess Hospital, Bergen, Norway*
[3]*Department of Pathology, Haukeland University Hospital, Bergen, Norway*
[4]*Department of Clinical Medicine (K1), University of Bergen, Bergen, Norway*
[5]*Department of Orthopaedic Surgery, Haukeland University Hospital, Bergen, Norway*
[6]*Department of Plastic Surgery, Haukeland University Hospital, Bergen, Norway*
[7]*Department of Haematology, Oslo University Hospital, Rikshospitalet, Oslo 0424, Norway*

Correspondence should be addressed to Synne Dragesund Rørvik; synne.dr@hotmail.no

Academic Editor: Masayuki Nagasawa

Introduction. Necrotizing soft tissue infections are rapidly progressing infections associated with severe inflammation and cytokine release. Early recognition and surgical intervention are key factors to secure survival. The current case presents a patient with multifocal necrotizing soft tissue infection as the initial presentation of severe aplastic anaemia. *Case Presentation.* A man in his fifties was admitted with septic shock with multiorgan failure and severe pancytopenia, after two days of malaise with high fever and right flank pain. The diagnosis streptococcal necrotizing myositis was significantly delayed due to atypical clinical findings. After initial surgical exploration, the decision was made to defer from surgical debridement due to extensive involvement of several muscle groups, grave pancytopenia, and suspected dismal prognosis. Surprisingly, the patient stabilized after antibiotics and intensive care treatment. Based on severe pancytopenia and hypocellular bone marrow, with no evidence of other bone marrow disorders, the patient was diagnosed with aplastic anaemia. Treatment for aplastic anaemia with antithymocyte globulin, cyclosporine, and eltrombopaq was started, and 2 months later, a partial haematological recovery was observed. The patient could be discharged from hospital without antibiotic treatment. *Conclusions.* This case illustrates the crucial role of a multidisciplinary approach on admission and further during the clinical course. Clinical improvement despite severe neutropenia and stabilization during immunosuppressive therapy suggest that immunological factors modulate clinical course in necrotizing soft tissue infections.

1. Introduction

Necrotizing soft tissue infections (NSTIs) are characterized by significant inflammation, multiorgan failure, morbidity, and mortality [1]. A dramatic increase in mortality is seen if surgery is delayed or surgical debridement is inadequate [2, 3]. Furthermore, the initial inflammatory response contributes to the early mortality as well as the prolonged recovery and late mortality [4, 5]. Although several studies have demonstrated that age, presence of chronic diseases, steroid use, previous blunt trauma, and a lower body mass index are risk factors for NSTIs [6, 7], the underlying pathophysiological mechanisms are poorly understood. However, experimental data suggest that bacterial pyrogenic exotoxin-induced immune activation contributes to muscle inflammation as well as compromised cellular and humoral immunity [8]. In the current article, we describe a patient with NSTI in several muscle groups as the initial presentation of aplastic anaemia (AA) with severe neutropenia. Despite a significant diagnostic delay, the patient improved gradually without extensive surgical intervention and response to immunosuppressive therapy did not exuberate the muscle disease.

2. Case Presentation

A 50-year-old male was admitted after two days of malaise, high fever, and right flank pain. His medical history included bilateral Calve-Legg-Perthes disease treated with left side total hip arthroplasty, gout, and hypothyroidism for which he received allopurinol, diclofenac, and levothyroxine, respectively. He had no known prior haematological diseases and had a normal haemoglobin level and peripheral white blood cell counts at his last routine examination, 18 months prior to admission. He denied having fever, with the exception of the days prior to admission, neither the skin nor mucosal bleeding, weight loss, or night sweats.

He was severely hypotensive at admission with a systolic blood pressure of 50 mmHg; he appeared drowsy and lethargic but responded adequately to questions and commands. Clinical examination revealed a bluish red discoloration on the right flank without additional prominent findings with no obvious signs of previous penetrating or blunt trauma. Arterial blood gas analysis showed a compensated metabolic acidosis with increased lactate level 4.2 mmol/L (normal level 0.9–1.7 mmol/L). Empiric antibiotic treatment with penicillin G plus gentamicin together with fluid resuscitation and noradrenaline-infusion was immediately initiated. The blood pressure subsequently stabilized at 100/60 mmHg. Initial blood sample testing showed the following results:

(i) A significant acute-phase response with a C-reactive protein (CRP) level of 592 mg/L (normal level <5 mg/L), procalcitonin 56.2 μg/L (<0.1 μg/L), and fibrinogen 8.6 g/L (1.9–4.0 g/L)

(ii) Severe pancytopenia with total peripheral blood leucocytes counts below 0.5×10^9/L ($3.5–11.0 \times 10^9$/L), neutrophils 0.1×10^9/L ($1.7–8.2 \times 10^9$/L), haemoglobin 6.1 g/dL (13.4–17.0 g/dL), reticulocytes 0.01×10^{12}/L ($0.03–0.1 \times 10^{12}$/L), and thrombocytes 3×10^9/L ($145–348 \times 10^9$/L). Activated partial thromboplastin time and international normalized ratio were both within normal reference values.

(iii) Severe renal failure with creatinine 430 μmol/L (60–105 μmol/L)

(iv) Evidence of myonecrosis with a myoglobin level of 6,486 μmol/L (<70 μmol/L), creatinine kinase level of 10,430 U/L (40–80 U/L), and lactate dehydrogenase 340 U/L (105–205 U/L)

A full-body computed tomography (CT) showed a subcutaneous haematoma of the right flank, but without signs of thickened fascia, gas in the soft tissue, or signs of injury to other organs or bone structures. The liver and spleen appeared normal. At this time point, the patient was transferred to the intensive care unit (ICU) at our university hospital, and progression of the skin lesion was noted at admission. The lesion now included a well-demarcated erythema involving the entire right half of the torso, abdomen, and gluteal region, but neither bulla nor skin necrosis was present. There was no crepitus formation, fluctuations, or pain on touch. The clinical picture was considered as possible deep tissue infection, but a watchful waiting strategy was chosen because of the high risk associated with major surgery in patients with severe pancytopenia and the absence of typical NSTI findings. Antibiotic treatment was changed to meropenem plus clindamycin. Ultrasound did not reveal presence of abscesses or gas. Gram stain of fluids aspirated from the affected areas was negative for bacteria, and cytological examination did not indicate that the subcutaneous fluid originated from a haematoma, as indicated by CT. Blood cultures at admission and during the subsequent clinical course were all negative.

Further diagnostic work-up was done to evaluate the cause of the bone marrow failure. The bone marrow smear showed a significantly hypocellular, almost acellular marrow. No megakaryocytes were present. There was no increase in blast cells, and hemophagocytosis was not present. The smear was dominated by mature lymphocytes and monocytes, and there were no clear signs of myelodysplasia. Immunophenotyping of peripheral blood and bone marrow aspirate (analysed according to standard EuroFlow protocol) showed no presence of lymphoma, leukaemia, myelodysplastic syndrome, or paroxysmal nocturnal haemoglobinuria. The levels of folic acid, cobalamin, zinc, lead, copper, selenium, mercury, cadmium, and metabolic hormones were within normal range. Serology of parvovirus, human immunodeficiency virus (HIV), hepatitis B and C, Epstein-Barr virus, and cytomegalovirus was negative. Based on initial findings, the diagnosis of severe aplastic anaemia was suspected, and treatment with granulocyte colony-stimulating factor (G-CSF) was therefore initiated while waiting for the results from cytogenetic bone marrow examination and bone biopsy.

Over the next 48 hours, vasoactive agents could be weaned off, lactate levels normalized, renal function improved, and myoglobin and creatinine kinase levels decreased significantly. The patient could be discharged from the ICU. However, the erythema on the right flank/hip increased and became more painful. A repeated CT of the right latissimus dorsi muscle (Figure 1(a)) suggested deep tissue infection with muscle necrosis, and a magnetic resonance tomography imaging (MRI) was also consistent with myonecrosis (Figures 1(b)). It was therefore decided to proceed to explorative surgery. Upon surgical exploration, the fascia of the right latissimus dorsi muscle was found to be greenish and thickened, and the underlying muscle was necrotic with an absence of bleeding and contractility upon stimulation (Figure 2), but without smell or gas release. The findings were regarded as diagnostic for necrotizing bacterial myositis. A complete debridement of the necrotic muscle would have resulted in a wound area reaching from the right shoulder through the entire dorsal area of the chest, abdomen, and gluteal region, and despite the severe bone marrow failure, the clinical condition was at this time stable

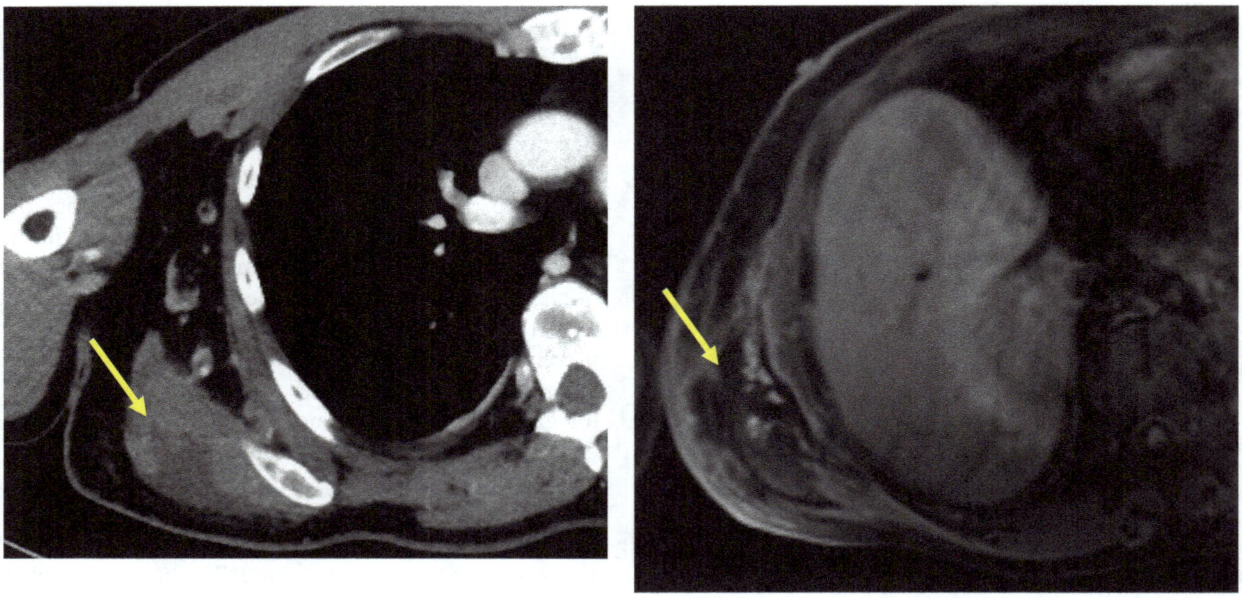

(a) (b)

Figure 1: (a) Coronal images from a contrast CT of the thorax showing right latissimus dorsi muscle suggestive of deep tissue infection with possible muscle necrosis. (b) Coronal images from a contrast MRI of the thorax showing myonecrosis of the right latissimus dorsi muscle.

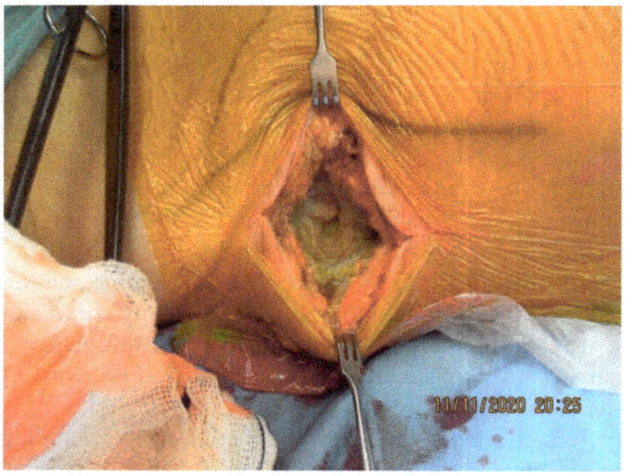

Figure 2: Intraoperative images of the right latissimus dorsi muscle. Thickened and greenish fascia with underlying necrotic muscle.

with a decrease of CRP levels. Further surgical debridement was therefore deferred. Perioperative tissue and fluid samples were obtained for microbiological and histopathological analyses. Microscopy of Gram-stained smears of the muscle biopsies revealed no microbes; however, due to the greenish discoloration of the fascia and muscle, *Pseudomonas* spp. was suspected, and tobramycin, later replaced by ciprofloxacin, was added to the antibacterial regimen. Finally, MRI of the head detected ischemic strokes in the right corona radiate and the left cerebellum, possibly caused by septic emboli, but transthoracic echocardiography showed normal cardiac function and no valve vegetation.

The trephine biopsy showed hypocellular bone marrow (only 5–10% cellularity, Figure 3(a)) with only a small number of lymphocytes and plasma cells, and complete absence of both megakaryocytes, myelopoiesis, and erythropoiesis. The number of blast cells was not increased, and there were no signs of marrow fibrosis or gelatinous transformation of the bone marrow. The chromosome analysis showed normal male karyotype. Next-generation sequencing genetic testing, covering over 300 different genes, including genes involving in hereditary bone marrow failure syndromes, was without any specific finding. These findings were consistent with aplastic anaemia, but a mitomycin C test was not possible due to the low lymphocyte level. Eltrombopaq treatment was therefore started, and the G-CSF dose was also doubled, but granulocyte transfusions were not available.

Histological examination of muscle biopsies showed colonies of Gram-positive cocci and extensive muscle necrosis. All bacterial cultures of the muscle biopsies were negative, but 16S-ribosomal RNA (16s-rRNA) gene sequencing performed on bacterial DNA from muscle biopsies identified *Streptococcus dysgalactiae* (SD) in 3 out of 4 samples. Thus, the diagnosis streptococcal necrotizing myositis was confirmed, and antimicrobial treatment with meropenem and clindamycin without ciprofloxacin was continued.

The clinical picture was surprisingly peaceful despite the severe NSTI with widespread necrosis. The patient had intermittent low-grade fever, the erythema regressed, and the CRP level decreased to 100 mg/L. NSTI is usually regarded as a surgical emergency where early and aggressive surgical debridement of the infected muscle and fascia is imperative to secure survival. This usually requires multiple surgeries with removal of the affected muscles and fascia followed by a prolonged period of wound management before closure of the skin is possible. During this time

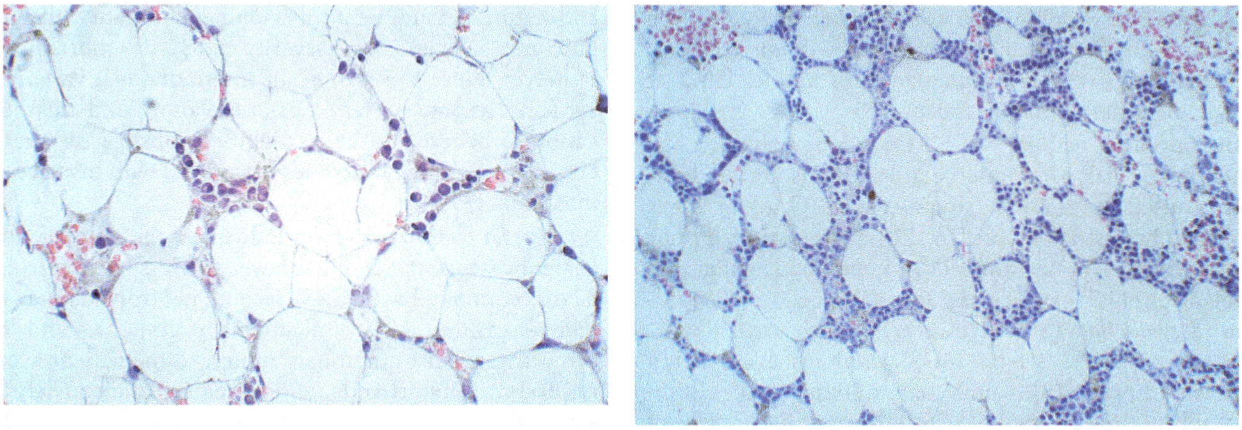

(a) (b)

FIGURE 3: (a) Trephine biopsy showing markedly hypocellular bone marrow, with 5–10% cellularity. (b) Trephine biopsy showing a significant increase of bone marrow cellularity after treatment with IST.

TABLE 1: Important aspect of the clinical course.

Timeline	Day 1	Day 3	Day 5	Day 7	Day 8	Day 17	Day 77	Day 90
	Transferred to ICU	Discharged from ICU						Discharged from hospital
C-reactive protein	592 mg/L					170 mg/L		1 mg/L
Antimicrobial therapy	Antibiotics initiated						Treatment discontinued	
CT scan or/and MRI	X		X					
Surgical exploration				X				
AA directed therapy					Eltrombopaq initiated	ATG and cyclosporine initiated		
Neutrophil count	0.1×10^9/L					0.0×10^9/L		0.6×10^9/L

period, adequate neutrophil and platelet function and counts are required to avoid superinfections and secure wound healing.

Severe AA requires treatment with allogenic stem cell transplantation or immunosuppressive therapy to improve the prognosis. AA left untreated incurs a high risk of death from infections. Since the clinical situation was stable, further surgery was deferred and intensive immunosuppressive therapy with horse antithymocyte globulin (ATG) and cyclosporine A combined with eltrombopaq was initiated. This had to be combined with ongoing antimicrobial therapy until neutrophil recovery was achieved. A summary of important clinical aspect is given in Table 1.

The patient was discharged from hospital after 3 months and was followed up weekly through outpatient care. Peripheral blood evaluation at discharge showed leucocytes 1.7×10^9/L, neutrophils 0.6×10^9/L, haemoglobin of 7.8 g/dL, reticulocytes 0.039×10^{12}/L, and a thrombocyte count of 14×10^9/L. A new bone marrow biopsy showed a significant increase of the cellularity with detectable haematopoiesis as signs of regeneration (Figure 3(b)).

3. Discussion

NSTIs are rapidly progressive infections associated with significant tissue destruction, systemic toxicity, and a high mortality rate if not treated early [9]. Timely identification and treatment including prompt surgery with extensive debridement are essential to secure survival [10, 11]. The current case presents a patient with severe multifocal NSTI as the initial presentation of severe AA; despite circulatory collapse, he stabilized after antibiotic and intensive care treatment and recovered without surgical debridement.

The patient fulfilled the generally accepted criteria for severe AA and had peripheral pancytopenia and bone marrow hypocellularity; the 1-year mortality rate if this disease is left untreated exceeds 80% and is mainly due to bacterial and fungal infections [12–15]. AA requires prompt treatment with either allogeneic stem cell transplantation (HSCT) or immunosuppressive therapy (IST) with ATG and cyclosporine to establish bone marrow function. Treatment in AA is individualized based on age, donor availability, comorbidities, and risk of infections. In the current case, standard IST in combination with eltrombopaq was the chosen first-line therapy, since there was no donor available, and the ongoing severe infection made him unfit for HSCT at the time of initiating the treatment.

The microbial aetiology of NSTIs can be polymicrobial or monomicrobial. Monomicrobial infections are predominantly caused by group A streptococcus (GAS) or other beta-haemolytic streptococci [16, 17]. The aetiology in our case was identified by 16S-rRNA gene sequencing that cannot distinguish between the two subspecies of *Streptococcus dysgalactiae* (SD). However, *Streptococcus dysgalactiae* subspecies *dysgalactiae* (SDSD) is almost exclusively a zoonotic pathogen [18], which makes *Streptococcus dysgalactiae* subspecies *equisimilis* (SDSE) the most likely cause of infection in our patient.

Reported risk factors for SDSE NSTIs are blunt trauma, age, male gender, and immune defects [1, 6, 7, 17, 19–21] that were all present in our patient. Furthermore, the patient's regular use of nonsteroidal anti-inflammatory drugs (NSAIDs) may have suppressed neutrophil functions and thereby masked early clinical signs and contributed to delayed diagnosis of NSTI [22, 23].

Neither clinical signs, radiological, nor laboratory findings can distinguish NSTIs from nonnecrotizing skin infections, and explorative surgery is required to establish the diagnosis [24]. Severe and localized pain is often the only early sign of infection in immunocompromised patients, but they may even experience less pain due to the inadequate immune response [25–27]. Hence, the diagnosis of NSTI can easily be overlooked and surgical exploration delayed [25]. This was also the case for our patient. Neutrophil migration to the site of infection is a crucial step in host defence [28]; the neutropenia may then have limited the endothelial injury and the overall systemic inflammatory response [29, 30] and thereby contributed to the successful outcome.

Streptococcal virulence factors are well-described contributors to the pathogenesis of NSTIs [10, 31, 32]. Putative virulence factors for SDSE include adhesins, toxins, and factors important for dissemination in human tissues and interference with the host immune responses. An example of such virulence factor is extracellular nuclease and streptodornase (DNase), which allows the bacteria to escape killing in neutrophil extracellular traps (NETs) [16, 33–37]. The extensive host inflammatory response to streptococcal infections, and especially neutrophil migration and degranulation, is considered to play a major role in tissue damage and systemic toxicity in these infections [4, 28]. Analysis of streptococcal NSTI patient tissue biopsies showed a strong correlation between bacterial load, neutrophil influx and degranulation markers, and tissue inflammation [38]. The mechanism behind neutrophil activation is incompletely understood, but streptococcal M-proteins have been shown to trigger activation and degranulation of neutrophils which contribute to vascular leakage and acute lung injury in the course of NSTI. Furthermore, streptococcal exotoxins may act as superantigens (SAgs) that can induce a broad and uncontrolled release of various cytokines [35]. Both tissue and serum measurements of cytokines correlate with clinical outcomes such as disease severity and 30-day mortality [38]. However, there is a significant interindividual variation in cytokine response after SAgs stimulation, and this observation is believed to be partially responsible for the heterogeneous clinical outcomes in patients with invasive GAS infections [39].

Several factors may have influenced the outcome in the current case. First, SDSE has fewer and less potent virulence factors compared with GAS. Second, neutropenia may have dampened the initial inflammatory response and been protective against pulmonary injury, so the patient avoided respiratory support and could be managed adequately with supportive care. Third, several studies have shown that T cell subsets are expanded and functionally abnormal in AA with abnormal response to immunological stimuli [40]. This might also have dampened both the early and late immunological responses.

Data on mortality and prognostic factors in NSTIs caused by SDSE are scarce. A 15-year retrospective survey in Western Norway found the 30-day mortality rate in SDSE NSTIs to be 31% [17]. Studies comparing invasive GAS and SD disease in general indicate that death among SD cases is more often related to age and comorbidity and more rarely to septic shock than in GAS infections [20, 41]. Bacteraemia is an independent predictor of mortality for NSTIs [42]. In the present case, repeated blood cultures were negative. Positive blood cultures are found in 40–60% of streptococcal NSTIs, and bacteraemia is more common in GAS NSTIs than in SDSE NSTIs [6, 43–45]. Although tissue biopsies showed Gram-positive cocci in the necrotic muscle, there was no growth in the tissue or fluid cultures. This was most likely due to the ongoing antibiotic therapy.

Early initiation of antibiotic treatment can limit the expansion of the total bacteria load and thereby improve prognosis [46]. Empirical antibiotic treatment of NSTIs is often inadequate. In a UK study, 92% of patients with severity class IV skin and soft tissue infections, including NSTIs, received antibiotics considered inappropriate compared to UK guidelines [47]. However, our patient received adequate broad-spectrum antibiotics (i.e., meropenem plus clindamycin) consistent with the recommendations for treatment of streptococcal beta-haemolytic NSTIs from admission [11]. Treatment including clindamycin has shown to be superior to beta-lactam antibiotics in two observational studies on streptococcal NSTIs [48, 49] and has a crucial role in controlling local inflammation by reducing local toxin production [50].

To the best of our knowledge, this is the first case report to describe a patient who presents with NSTI as the initial presentation of AA that successfully could be treated with IST. Ugarte-Torres et al. present a patient with relapsed AA that developed bilateral lower extremity necrotizing fasciitis caused by multidrug-resistant *Aeromonas hydrophilia*. As with our patient, IST with ATG and cyclosporine A was initiated, but the patient passed away after subsequent surgery [26].

4. Conclusion

The current case illustrates that the clinical course of NSTI in severely neutropenic patient can be atypical and easily overlooked. The clinical improvement despite severe neutropenia and stabilization during immunosuppressive therapy suggests that tissue damage in NSTI may in part be caused by secondary immunological factors.

Abbreviations

AA: Aplastic anaemia
GAS: Group A streptococcus
MRI: Magnetic resonance tomography imaging
NSTI: Necrotizing soft tissue infections
SDSE: *Streptococcus dysgalactiae* subspecies *equisimilis*.

Consent

Written informed consent was obtained from the patient for publication of this case report, including images and any potentially identifying information.

Authors' Contributions

SDR and THAT were responsible for the draft of the manuscript and coordinated the final version of the manuscript. All authors wrote, revised, and approved the final manuscript.

References

[1] D. L. Stevens and A. E. Bryant, "Necrotizing soft-tissue infections," *New England Journal of Medicine*, vol. 378, no. 10, p. 971, 2018.
[2] M. Sartelli, X. Guirao, T. C. Hardcastle et al., "2018 WSES/SIS-E consensus conference: recommendations for the management of skin and soft-tissue infections," *World Journal of Emergency Surgery*, vol. 13, no. 1, p. 58, 2018.
[3] D. L. Stevens, A. L. Bisno, H. F. Chambers et al., "Executive summary: practice guidelines for the diagnosis and management of skin and soft tissue infections: 2014 update by the infectious diseases society of America," *Clinical Infectious Diseases*, vol. 59, no. 2, pp. 147–159, 2014.
[4] M. B. Hansen, fnm au, L. S. Rasmussen et al., "Association between cytokine response, the LRINEC score and outcome in patients with necrotising soft tissue infection: a multicentre, prospective study," *Scientific Reports*, vol. 7, no. 1, Article ID 42179, 2017.
[5] M. B. Hansen, "Biomarkers of necrotising soft tissue infections aspects of the innate immune response," *Danish medical journal*, vol. 64, no. 7, 2017.
[6] T. Bruun, E. Rath, M. B. Madsen et al., "Risk factors and predictors of mortality in streptococcal necrotizing soft-tissue infections: a multicenter prospective study," *Clinical Infectious Diseases*, vol. 72, no. 2, pp. 293–300, 2021.
[7] Z. B. Nuwayhid, D. M. Aronoff, and Z. D. Mulla, "Blunt trauma as a risk factor for group A streptococcal necrotizing fasciitis," *Annals of Epidemiology*, vol. 17, no. 11, pp. 878–881, 2007.
[8] S. N. Shishido, S. Varahan, K. Yuan, X. Li, and S. D. Fleming, "Humoral innate immune response and disease," *Clinical Immunology*, vol. 144, no. 2, pp. 142–158, 2012.
[9] J. A. Majeski and J. F. John Jr., "Necrotizing soft tissue infections: a guide to early diagnosis and initial therapy," *Southern Medical Journal*, vol. 96, no. 9, pp. 900–905, 2003.
[10] D. A. Anaya and E. P. Dellinger, "Necrotizing soft-tissue infection: diagnosis and management," *Clinical Infectious Diseases: An Official Publication of the Infectious Diseases Society of America*, vol. 44, no. 5, pp. 705–710, 2007.
[11] D. L. Stevens, A. L. Bisno, H. F. Chambers et al., "Practice guidelines for the diagnosis and management of skin and soft tissue infections: 2014 update by the Infectious Diseases Society of America," *Clinical Infectious Diseases*, vol. 59, no. 2, pp. e10–e52, 2014.
[12] R. A. Brodsky and R. J. Jones, "Aplastic anaemia," *The Lancet*, vol. 365, no. 9471, pp. 1647–1656, 2005.
[13] H. A. Torres, G. P. Bodey, K. V. I. Rolston, H. M. Kantarjian, I. I. Raad, and D. P. Kontoyiannis, "Infections in patients with aplastic anemia," *Cancer*, vol. 98, no. 1, pp. 86–93, 2003.
[14] M. Weinberger, I. Elattar, D. Marshall et al., "Patterns of infection in patients with aplastic anemia and the emergence of Aspergillus as a major cause of death," *Medicine (Baltimore)*, vol. 71, no. 1, pp. 24–43, 1992.
[15] K. Vaht, M. Göransson, K. Carlson et al., "Incidence and outcome of acquired aplastic anemia: real-world data from patients diagnosed in Sweden from 2000-2011," *Haematologica*, vol. 102, no. 10, pp. 1683–1690, 2017.
[16] T. Bruun, B. R. Kittang, B. J. de Hoog et al., "Necrotizing soft tissue infections caused by Streptococcus pyogenes and Streptococcus dysgalactiae subsp. equisimilis of groups C and G in western Norway," *Clinical Microbiology and Infections*, vol. 19, no. 12, pp. E545–E550, 2013.
[17] O. Oppegaard, H. Mylvaganam, and B. R. Kittang, "Beta-haemolytic group A, C and G streptococcal infections in Western Norway: a 15-year retrospective survey," *Clinical Microbiology and Infections*, vol. 21, no. 2, pp. 171–178, 2015.
[18] V. V. Vieira, L. M. Teixeira, V. Zahner et al., "Genetic relationships among the different phenotypes of Streptococcus dysgalactiae strains," *International Journal of Systematic Bacteriology*, vol. 48, no. 4, pp. 1231–1243, 1998.
[19] T. Ikebe, S. Murayama, K. Saitoh et al., "Surveillance of severe invasive group-G streptococcal infections and molecular typing of the isolates in Japan," *Epidemiology and Infection*, vol. 132, no. 1, pp. 145–149, 2004.
[20] K. Ekelund, P. Skinhøj, J. Madsen, and H. B. Konradsen, "Invasive group A, B, C and G streptococcal infections in Denmark 1999-2002: epidemiological and clinical aspects," *Clinical Microbiology and Infections*, vol. 11, no. 7, pp. 569–576, 2005.
[21] M. Hindsholm and H. C. Schønheyder, "Clinical presentation and outcome of bacteraemia caused by beta-haemolytic streptococci serogroup G," *Acta Pathologica, Microbiologica et Immunologica Scandinavica: Acta Pathologica Microbiologica et Immunologica Scandinavica*, vol. 110, no. 7-8, pp. 554–558, 2002.
[22] D. L. Stevens, "Could nonsteroidal antiinflammatory drugs (NSAIDs) enhance the progression of bacterial infections to toxic shock syndrome?" *Clinical Infectious Diseases*, vol. 21, no. 4, pp. 977–980, 1995.

[23] C. Souyri, P. Olivier, S. Grolleau, and M. Lapeyre-Mestre, "Severe necrotizing soft-tissue infections and nonsteroidal anti-inflammatory drugs," *Clinical and Experimental Dermatology*, vol. 33, no. 3, pp. 249–255, 2008.
[24] T. Goh, L. G Goh, C. H Ang, and C. H Wong, "Early diagnosis of necrotizing fasciitis," *British Journal of Surgery*, vol. 101, no. 1, pp. e119-25, 2014.
[25] E. Z. Keung, X. Liu, A. Nuzhad, C. Adams, S. W. Ashley, and R. Askari, "Immunocompromised status in patients with necrotizing soft-tissue infection," *JAMA Surgery*, vol. 148, no. 5, pp. 419–426, 2013.
[26] A. Ugarte-Torres, S. Perry, A. Franko, and D. L. Church, "Multidrug-resistant Aeromonas hydrophila causing fatal bilateral necrotizing fasciitis in an immunocompromised patient: a case report," *Journal of Medical Case Reports*, vol. 12, no. 1, p. 326, 2018.
[27] B. W. Duncan, N. S. Adzick, A. A. deLorimier et al., "Necrotizing fasciitis in two children with acute lymphoblastic leukemia," *Journal of Pediatric Surgery*, vol. 27, no. 5, pp. 668–671, 1992.
[28] E. Kolaczkowska and P. Kubes, "Neutrophil recruitment and function in health and inflammation," *Nature Reviews Immunology*, vol. 13, no. 3, pp. 159–175, 2013.
[29] S. M. Opal and T. van der Poll, "Endothelial barrier dysfunction in septic shock," *Journal of Internal Medicine*, vol. 277, no. 3, pp. 277–293, 2015.
[30] M. Bosmann and P. A. Ward, "The inflammatory response in sepsis," *Trends in Immunology*, vol. 34, no. 3, pp. 129–136, 2013.
[31] T. W. Hakkarainen, N. M. Kopari, T. N. Pham, and H. L. Evans, "Necrotizing soft tissue infections: review and current concepts in treatment, systems of care, and outcomes," *Current Problems in Surgery*, vol. 51, no. 8, pp. 344–362, 2014.
[32] T. Calandra, J. Cohen, and I. C. U.C.C., "The international sepsis forum consensus conference on definitions of infection in the intensive care unit," *Critical Care Medicine*, vol. 33, no. 7, pp. 1538–1548, 2005.
[33] Y. Shimomura, K. Okumura, S. Y. Murayama et al., "Complete genome sequencing and analysis of a Lancefield group G Streptococcus dysgalactiae subsp. equisimilis strain causing streptococcal toxic shock syndrome (STSS)," *BMC Genomics*, vol. 12, no. 1, p. 17, 2011.
[34] S. Hashikawa, Y. Iinuma, M. Furushita et al., "Characterization of group C and G streptococcal strains that cause streptococcal toxic shock syndrome," *Journal of Clinical Microbiology*, vol. 42, no. 1, pp. 186–192, 2004.
[35] S. Watanabe, N. Takemoto, K. Ogura, and T. Miyoshi-Akiyama, "Severe invasive streptococcal infection by Streptococcus pyogenes and Streptococcus dysgalactiae subsp. equisimilis," *Microbiology and Immunology*, vol. 60, no. 1, pp. 1–9, 2016.
[36] C. M. Brandt and B. Spellerberg, "Human infections due toStreptococcus dysgalactiaeSubspeciesequisimilis," *Clinical Infectious Diseases*, vol. 49, no. 5, pp. 766–772, 2009.
[37] J. T. Buchanan, A. J. Simpson, R. K. Aziz et al., "DNase expression allows the pathogen group A Streptococcus to escape killing in neutrophil extracellular traps," *Current Biology*, vol. 16, no. 4, pp. 396–400, 2006.
[38] L. Johansson, P. Thulin, D. E. Low, and A. Norrby-Teglund, "Getting under the skin: the immunopathogenesis ofStreptococcus pyogenesDeep tissue infections," *Clinical Infectious Diseases*, vol. 51, no. 1, pp. 58–65, 2010.
[39] A. Norrby-Teglund, S. Chatellier, D. E. Low, A. McGeer, K. Green, and M. Kotb, "Host variation in cytokine responses to superantigens determine the severity of invasive group A streptococcal infection," *European Journal of Immunology*, vol. 30, no. 11, pp. 3247–3255, 2000.
[40] S. Kordasti, B. Costantini, T. Seidl et al., "Deep phenotyping of Tregs identifies an immune signature for idiopathic aplastic anemia and predicts response to treatment," *Blood*, vol. 128, no. 9, pp. 1193–1205, 2016.
[41] S. Rantala, J. Vuopio-Varkila, R. Vuento, H. Huhtala, and J. Syrjänen, "Predictors of mortality in beta-hemolytic streptococcal bacteremia: a population-based study," *Journal of Infection*, vol. 58, no. 4, pp. 266–272, 2009.
[42] K.-F. Huang, M.-H. Hung, Y.-S. Lin et al., "Independent predictors of mortality for necrotizing fasciitis: a retrospective analysis in a single institution," *The Journal of Trauma, Injury, Infection, and Critical Care*, vol. 71, no. 2, pp. 467–473, 2011.
[43] R. Kaul, A. McGeer, D. E. Low, K. Green, B. Schwartz, and A. E. Simor, "Population-based surveillance for group A streptococcal necrotizing fasciitis: clinical features, prognostic indicators, and microbiologic analysis of seventy-seven cases," *The American Journal of Medicine*, vol. 103, no. 1, pp. 18–24, 1997.
[44] C. Hua, E. Sbidian, F. Hemery et al., "Prognostic factors in necrotizing soft-tissue infections (NSTI): a cohort study," *Journal of the American Academy of Dermatology*, vol. 73, no. 6, pp. 1006-1012, 2015.
[45] A. Sharkawy, D. E. Low, R. Saginur et al., "Severe group a streptococcal soft-tissue infections in Ontario: 1992-1996," *Clinical Infectious Diseases*, vol. 34, no. 4, pp. 454–460, 2002.
[46] A. Kumar, C. Haery, B. Paladugu et al., "The duration of hypotension before the initiation of antibiotic treatment is a critical determinant of survival in a murine model ofEscherichia coliSeptic shock: association with serum lactate and inflammatory cytokine levels," *The Journal of Infectious Diseases*, vol. 193, no. 2, pp. 251–258, 2006.
[47] C. Marwick, J. Broomhall, C. McCowan et al., "Severity assessment of skin and soft tissue infections: cohort study of management and outcomes for hospitalized patients," *Journal of Antimicrobial Chemotherapy*, vol. 66, no. 2, pp. 387–397, 2011.
[48] J. Zimbelman, A. Palmer, and J. Todd, "Improved outcome of clindamycin compared with beta-lactam antibiotic treatment for invasive Streptococcus pyogenes infection," *The Pediatric Infectious Disease Journal*, vol. 18, no. 12, pp. 1096–1100, 1999.
[49] Z. D. Mulla, P. E. Leaverton, and S. T. Wiersma, "Invasive group A streptococcal infections in Florida," *Southern Medical Journal*, vol. 96, no. 10, pp. 968–973, 2003.
[50] D. L. Stevens, A. E. Bryant, and S. P. Hackett, "Antibiotic effects on bacterial viability, toxin production, and host response," *Clinical Infectious Diseases*, vol. 20, pp. S154–S157, 1995.

30

Spontaneous Spinal Epidural Hematoma in a Patient on Apixaban for Nonvalvular Atrial Fibrillation

Ahmad El Alayli, Logeswari Neelakandan, and Hicham Krayem

Detroit Medical Center Sinai Grace Hospital, Detroit, MI, USA

Correspondence should be addressed to Ahmad El Alayli; ahmadelalayli@gmail.com

Academic Editor: Håkon Reikvam

Background. With the rise in the use of direct oral anticoagulants (DOACs), more hemorrhagic complications are being encountered. Since the first description of a case of spontaneous spinal epidural hematoma (SSEH) related to the utilization of DOACs in 2012, there have been few reports describing a similar association. However, no cases so far have reported an association between SSEHs and apixaban. *Case Description*: A 76-year-old lady, with a history of nonvalvular atrial fibrillation, presented with a new onset of progressive left lower and upper extremity weakness. She reported back pain and numbness in the left leg up to the knee along with numbness in the left arm up to the shoulder. A CT scan of the neck was suggestive of an epidural hematoma extending from C2-C3 level to C6-C7. As the patient was on apixaban at the time, surgical treatment was delayed for two days to decrease the risk of intraoperative bleeding. Nine days later, she was discharged. Her physical exam was almost unchanged from that on presentation, except for resolution of pain and minimal improvement in motor power in her left lower extremity from 1/5 to 2/5 distally. *Conclusions.* Spinal hematomas represent surgical emergencies with earlier intervention portending better outcome. Based on the few case reports that point to DOACs as a potential culprit, it appears that a high suspicion index resulting in earlier SSEH diagnosis and intervention is crucial for improved neurological outcome and recovery. Prompt diagnosis remains a challenge, especially that SSEH can mimic cerebrovascular accidents.

1. Background

Since the first description of a case of SH associated with the use of a DOAC (rivaroxaban) in 2012 [1], there have been a total of 10 other reports describing both SSEH and spinal subdural hematomas (SSDHs) in association with different DOACs [2–9]. As the use of DOACs continues to increase [10], more similar cases are expected to complicate treatment with these agents. SSEH represents the vast majority of cases of SH [11]. However, no cases so far have been reported about an association between apixaban and SSEH (Table 1). Despite reports of successful medical management [13, 14], surgical decompression remains the cornerstone of management of these patients with earlier intervention correlating with better outcome [15]. However, even with the recent FDA approval of idarucizumab as a reversal agent for dabigatran and andexanet alfa for apixaban and rivaroxaban [16], the limited availability and experience with these agents complicates the timing of surgery. We hope that this case report and literature review will help in establishing a better idea about the optimal management of these patients and raise awareness about the importance of having a high index of suspicion for this condition when encountering a patient on DOACs.

2. Case Report

A 76-year-old African American lady presented to the hospital with new onset weakness and back pain. Her medical history consisted of essential hypertension, atrial fibrillation, abdominal aortic aneurysm, sick sinus syndrome, asthma, and gout. She reported that her back pain started after she came back from the bathroom at 4 : 00 a.m. while trying to sit down on the bed. The patient described the pain as shooting in nature, severe in intensity, and radiating

Table 1: Cases of SSDH and SSEH associated with the use of DOACs described in the literature.

Study	Age of the patient (Years), gender	Presenting symptoms	DOAC used	Site (epidural/ subdural)	Radiographic findings	Intervention used	Time from last DOAC dose to procedure (>24 hours)	Onset of neurologic deficit symptoms to intervention (>24 hours)	Reversal agent used	Recovery/ marked improvement
This case	76, F	Severe back pain and progressing LUE and LLE weakness and numbness	Apixaban	Epidural	CT: epidural hematoma from C2-C3 to C6-C7	C2–C7 laminectomy and hematoma evacuation	Yes	Yes	None	No
Jaeger et al. [1]	61, F	Severe back pain with bilateral LE weakness and numbness	Rivaroxaban	Epidural	MRI: epidural hematoma C2–T8	None	N/A	N/A	None	Yes
Bamps et al. [2]	70, M	Severe cervical pain, tetraplegia, sensory loss, and severe autonomic instability	Dabigatran	Epidural	CT: C2–C4 epidural hematoma	C2–C4 laminectomy and hematoma evacuation	No	No	Prothrombin complex concentrate	Yes
Ozel et al. [3]	69, F	Severe cervical pain followed by quadriplegia	Rivaroxaban	Epidural	CT: C2–C4 epidural hematoma	None	N/A	N/A	None	Yes
Ismail et al. [4]	72, M	Severe back pain, bilateral lower extremities weakness and numbness, and urinary incontinence	Rivaroxaban	Epidural	MRI: T11-L2 epidural hematoma	T11–L2 laminectomy and hematoma evacuation	No	No	Fresh frozen plasma	Yes
Goldfine et al. [5]	74, M	Gradual onset neck pain and waxing and waning paralysis of all extremities with fecal incontinence	Rivaroxaban	Epidural	MRI: foramen magnum-C7 epidural hematoma	Surgery and hematoma evacuation	Yes	No	None	U/K
Zaarour et al. [6]	58, M	Sudden back pain with progressive numbness in bilateral lower extremities followed by progressive weakness	Rivaroxaban	Subdural	MRI: C7-T2 subdural hematoma with edema	Steroids followed by laminectomy and evacuation	Yes	Yes	Aminocaproic acid	Yes

Table 1: Continued.

Study	Age of the patient (Years), gender	Presenting symptoms	DOAC used	Site (epidural/ subdural)	Radiographic findings	Intervention used	Time from last DOAC dose to procedure (>24 hours)	Onset of neurologic deficit symptoms to intervention (>24 hours)	Reversal agent used	Recovery/ marked improvement
Castillo et al. [7]	69, M	Excruciating back pain with progressing lower extremities weakness leading to paraplegia and bowel and bladder dysfunction	Rivaroxaban	Subdural	MRI: T3-Conus medullaris subdural hematoma	Cervical and lumbar CSF drains	Yes	Yes	None	No
Dargazanli et al. [8]	72, M	Back pain, flaccid paraplegia, positive Babinski, thermalogic hypoesthesia, absent knee and ankle reflexes, and decreased anal tone	Rivaroxaban	Subdural	MRI: T6–T8 subdural hematoma	T6–T8 laminectomy with hematoma evacuation, received IV steroids after surgery	Yes	Yes	Prothrombin complex concentrate	No
Colell et al. [9]	75, F	Paraparesis, hyperreflexia, hypoesthesia, no plantar reflex on the left	Dabigatran switched to apixaban before episode	Subdural	MRI: large subdural hemorrhage with discontinuous cervical-dorsal-lumbosacral involvement with secondary spinal cord compression	D1–D3 vertebral laminectomy with hematoma evacuation followed by D4–D7 laminectomy with hematoma evacuation 1 week later	Yes	Yes	None	Yes
Radcliff et al. [12]	53, F	Pain in the right buttock and leg, numbness in bilateral buttock and sensation of incomplete bladder emptying	Rivaroxaban	Epidural	MRI: spinal epidural hematoma at right L4-L5	L4-L5 laminectomy and evacuation of hematoma	U/K	No	None	Yes

down her left arm with no clear exacerbating or relieving factors. Over the following few minutes, she developed progressive weakness in her left lower and upper extremities and later on became unable to move her left leg which led to her being transferred to the Medical Intensive Care Unit. She also developed numbness in her left leg up to the level of the knee and in her left arm up to the level of the shoulder. There was no history of any urinary or stool incontinence or retention or any previous similar episodes.

The patient had been recently diagnosed with atrial fibrillation one month prior to presentation in an outside hospital and had since been maintained on apixaban 1 tablet 5 mg twice daily. Her other home medications included alprazolam, allopurinol, losartan, hydrochlorothiazide, and metoprolol. She reported full compliance with her medications prior to presentation. A dual chamber pacemaker was inserted 11 days before this visit in an outside hospital, and her other surgical history included a hysterectomy several years ago for uterine fibroids. She denied any history of smoking, alcohol abuse, or illicit substances usage. The patient did not have previous bleeding history.

The patient's vital signs on presentation were within normal limits, and her neurological exam showed a patient alert and oriented to time, place, and person with intact speech. Her motor power was 5/5 in her right upper extremity proximally and 4/5 distally and 3/5 in her left upper extremity proximally and 1/5 distally. In her lower extremities, the motor power was 5/5 on the right and 1/5 all over on the left. She had decreased sensation to light touch in her left upper and lower extremities. She had no clonus, and Hoffman and Babinski signs were negative bilaterally. Her reflexes were 2+ all over and symmetric.

Initial lab tests were significant for hypokalemia (3.1 mmol/L), leukocytosis (12700 WBCs per microliter), and slight anemia with a hemoglobin level of 9.3 g/dl with unknown baseline. Her other lab tests including liver function and renal function were within normal limits.

Given her presentation of acute focal neurological deficit, a noncontrast head CT scan was ordered and showed signs of chronic vascular ischemic disease only. The patient continued to have severe back pain, and having a history of abdominal aortic aneurysm, an acute aortic dissection was suspected, and hence, a CT angiogram of the abdomen, pelvis, and thorax was ordered. The CT angiogram did not show any signs of aortic dissection. A CT scan of the neck was performed to investigate the cause of the left upper extremity weakness and numbness. It showed an epidural soft tissue density extending along the left aspect of the spinal canal causing compression and marked rightward deviation of the cord concerning for an epidural hematoma extending from C2-C3 level to C6-C7 (Figure 1).

As the patient was on apixaban at the time, a decision was made to delay surgical treatment for 2 days to decrease the risk of intraoperative bleeding. A C2-C7 laminectomy, hematoma exclusion, and spinal fusion were then performed. On discharge, 9 days later, her physical exam was mostly unchanged from that on presentation except for the resolution of pain and improvement in motor power in her left lower extremity from 1/5 to 2/5 distally.

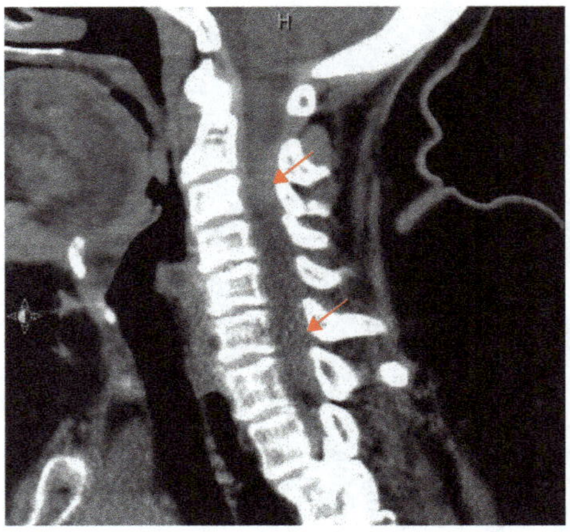

FIGURE 1: Sagittal CT scan image showing posterior epidural hematoma.

3. Discussion and Conclusions

Spinal hematomas represent surgical emergencies with earlier intervention portending better outcome [15]. The acute presentation, however, represents an important diagnostic challenge [15] especially as a mimicker of cerebrovascular accidents [18]. Even though no direct trauma is involved in spontaneous spinal hematomas, some activities have been associated with onset such as stretch exercises [19] and Valsalva maneuvers during trumpet playing [20] and defecation [3], for example, which might have been the case in our patient as well. Even though new reversal agents have been recently approved for dabigatran, apixaban, and rivaroxaban [16], the lack of their widespread use makes it essential to identify the best evidence-supported choice for surgical timing of evacuation. Based on the few case reports that have been published so far, it seems that the benefit of earlier intervention outweighs the risk of surgical bleed.

According to our literature review, 4 patients underwent surgical intervention within 24 hours of symptoms onset, and 3 of these 4 patients (75%) had excellent outcomes with unknown outcome in the third one [2, 4, 5]. Preceding the emergent surgical interventions, prothrombin complex concentrate was given to one patient and fresh frozen plasma to the other which has been shown in some previous studies to be an effective reversal method for factor X inhibitors [21]. There was no associated bleeding with either surgical intervention. On the other hand, 5 cases (including this report) had delayed surgical intervention (>24 hours) [5–9]. Among these cases, only 2 had good recovery (40%), and 3 had bad outcomes. No perioperative bleed was reported in any of the cases. The short follow-up period in most of these articles including ours (9 days) represent a major limiting factor in most of these reports.

The number of cases reported is insufficient to reach any statistically significant result, but seems to be pointing towards the importance of early surgical intervention for neurologic recovery. With the development of new reversal agents and increased experience with the current ones, earlier surgical intervention is most likely to increase in frequency as surgeons become more comfortable operating on these patients leading hopefully to less neurologic deficit. This means that a high suspicion index leading to earlier diagnosis is key for timely intervention, and we hope that this article will help in raising awareness about this condition as a potential complication of DOACs use, especially with the significant and continuous increase in their utilization.

Abbreviations

DOACs: Direct oral anticoagulants
SH: Spinal hematoma
SSEH: Spontaneous spinal epidural hematoma
SSDH: Spinal subdural hematoma.

Consent

A consent form was obtained and signed by the patient and kept in her medical records.

Authors' Contributions

AE reviewed the literature, collected and analyzed the data, and wrote the manuscript. LN gathered the history, examined the patient, and reviewed and edited the manuscript. HK reviewed and edited the manuscript.

References

[1] M. Jaeger, B. Jeanneret, and S. Schaeren, "Spontaneous spinal epidural haematoma during Factor Xa inhibitor treatment (Rivaroxaban)," *European Spine Journal*, vol. 21, no. Suppl 4, pp. S433–S435, 2012.

[2] S. Bamps, T. Decramer, N. Vandenbussche et al., "Dabigatran-associated spontaneous acute cervical epidural hematoma," *World Neurosurgery*, vol. 83, no. 2, pp. 257-258, 2015.

[3] O. Ozel, E. Demircay, A. Kircelli, and T. Cansever, "Atypical presentation of an epidural hematoma in a patient receiving rivaroxaban after total hip arthroplasty," *Orthopedics*, vol. 39, no. 3, pp. e558–e560, 2015.

[4] R. Ismail, E. Zaghrini, and E. Hitti, "Spontaneous spinal epidural hematoma IN a patient ON rivaroxaban: case report and literature review," *The Journal of Emergency Medicine*, vol. 53, no. 4, pp. 536–539, 2017.

[5] C. Goldfine, C. Glazer, and R. Ratzan, "Spontaneous spinal epidural hematoma from rivaroxaban," *Clinical Practice and Cases in Emergency Medicine*, vol. 2, no. 2, pp. 151–154, 2018.

[6] M. Zaarour, S. Hassan, N. Thumallapally, and Q. Dai, "Rivaroxaban-induced nontraumatic spinal subdural hematoma: an uncommon yet life-threatening complication," *Case Reports in Hematology*, vol. 2015, Article ID 275380, 5 pages, 2015.

[7] J. M. Castillo, H. F. Afanador, E. Manjarrez, and X. A. Morales, "Non-traumatic spontaneous spinal subdural hematoma in a patient with non-valvular atrial fibrillation during treatment with rivaroxaban," *American Journal of Case Reports*, vol. 16, pp. 377–381, 2015.

[8] C. Dargazanli, N. Lonjon, and G. Gras-Combe, "Non-traumatic spinal subdural hematoma complicating direct factor Xa inhibitor treatment (rivaroxaban): a challenging management," *European Spine Journal*, vol. 25, no. Suppl 1, pp. S100–S103, 2016.

[9] A. Colell, A. Arboix, F. Caiazzo, and E. Grivé, "Iatrogenic spinal subdural hematoma due to apixaban: a case report and review of the literature," *Case Reports in Hematology*, vol. 2018, Article ID 4507638, 5 pages, 2018.

[10] E. Biggs, V. Allan, and S. Vermes, "Noacs versus warfarin use IN the management of atrial fibrillation patients," *Journal of the American College of Cardiology*, vol. 69, no. 11, p. 345, 2017.

[11] D. Kreppel, G. Antoniadis, and W. Seeling, "Spinal hematoma: a literature survey with meta-analysis of 613 patients," *Neurosurgical Review*, vol. 26, no. 1, pp. 1–49, 2003.

[12] K. E. Radcliff, A. Ong, J. Parvizi, Z. Post, and F. Orozco, "Rivaroxaban-induced epidural hematoma and cauda equina syndrome after total knee arthroplasty: a case report," *Orthopaedic Surgery*, vol. 6, no. 1, pp. 69–71, 2014.

[13] S. A. Borkar, G. L. Prasad, G. D. Satyarthee, and A. K. Mahapatra, "Spontaneous spinal extradural hematoma in a child with hemophilia B, surgery or medical management—a dilemma?" *Journal of Pediatric Neurosciences*, vol. 6, pp. 131–133, 2011.

[14] S. J. Hentschel, A. R. Woolfenden, and D. J. Fairholm, "Resolution of spontaneous spinal epidural hematoma without surgery," *Spine*, vol. 26, no. 22, pp. E525–E527, 2001.

[15] M. T. Lawton, R. W. Porter, J. E. Heiserman, R. Jacobowitz, V. K. H. Sonntag, and C. A. Dickman, "Surgical management of spinal epidural hematoma: relationship between surgical timing and neurological outcome," *Journal of Neurosurgery*, vol. 83, no. 1, pp. 1–7, 1995.

[16] P. Gelosa, L. Castiglioni, M. Tenconi et al., "Pharmacokinetic drug interactions of the non-vitamin K antagonist oral anticoagulants (NOACs)," *Pharmacological Research*, vol. 135, pp. 60–79, 2018.

[17] M. Messerer, J. Dubourg, S. Diabira, T. Robert, and A. Hamlat, "Spinal epidural hematoma," *European Journal of Emergency Medicine*, vol. 19, no. 1, pp. 2–8, 2012.

[18] T. Akimoto, T. Yamada, S. Shinoda, Y. Asano, and D. Nagata, "Spontaneous spinal epidural hematoma as a potentially important stroke mimic," *Journal of Central Nervous System Disease*, vol. 6, pp. 15–20, 2014.

[19] T. Abe, Y. Nagamine, S. Ishimatsu, and Y. Tokuda, "Spinal epidural hematoma after stretch exercise: a case report," *American Journal of Emergency Medicine*, vol. 27, pp. 902.e1-902.e2, 2009.

[20] S. David, R. F. Salluzzo, J. M. Bartfield, and E. T. Dickinson, "Spontaneous cervicothoracic epidural hematoma following prolonged Valsalva secondary to trumpet playing," *The American Journal of Emergency Medicine*, vol. 15, no. 1, pp. 73–75, 1997.

[21] M. N. Smith, L. Deloney, C. Carter, K. A. Weant, and E. A. Eriksson, "Safety, efficacy and cost of four-factor prothrombin complex concentrate (4F-PCC) in patients with factor Xa inhibitor-related bleeding: a retrospective study," *Journal of Thrombosis and Thrombolysis*, vol. 48, no. 2, pp. 250–255, 2019.

31

Inherited Moderate Factor X Deficiency Presenting as Cardiac Tamponade

Tamer Othman,[1] **Ayman Abdelkarim**,[1] **Karen Huynh**,[1] **An Uche**,[2] **and Jennifer Lee**[2]

[1]*Department of Internal Medicine, Harbor-UCLA Medical Center, Torrance, CA, USA*
[2]*Division of Hematology and Medical Oncology, Harbor-UCLA Medical Center, Torrance, CA, USA*

Correspondence should be addressed to Tamer Othman; tothman2@dhs.lacounty.gov

Academic Editor: Eduardo Arellano-Rodrigo

Factor X deficiency is a rare bleeding disorder that varies in the severity of its clinical manifestations. The symptoms of this disorder can occur at any age, although most severe cases appear in childhood. The rarity of this condition has not allowed for the establishment of evidence-based management guidelines, and thus, individuals afflicted with factor X deficiency are treated based on limited literature and the opinions of clinicians with extensive experience. In this case report, we discuss a unique presentation of a 38-year-old male who was found to have cardiac tamponade as a result of his newly diagnosed inherited moderate factor X deficiency. This was discovered by obtaining a factor X activity assay and confirmed with genetic testing which demonstrated a missense variant on the factor X gene on chromosome 13. His management involved correction of his factor X deficiency with fresh frozen plasma, a pericardiocentesis, and placement of a pericardial window. He has been asymptomatic and without hemorrhagic episodes for the 10 months following his discharge.

1. Introduction

Factor X is a vitamin K-dependent coagulation factor that is produced by the liver and is responsible for converting prothrombin to thrombin [1]. Factor X deficiency can be acquired or inherited. Inherited factor X deficiency is a very rare autosomal recessive coagulation disorder that affects 1 in every 1 million people and accounts for 10% of all rare bleeding diseases [2]. Individuals with homozygous factor X deficiency generally present early in life with severe bleeding symptoms, whereas heterozygotes, though typically clinically asymptomatic, may experience major bleeding if they undergo a major surgery or traumatic injury [3]. Acquired factor X deficiency is also rare, but when it occurs it is usually in the setting of amyloidosis.

2. Case Summary

A 38-year-old Hispanic male, born in Mexico, with no known chronic medical problems presented with a 4-day history of dyspnea on exertion and orthopnea, along with positional and pleuritic chest pain. He also endorsed a dry cough that had been ongoing for months without hemoptysis. He denied fevers, chills, night sweats, unintentional weight loss, or recent trauma. He was not seen in a healthcare setting for years. He was not taking any medications at home and had no recent exposure to anticoagulants. There was no family history of bleeding disorders. He endorsed some episodes of epistaxis during the summer months and waking up in the morning with his face covered in blood in the past, but denied a personal history of bleeding from other mucosal surfaces such as gum bleeding, hematuria, hematochezia, melena, prolonged bleeding after dental procedures and a tooth extraction, swelling in joints, and spontaneous skin bruising. He had an appendectomy 14 years prior and recalls complications, such as prolonged bleeding that required blood product transfusions and a second surgery; however, details from that hospitalization are unknown. Physical exam was only remarkable for obesity, trace bilateral pretibial pitting edema, and an old appendectomy scar. Initial labs revealed a platelet count of 477 and a coagulation profile that is summarized in Table 1.

TABLE 1: Coagulation profile and mixing studies of the patient.

Prothrombin time (seconds)	69.3 (reference range: 12–14.2)
International normalized ratio	8.10 (reference range: 0.90–1.11)
Activated partial thromboplastin time (seconds)	70.5 (reference range: 24.7–35.3)
Thrombin time (seconds)	15.4 (reference range: 14.5–18.5)
PT 50/10 mixing study (seconds)	13.5 (reference range: 12–14.2)
aPTT 50/50 mixing study (seconds)	28.5 (reference range: 24.7–35.3)

A bedside ultrasound of the heart revealed a large circumferential pericardial effusion and right atrial collapse. A subsequent transthoracic echo (TTE) confirmed the large, circumferential pericardial effusion along with echo and Doppler evidence of tamponade (Figure 1). Further laboratory workup of coagulopathy revealed a factor X level of 1%. The rest of his tested factor activity levels are summarized in Table 2.

The patient received a one-time dose of aspirin 324 mg in the emergency room, and was then started on colchicine 0.6 mg twice daily for treatment of pericarditis. Nonsteroidal anti-inflammatory drugs were not administered during his hospital course due to his high risk of bleeding. The initial plan to correct his factor X deficiency in preparation for a pericardiocentesis was to administer 20 mL/kg of fresh frozen plasma (FFP) [4], but after receiving 1 unit of fresh FFP on day 4 of admission, he developed a urticarial transfusion reaction, so the transfusion was stopped and he was given famotidine 20 mg and diphenhydramine 25 mg. Due to this transfusion reaction, he was slowly administered FFP to correct his factor X deficiency over the next few days, receiving 1 more unit on day 5 and 2 more units on day 6, which he tolerated well. A pericardiocentesis with pericardial drain tube placement was performed on day 6 of admission with significant hemorrhagic drainage over the subsequent days. As a result, he received 3 more units of FFP on day 8, 4 units of FFP on day 9, and 2 units of FFP on day 10 prior to undergoing a pericardial window procedure. Postoperative TTE revealed a residual, but stable pericardial effusion without evidence of tamponade. The decision to administer FFP during his hospital course was based on his continuous hemorrhagic drainage rather than a goal factor X activity level due to his transfusion reaction and was only guided by his internationalized normal ratio (INR) prior to undergoing a procedure. He underwent reversal of his coagulopathy with oral vitamin K 10 mg for 5 days, and 13 units of FFP total. As a result, his factor X activity level rose to as high as 15%. Other options that were considered to reverse his coagulopathy were prothrombin complex concentrates (PCCs) and high-purity, plasma-derived factor X concentrate (pdFX). PCC was not administered due to a factor IX activity level above the upper limit of normal and the risk of thrombotic complications, and pdFX was not readily available at our institution. The etiology of his tamponade was thought to be related to pericarditis, with coagulopathy due to factor X deficiency leading to hemopericardium. Evaluation for amyloidosis, which included a serum protein electrophoresis (SPEP), a urine protein electrophoresis (UPEP), serum light chains, cytology of the pericardial fluid, and pathology of the surgical sample of his pericardium, was unremarkable. The patient was discharged without active bleeding or reaccumulation of the pericardial effusion. Repeat factors VII and X levels 10 months after discharge were 110% and 2%, respectively. Outpatient genetic testing revealed a homozygous missense variant that resulted in a single amino acid substitution of glycine to arginine at codon 21 in exon 1 of the factor X gene product.

3. Discussion

Factor X is a vitamin K-dependent serine protease that is positioned at the convergence of the extrinsic and intrinsic pathways of the clotting cascade and plays a crucial role in the coagulation pathway as the first enzyme in the common pathway to cross-linked fibrin clot formation [5, 6]. Factor X deficiency can be either inherited in an autosomal recessive manner or acquired. Acquired factor X deficiency is usually associated with amyloidosis but may also be due to anticoagulant therapy, underlying liver disease, medications (such as phenytoin), and paraproteinemia [1, 3].

The presentation of factor X deficiency is highly variable and symptoms can develop at any age. Generally, however, the more severe disorders present earlier on in life. Another case report demonstrates that moderate factor X deficiency does not necessarily present early in life or as a spontaneous hemorrhage as in our patient [7].

Patients with factor X deficiency are classified into 3 groups depending on the functional assay level: mild if it ranges from 6 to 10%, moderate if it ranges from 1 to 4%, and severe if it is <1% [1]. Our patient was diagnosed with moderate factor X deficiency as his initial factor X activity level was 1% in the acute bleeding setting and increased to 2% upon recovery 2 months later, which is likely a more accurate representation of his baseline physiological factor X activity level. His history and medical workup were negative for an acquired etiology, and genetic testing confirmed a hereditary etiology of factor X deficiency. In general, a diagnosis of inherited factor X deficiency is based upon identification of characteristic symptoms, a detailed patient and family history, a thorough clinical evaluation, and a variety of specialized tests, such as the factor X functional activity assay. Molecular genetic testing can confirm a diagnosis of inherited factor X deficiency, but is usually not necessary. In a clinical setting, molecular genetic testing can be challenging due to costs and the limited availability of the test as it is only available as a diagnostic service at specialized laboratories. Thus, the decision to pursue molecular genetic testing for factor X deficiency would be left to the discretion of the clinician.

One study looked at several important registries to summarize the bleeding symptoms reported as a result of

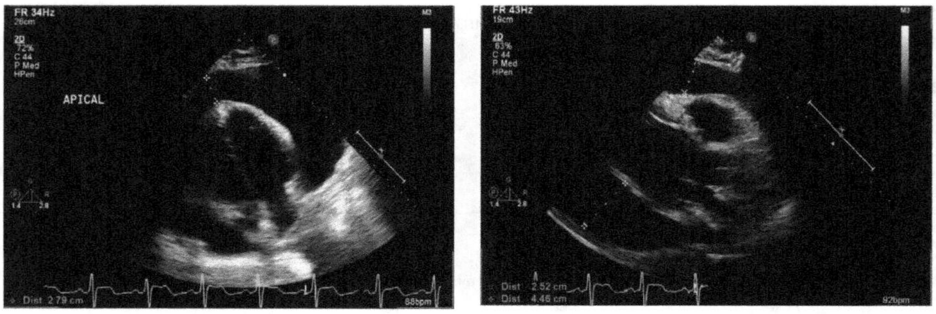

(a) (b)

Figure 1: Apical (a) and parasternal (b) long axis views of the hemorrhagic pericardial effusion on presentation.

Table 2: Factor activity assays of the patient.

Factor II activity (%)	116 (reference range: 70–150)
Factor V activity (%)	71 (reference range: 65–150)
Factor VII activity (%)	43 (reference range: 60–150)
Factor IX activity (%)	173 (reference range: 60–150)
Factor X activity (%)	1 (reference range: 60–150)

factor X deficiency. The registries examined were the Greifswald Registry of Factor X Deficiency in Europe and Latin America, the Rare Bleeding Disorder Registry in North America, population registries of inherited bleeding disorders from the UK Hemophilia Centre Directors' Organization, and the Hemophilia Surveillance System in Iran [6]. The symptoms described included easy bruising, epistaxis, gum bleeding, menorrhagia, hematuria, hematomas, hemarthrosis, GI bleeding, intracranial hemorrhage, and umbilical cord bleeding. To our knowledge, a hemorrhagic pericardial effusion causing cardiac tamponade has not been reported as a manifestation of factor X deficiency, thus making our patient's presentation unique.

Factor X deficiency is typically suspected when both prothrombin time and activated partial thromboplastin time are elevated and correct with a mixing study. Factor X deficiency can be investigated by either a functional activity assay, an immunological assay, or a chromogenic assay. Immunologic and chromogenic assays can miss dysfunctional factor X activity and thus should not be used to screen for factor X deficiency [6].

There are currently no evidence-based management guidelines for factor X deficiency due to the rarity of this condition. Guidelines for management of factor X deficiency have been published by the United Kingdom Haemophilia Centre Doctors' Organization based on the available literature and extensive clinical experience [8]. Minor bleeding symptoms may be managed by topical therapies and antifibrinolytic agents, such as tranexamic acid or epsilon-aminocaproic acid. More severe bleeding symptoms may require factor X replacement with FFP. Alternative agents that may be used to reverse the coagulopathy from factor X deficiency include PCC and pdFX [9, 10]. Adverse events associated with FFP include allergic reactions and transfusion-related acute lung injury, while PCC is associated with hypercoagulable complications, such as disseminated intravascular coagulation (DIC) and venous thromboembolism (VTE) [6]. Investigations of the efficacy and safety of pdFX have shown no serious adverse events related to its administration [10, 11].

For patients undergoing surgery or require treatment for active bleeding, a target factor X activity level has not been established. A factor X activity level of 1–40% may be adequate for hemostasis and should not exceed 50% due to an increased risk of VTE [1, 6]. Prophylactic factor replacement therapy has been used in patients with hemophilia A and B to prevent recurrent hemarthrosis and reduce joint damage [12, 13], but there are no clear guidelines regarding prophylactic factor replacement therapy in factor X deficiency [6].

Since our patient's factor IX level was above the upper limit of normal, he was treated with FFP rather than PCC due to its association with VTE. pdFX is not readily available at our institution. FFP was given until the hemorrhagic drainage from his pericardial drain resolved. Hemostasis was achieved for this patient at a factor X activity level of 15%. Since the patient was stable with no significant bleeding, close monitoring was favored over prophylactic replacement therapy.

Of note, our patient had a factor VII level of 43% in the setting of an acute bleed. Patient's with factor VII levels >10% generally do not exhibit bleeding symptoms [14]. Therefore, the thought was that the factor X deficiency was responsible for his presentation and was thus the target of his diagnostic workup. To confirm a factor VII deficiency diagnosis however, the factor VII assay should be repeated at least once [15]. The repeat factor VII level for our patient once his bleeding resolved was 110%, which is likely a more accurate representation of his baseline physiologic factor VII activity. The mild decrease in his factor VII activity level was possibly due to consumption of his factor VII due to his ongoing bleeding on presentation, which was restored to normal limits with resolution of his bleeding.

A combined factor VII and X deficiency has been reported in the literature; however [16], this combined factor deficiency may be due to coincidental inheritance of separate coagulation factor deficiencies, such as a missense variation in both factor VII and factor X genes or a large deletion on the long arm of chromosome 13 involving both the factor VII and factor X gene. Determining the mechanism of a combined factor VII and factor X deficiency has clinical ramifications. Firstly, it can change management in certain circumstances that require coagulation factor repletion, as not all PCC preparations contain factor VII [17]. Additionally, it can assist with predicting patterns of inheritance and genetic counseling. As the patient's family denied bleeding symptoms, there are no plans for genetic testing of other family members, and as explained previously is usually not necessary to diagnose inherited factor X deficiency, but the patient was educated on the inheritance pattern of his disorder and the possibility of other family members inheriting this rare disorder. Family members may benefit from screening of coagulation studies, namely PTT, for risk stratification prior to surgical procedures.

In conclusion, factor X deficiency is a very rare disease, and as a result, not all potential bleeding complications have been reported, such as a hemorrhagic pericardial effusion causing cardiac tamponade. Furthermore, a lack of evidence-based management guidelines for this disease is due to the rarity of this condition and thus, management is based primarily on limited literature and clinical experience. This case report highlights a unique presentation of factor X deficiency and our management plan for this patient in the absence of evidence-based guidelines. Determining management by assessing clinical symptoms as opposed to laboratory values may be a valid strategy in the treatment of other rare disorders that lack evidence-based management guidelines.

References

[1] T. Chatterjee, J. Philip, V. Nair et al., "Inherited factor X (stuart-prower factor) deficiency and its management," *Medical Journal Armed Forces India*, vol. 71, no. 1, pp. S184–S186, 2015.

[2] M. Menegatti and F. Peyvandi, "Factor X deficiency," *Seminars in Thrombosis and Hemostasis*, vol. 35, no. 4, pp. 407–415, 2009.

[3] J. Uprichard and D. J. Perry, "Factor X deficiency," *Blood Reviews*, vol. 16, no. 2, pp. 97–110, 2002.

[4] P. M. Mannucci, S. Duga, and F. Peyvandi, "Recessively inherited coagulation disorders," *Blood*, vol. 104, no. 5, pp. 1243–1252, 2004.

[5] D. J. Perry, "Factor X and its deficiency states," *Haemophilia*, vol. 3, no. 3, pp. 159–172, 1997.

[6] D. L. Brown and P. A. Kouides, "Diagnosis and treatment of inherited factor X deficiency," *Haemophilia*, vol. 14, no. 6, pp. 1176–1182, 2008.

[7] M.-A. van Dievoet, I. Leclercq, C. Hermans et al., "Does haemophilia slow down the development of liver fibrosis?," *Haemophilia*, vol. 25, no. 1, pp. e32–e35, 2019.

[8] P. H. B. Bolton Maggs, D. J. Perry, E. A. Chalmers et al., "The rare coagulation disorders—review with guidelines for management from the United Kingdom haemophilia centre doctors' organisation," *Haemophilia*, vol. 10, no. 5, pp. 593–628, 2004.

[9] A. J. Siddon and C. A. Tormey, "Successful use of four factor-prothrombin complex concentrate for congenital factor X deficiency in the setting of neurosurgery," *Laboratory Medicine*, vol. 47, no. 3, pp. e35–e37, 2016.

[10] M. A. Escobar, G. Auerswald, S. Austin, J. N. Huang, M. Norton, and C. M. Millar, "Experience of a new high-purity factor X concentrate in subjects with hereditary factor X deficiency undergoing surgery," *Haemophilia*, vol. 22, no. 5, pp. 713–720, 2016.

[11] S. K. Austin, K. Kavakli, M. Norton, F. Peyvandi, A. Shapiro, and The FX Investigators Group, "Efficacy, safety and pharmacokinetics of a new high-purity factor X concentrate in subjects with hereditary factor X deficiency," *Haemophilia*, vol. 22, no. 3, pp. 419–425, 2016.

[12] J. Oldenburg, "Optimal treatment strategies for hemophilia: achievements and limitations of current prophylactic regimens," *Blood*, vol. 125, no. 13, pp. 2038–2044, 2015.

[13] G. Castaman, "The benefits of prophylaxis in patients with hemophilia B," *Expert Review of Hematology*, vol. 11, no. 8, pp. 673–683, 2018.

[14] F. Benlakhal, T. Mura, J.-F. Schved, and M. Giansily-Blaizot, "A retrospective analysis of 157 surgical procedures performed without replacement therapy in 83 unrelated factor VII-deficient patients," *Journal of Thrombosis and Haemostasis*, vol. 9, no. 6, pp. 1149–1156, 2011.

[15] M. Napolitano, S. Siragusa, and G. Mariani, "Factor VII deficiency: clinical phenotype, genotype and therapy," *Journal of Clinical Medicine*, vol. 6, no. 4, p. 38, 2017.

[16] A. Pavlova, B. Preisler, J. Driesen et al., "Congenital combined deficiency of coagulation factors VII and X—different genetic mechanisms," *Haemophilia*, vol. 21, no. 3, pp. 386–391, 2015 May.

[17] M. Franchini and G. Lippi, "Prothrombin complex concentrates: an update," *Journal of Blood Transfusion*, vol. 8, no. 3, pp. 149–154, 2010.

32

Severe Thrombocytopenia Associated with Dengue Fever: An Evidence-Based Approach to Management of Thrombocytopenia

Sulagna Das,[1] **Charles Abreu**,[1] **Micah Harris**,[2] **John Shrader**,[1] **and Satish Sarvepalli**[1]

[1]*Department of Medicine, Kettering Health, Dayton, OH, USA*
[2]*Boonshoft School of Medicine, Wright State University, Dayton, OH, USA*

Correspondence should be addressed to Charles Abreu; charles.abreu@ketteringhealth.org

Academic Editor: Håkon Reikvam

Dengue is a mosquito-borne viral illness common in tropical and subtropical countries but very rare in the United States. Patients infected with dengue often present with thrombocytopenia. In the setting of dengue, platelet transfusions as a treatment for thrombocytopenia have no clear benefits in reduction of severe bleeding or improvement of the platelet count. Here, we present a case of a traveler infected with dengue virus and discuss the approach to treat thrombocytopenia.

1. Introduction

The dengue virus (DENV) is the most common arbovirus in the world transmitted by the Aedes aegypti mosquito. The virus belongs to the Flaviviridae family, and the disease can be spread by one of the four types: DENV-1, DENV-2, DENV-3, and DENV-4. Dengue is rare in the United States and is often described as the "fever in the returned traveler" due to its common presentation in travelers returning from an endemic region such as the tropical areas of Southeast Asia and the Caribbean [1, 2].

The course of illness ranges from asymptomatic to life-threatening, and incubation typically lasts three to fourteen days. Secondary infection with a second serotype often results in a worse prognosis. The three phases of infection include febrile, critical, and recovery. The febrile phase begins around day four to seven of infection and lasts around three to seven days. Fever is sudden during onset and typically high (greater than 40°C), lasting two to seven days. It can be accompanied by myalgias, arthralgias, nausea, vomiting, diarrhea, abdominal pain, lymphadenopathy, hepatomegaly, maculopapular rash, leukopenia, thrombocytopenia, and transaminitis [3]. The critical phase of infection can be followed after defervescence and is more common in patients with secondary infection and other comorbidities [4]. Thrombocytopenia is common and can occur with vascular leakage, shock, and organ impairment [5]. Theorized mechanisms for thrombocytopenia include platelet activation, which causes attachment to the vascular wall forming thrombi and removal from circulation, immune cytotoxic effects through opsonization of platelets and direct infection of platelets, and megakaryocytes by the virus [6]. The recovery phase occurs with resolution and stabilization of vitals. Diagnosis is with serology of antidengue IgM, and treatment is supportive [3].

Given the rarity of dengue in the United States, physicians should start to consider dengue when patients present with a history of travel from an endemic region and suggestive clinical symptoms. Here, we describe a case of dengue fever in a traveler from an endemic region presenting with severe thrombocytopenia.

2. Case

A 47-year-old Asian Indian male with no significant past medical history, who came from India four days prior to admission, presented with fever with diffuse body aches to hospital in the Midwestern United States. He stated that he was fully vaccinated for COVID-19. As stagnant water is a breeding source for mosquitoes when asked, the patient did mention having air conditioning (AC) in his house, a common source for stagnant water. He stated that he turned his AC on a few times this year, and then, for the last two months, it had been off. The patient's mother was diagnosed with dengue recently in India. The patient also reported that since it is very common to get mosquito bites in India, he did not pay attention and was not sure if he recently noticed increased mosquito bites. The patient denied any petechiae, hematuria, hematemesis, or melena. On admission, his labs were significant for creatine kinase 999 U/L, lactate dehydrogenase 663 U/L, platelet count 41 K/μL, D-dimer 2664 ng/mL, and aspartate aminotransferase (AST) 141 U/L. Peripheral smear was negative for malaria, and Lyme serology was negative. On day 2 of admission, the platelet count dropped to 11 K/μL, and he received 1 unit of platelet transfusion with improvement of his platelet count to 18 K/μL, but within the next 6 hours, the platelet count dropped to 10 K/μL. Infectious disease and hematology-oncology were consulted, and the recommendation was given to not transfuse platelets anymore unless platelets dropped below 10 K/μL as it could increase the risk of volume overload. On day three, the patient was noted to have petechiae on his lower extremities (Figure 1). Over the next few days, the platelet counts continued to fluctuate between 11 K/μL and 18 K/μL. From day five, continued improvement was noted in the platelet count, and the creatinine kinase level came down to reference range levels. Petechiae resolved by day seven, and the patient's appetite continued to improve. The patient was discharged on day seven when his platelet was 35 K/μL, and he had no episodes of bleeding. On outpatient follow-up two days later, his platelet count had improved to 172 K/μL. Two weeks later, his dengue fever antibody IgG resulted positive with a titer of 7.07 ISR.

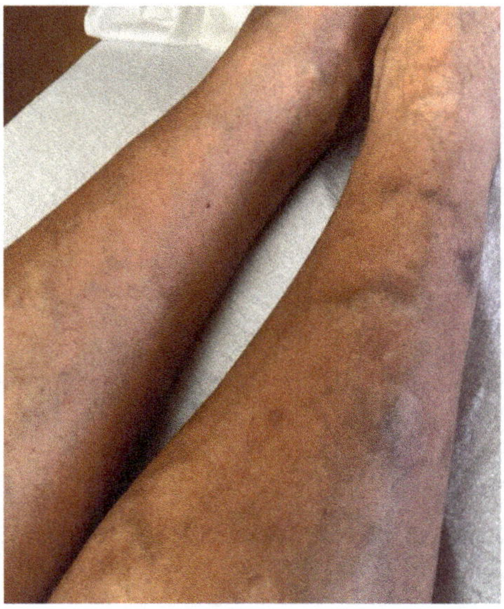

Figure 1: Petechiae.

3. Discussion

Thrombocytopenia is a very common clinical manifestation in dengue. Although there are several hypotheses, the mechanisms involved in thrombocytopenia and bleeding manifestation during DENV infection are not fully understood. By interrupting their function, DENV could directly or indirectly affect bone marrow progenitor cells [7] to reduce the proliferative capacity of hematopoietic cells [8]. Evidence suggests that DENV can induce bone marrow hypoplasia during the acute phase of the disease [9]. Thrombocytopenia in dengue may arise either from decreased production of cells from the bone marrow or from increased peripheral destruction of platelets and clearance from peripheral blood. A high mean platelet volume (MPV) indicates enhanced platelet destruction in patients. MPV is usually either high or normal in dengue patients; therefore, excessive platelet destruction could be the main reason for thrombocytopenia in dengue patients.

The cross-reactive antibodies anti-NS1, prM, and E viral proteins against platelets, endothelial cells, or coagulatory molecules may cause platelet dysfunction, endothelial cell damage, coagulation defects, and macrophage activation. Hemorrhage and plasma leakage in dengue hemorrhagic fever result from vascular fragility due to impaired platelet functions. Several studies showed that the platelet count in dengue hemorrhagic fever (DHF)/dengue fever showed a significant decrease on the fourth day of the illness. In fact, previous studies reported DHF in adults without shock, in which platelet counts mildly to moderately decreased on the third day until the seventh day of illness and reached normal levels on the eighth or ninth day [10–12]. In our case, the platelet count started to improve from day seven and came to normal by day ten.

According to clinical guidelines, platelet transfusions should be given to patients who develop serious hemorrhagic manifestations or have very low platelet counts, platelet counts falling below $10–20 \times 10^9$/L. In a study of 106 pediatric patients with dengue with thrombocytopenia and coagulopathy, there was no significant difference in hemorrhage between patients who received preventive transfusions compared to those who did not. Patients who received transfusion had a higher frequency of pulmonary edema and the increased length of hospitalization [13]. There were significant side effects with platelet transfusions, and it did not prevent the development of severe bleeding or shorten the time to bleeding cessation. Thus, according to the authors, platelet transfusions should not be routinely performed in the management of dengue [14, 15].

4. Conclusion

Since dengue viral illness is quite rare in the United States, clinicians should always consider dengue in their differentials if travelers from tropical countries present with suggestive symptoms. Thrombocytopenia is a very common clinical manifestation in dengue. The platelet count may drop very abruptly, but most of the time it follows its own clinical course and should be managed conservatively. It is very important for clinicians to know that platelet transfusions have no benefit in treating thrombocytopenia in dengue and should be avoided as they may cause significant side effects.

References

[1] S. Bhatt, P. W. Gething, O. J. Brady et al., "The global distribution and burden of dengue," *Nature*, vol. 496, no. 7446, pp. 504–507, 2013.

[2] L. E. Adams, S. W. Martin, N. P. Lindsey et al., "Epidemiology of dengue, chikungunya, and zika virus disease in U.S. States and territories, 2017," *The American Journal of Tropical Medicine and Hygiene*, vol. 101, no. 4, pp. 884–890, 2019.

[3] J. Whitehorn and J. Farrar, "Dengue, British Medical Bulletin," *Dengue*, vol. 95, no. 1, pp. 161–173, 2010.

[4] M. A. M. Khalil, J. Tan, M. A. U. Khalil, S. Awan, and M. Rangasami, "Predictors of hospital stay and mortality in dengue virus infection-experience from Aga Khan University Hospital Pakistan," *BMC Research Notes*, vol. 7, no. 1, p. 473, 2014.

[5] T. Adane and S. Getawa, "Coagulation abnormalities in Dengue fever infection: a systematic review and meta-analysis," *PLoS Neglected Tropical Diseases*, vol. 15, no. 8, Article ID e0009666, 2021.

[6] M. Raadsen, J. Du Toit, T. Langerak, B. van Bussel, E. van Gorp, and M. Goeijenbier, "Thrombocytopenia in virus infections," *Journal of Clinical Medicine*, vol. 10, no. 4, p. 877, 2021.

[7] B. Murgue, O. Cassar, M. Guigon, and E. Chungue, "Dengue virus inhibits human hematopoietic progenitor growth in vitro," *The Journal of Infectious Diseases*, vol. 175, no. 6, pp. 1497–1501, 1997.

[8] A. Basu, P. Jain, S. V. Gangodkar, S. Shetty, and K. Ghosh, "Dengue 2 virus inhibits in vitro megakaryocytic colony formation and induces apoptosis in thrombopoietin-inducible megakaryocytic differentiation from cord blood CD34+ cells," *FEMS Immunology and Medical Microbiology*, vol. 53, no. 1, pp. 46–51, 2008.

[9] S. Nakao, C.-J. Lai, and N. S. Young, "Dengue virus, a flavivirus, propagates in human bone marrow progenitors and hematopoietic cell lines," *Blood*, vol. 74, no. 4, pp. 1235–1240, 1989.

[10] C. Mitrakul, "Bleeding problem in dengue haemorrhagic fever: platelets and coagulation changes," *Southeast Asian Journal of Tropical Medicine & Public Health*, vol. 18, no. 3, pp. 407–412, 1987.

[11] T. Srichaikul and S. Nimmannitya, "Haematology in dengue and dengue haemorrhagic fever," *Best Practice & Research Clinical Haematology*, vol. 13, no. 2, pp. 261–276, 2000.

[12] F. R. F. G. Azin, R. P. Gonc¸alves, M. H. D. S. Pitombeira, D. M. Lima, and I. C. Branco, "Dengue: profile of hematological and biochemical dynamics," *Revista Brasileira de Hematologia e Hemoterapia*, vol. 34, no. 1, pp. 36–41, 2011.

[13] L. C. S. Lum, M. E.-A. Abdel-Latif, A. Y. T. Goh, P. W. K. Chan, and S. K. Lam, "Preventive transfusion in dengue shock syndrome—is it necessary?" *The Journal of Pediatrics*, vol. 143, no. 5, pp. 682–684, 2003.

[14] M. I. H. Khan, E. Anwar, A. Agha et al., "Factors predicting severe dengue in patients with dengue fever," *Mediterranean Journal of Hematology and Infectious Diseases*, vol. 5, no. 1, 2013.

[15] P. Kaur and G. Kaur, "Transfusion support in patients with dengue fever," *International Journal of Applied and Basic Medical Research*, vol. 4, no. 3, p. 8, 2014.

33

Atypical Thrombotic Thrombocytopenic Purpura Presenting as Stroke

Pradeepthi Badugu and Modupe Idowu

Division of Hematology, Department of Internal Medicine, McGovern Medical School, The University of Texas Health Science Center at Houston, 6411 Fannin Street, Houston 77030, USA

Correspondence should be addressed to Modupe Idowu; modupe.idowu@uth.tmc.edu

Academic Editor: Gergely Feher

Here we report a case of atypical thrombotic thrombocytopenic purpura that presented as an ischemic cerebrovascular accident. A 56-year-old man with multiple cardiovascular risk factors presented with sudden left-sided weakness, slurred speech, and left facial droop. He showed mild improvement when he was treated with thrombolytic therapy according to the hospital stroke protocol. Later in the course, he developed thrombocytopenia followed by schistocytes revealed by peripheral blood smear and other lab abnormalities. Thrombotic thrombocytopenic purpura (TTP) was suspected, and he was treated with total plasma exchange that improved his condition significantly. This case shows that TTP can have unusual and atypical presentations either with the first episode or upon relapse, making diagnosis extremely difficult. Because patients may not present the expected clinical findings, it is important to be aware of variant presentations. In the early stages of the disease, platelet aggregation and thrombus formation may not be widespread, and thrombocytopenia and microangiopathic hemolytic anemia may not be clinically evident. Patients can present soon after the onset of symptoms when the typical laboratory abnormalities may not have had ample time to manifest. Although most other similar cases in the literature had a previous typical presentation of the disease before an atypical presentation, our patient's first presentation was atypical. An atypical presentation of disease in a patient with cardiovascular risk factors may therefore be extremely difficult to diagnose. We believe that TTP should be considered for any patient presenting with stroke and thrombocytopenia.

1. Introduction

Thrombotic thrombocytopenic purpura (TTP) is often described as a pentad of thrombocytopenia, anemia, fever, renal dysfunction, and neurological abnormalities caused by unregulated von Willebrand factor- (VWF-) dependent platelet thrombosis [1]. ADAMTS13 is a metalloprotease that inhibits VWF-dependent platelet aggregation. Lack of this enzyme leads to persistent microvascular thrombi in multiple organs that in turn leads to the characteristic clinical presentations of TTP. Microthrombi exert a shearing force on the blood vessels and break red blood cells, resulting in schistocytes in peripheral smears. Clinical presentations of TTP can be typical or atypical either on initial presentation or upon relapse. Gastrointestinal, neurological, and bleeding manifestations are the most common presenting features of TTP [2]. "Atypical TTP" is the term used when clinical features at the time of admission are not typical of TTP but patients are later diagnosed with the disease. In atypical presentations, the manifestations of thrombosis may precede overt thrombotic microangiopathy and hemolytic anemia by days to months [3]. Here, we describe a case of atypical TTP that presented as an ischemic cerebrovascular accident without any hematological changes initially but later developed into thrombocytopenia and microangiopathic hemolytic anemia (MAHA). The patient was treated with fibrinolytics at presentation as part of a standard stroke protocol. However, his neurological symptoms improved only upon total plasma exchange.

2. Case

A 56-year-old man with a history of dyslipidemia, multiple transient ischemic attacks (TIAs), and a 40 pack-year smoking history presented to the local hospital with sudden left-sided weakness, slurred speech, and left facial droop. His family history was significant for stroke and diabetes in multiple family members. He was on atorvastatin for dyslipidemia. He had no history of connective tissue or autoimmune disease. He was diagnosed with acute ischemic cerebrovascular accident and was given tissue plasminogen activator (tPA). The patient received a single dose of atorvastatin 80 mg and aspirin 325 mg orally during the admission; he never received clopidogrel or ticlopidine therapy. The symptoms improved gradually, but he developed thrombocytopenia that worsened over the next few days. The team discontinued statin and aspirin therapy once they observed low platelets. The patient was managed conservatively, but his platelet counts reached a nadir at 16,000 per cubic mm. His peripheral blood smear showed no schistocytes in high-power fields. He was given a platelet transfusion with no improvement. He was then transferred to our hospital, and the inpatient hematology team was consulted. At the time of presentation, the patient complained of clumsiness in his left arm, although he was able to carry out daily activities with minimal difficulty. He was stable, the facial droop had resolved and speech slightly improved with residual dysarthria and expressive aphasia, and his motor power was better. A review of outside laboratory results revealed that 2 days before his transfer, his platelet count was 115,000 per cubic mm, BUN was 16, and his creatinine was 1.3. His initial lab values on arrival at our hospital were as follows: platelets 26,000 cells per cubic mm, hemoglobin (Hb) 10.7 g/dl, hematocrit (Hct) 31.2/L, leucocytes 16,300 cells per cubic mm, blood urea nitrogen 35, blood urea nitrogen/creatinine 27, lactic acid dehydrogenase of 794 (98–192), bilirubin 0.9, and reticulocyte count 2.8. During admission, B12 and folic acid levels, antiphospholipid panel, disseminated intravascular coagulation panel, coagulation panel, antinuclear antibodies, and rheumatoid factor were measured and found to be within normal limits. HIV, hepatitis B, and direct Coombs tests were negative. However, his peripheral blood smear showed 5-6 schistocytes/high-power field. Neither the patient nor his family members underwent any screening for connective tissue or autoimmune disorders.

The patient was immediately started on a daily total plasma exchange (TPE). On day 3, his neurological symptoms improved significantly, and his platelet count normalized to 167,000 per cubic mm. Despite the improved platelet count, TPE was continued for 2 more days. By day 5, his speech was clear and his expressive aphasia resolved. He recovered full strength in his right extremities and TPE was stopped. Blood samples were sent to the Blood Center of Wisconsin, Milwaukee, for measurement of ADAMTS13 levels, and we got the results 5 days later. ADAMTS13 activity measured using FRETS-VWF73 substrate was <5% (reference range ≥67%). ADAMTS13 inhibitor was measured using mixing studies with standard pooled plasma, and residual ADAMTS13 activity measured using FRETS-VWF73 substrate was <0.4 inhibitor units (reference range ≤0.4). Platelet count remained stable throughout the patient's stay. At the time of discharge, his counts and Hb/Hct remained stable, lactate dehydrogenase (LDH) was 249, and no schistocytes were present in peripheral blood smears. Because of his atypical presentation of TTP, he was advised to seek medical attention immediately if his neurological symptoms worsen to evaluate TTP relapse. After discharge, he was evaluated twice weekly with a CBC and LDH measurements after discharge for 2 weeks and once a week afterward. Higher levels of LDH were noticed subsequently normalized in 2 months. He complained of intermittent left facial numbness and tingling of the left hand during follow-up visits. The patient remained in remission without a relapse for 2 years after his initial presentation.

3. Literature Review

There are a few similar cases in the literature that are atypical presentations of TTP that presented as cerebrovascular accident (CVA). One is a 40-year-old woman with chronic relapsing TTP presented with facial numbness, left upper quadrant weakness, dysarthria, and diplopia. On admission, her Hb was 9.3 g/dl, PLT-239/cubic mm, and LDH-296 U/l (N = 68–239 u/l) and rare schistocytes were observed on a peripheral blood smear. A brain MRI showed acute right hemisphere infarction. Because of her significant history, TTP was considered as the etiology of her stroke, and she was started on TPE. After 12 hours of TPE, her hand and leg strength increased, and her dysarthria improved. Her neurological status significantly improved after 7 TPE treatments. Her ADAMTS13 level was 13% at the time of presentation, and ADAMTS13 inhibitor was detected [4]. Another case described by the same author is of a 42-year-old woman with a chronic history of relapsing TTP and a history of strokes in the setting of TTP. Her fourth episode of stroke was associated with motor weakness, dysphagia, and confusion, without lab findings for TTP. A magnetic resonance angiogram MRA showed an acute infarct in the left basal ganglia and old cerebral infarcts. Because of her history and stroke in the setting of TTP, she was immediately started on TPE. Her ADAMTS13 levels were 12% on admission, and she had ADAMTS13 IgG antibody. Her neurological symptoms significantly improved before the discontinuation of TPE, but she had multiple relapses in the following 3 years [4]. Tsai and Shulman [5] described a case of a 36-year-old African American woman with a first episode of TTP at the age of 27. She did well for 8 years, after which she experienced a stroke with motor deficits and dysarthria. Her platelet count, bilirubin, and LDH were normal, and no schistocytes were detected on the peripheral blood smear at the time of presentation. Three weeks later, she had an overt episode of TTP with PLT count 6 per cubic mm and schistocytes on the peripheral blood smear. Her neurological status and counts improved with TPE and prednisone. Idowu and Reddy [6] describe a case of a 45-year-old African American woman with a baseline of mild dysarthria, minimal expressive aphasia, and right upper extremity weakness and spasticity from a CVA and TTP 6 years previously. She now presented to the emergency department with left facial droop, left hemiparesis, and aphasia suggestive of stroke. She was diagnosed with acute stroke involving the right middle cerebral artery and started on tPA. Intra-arterial thrombolysis and thrombectomy were also performed but did not produce any improvement. Her hemoglobin count was normal with a slightly decreased platelet count, LDH was mildly elevated, and renal function was normal. A peripheral blood smear did not show any schistocytes. On the third day of hospitalization, her platelet count decreased from 113,000 to 97,000 cells per cubic mm, and hemoglobin dropped from 13.2 to 11.1 g/dl, without microangiopathic blood smear. TPE was started immediately. ADAMTS13 activity measured 16%, and mixing studies and ELISA assay were negative for ADAMTS13 inhibitor and IgG antibody. After 5 TPE treatments, she showed significant neurological recovery, stable Hb/Hct, and normal LDH, and her platelet count improved to 225,000 per cubic mm.

4. Discussion

The incidence of TTP is approximately 3.7 per million per year [7, 8]. Most cases are idiopathic, but some are associated with HIV, pregnancy, autoimmune diseases, infections, bone marrow transplantation, and use of drugs like cyclosporine, mitomycin, and ticlopidine [8]. In most cases, TTP is caused by deficiency of ADAMTS13. VWF is naturally secreted in ultralarge multimeres from endothelial cells. ADAMTS13 is a disintegrin and metalloprotease with thrombospondin type 1 motifs occurring in plasma that cleaves VWF at the Tyr 1605-Met 1606 bond in the central A2 subunit and prevents the accumulation of these large multimers that cause platelet aggregation and microvascular thrombosis [8]. A complete protease deficiency due to missense or frameshift mutations in the ADAMTS13 gene in the absence of an inhibitor is seen in familial TTP (Upshaw–Schulman syndrome). Patients with nonfamilial TTP have an acquired deficiency due to autoantibodies inhibiting the activity of the enzyme that accounts for most of the cases [7, 9, 10]. Deficiency of ADAMTS13 alone may not be the cause of TTP because it is observed that even with very low levels of the enzyme, the disease never manifested; hence, environmental factors play an important role in the development of the disease [3, 7, 11]. In the presence of ADAMTS13 deficiency, the tendency for VWF and platelets to form microthrombi is dependent on the platelet count and the conformational response of VWF to shear stress. Factors that increase shear stress activate VWF by causing conformational changes in the molecule. Environmental factors such as infections, inflammation, surgery, and pregnancy may decrease plasma ADAMTS13 activity by affecting its synthesis or by increasing its inactivation [11].

Clinical presentations of TTP are due to the microthromboses, constituting platelets, and VWF in the small vessels. Microthrombi cause shearing of the red blood cells resulting in schistocytes in peripheral smear, increased LDH, and decreased haptoglobin [3]. Although the disease is described as a pentad, the initial symptoms of TTP are nonspecific and variable [12, 13]. It is therefore risky to wait for the entire pentad to develop. Moreover, the classic pentad is not relevant to current practice. Often patients present with a range of neurological symptoms, including confusion, headaches, seizures, blurred vision, focal abnormalities, aphasia, stroke, and coma, due to the diffuse involvement of microcirculation in the brain [2, 3]. Some patients develop gastrointestinal symptoms such as abdominal pain, nausea, vomiting, and diarrhea that may be related to intestinal ischemia [2]. Renal abnormalities such as oliguria, microscopic hematuria, albuminuria, and acute renal failure may be involved [7]. Other possible symptoms are skin and mucosal bleeding, fatigue, dyspnea, and chest pain [2]. Thrombocytopenia with MAHA without an apparent cause is now sufficient to establish diagnosis and initiate treatment [2, 12]. In the early stages of the disease, platelet aggregation and thrombus formation may not be widespread, and thrombocytopenia and MAHA may not be clinically evident [4]. Patients can present soon after the onset of symptoms before classic laboratory abnormalities such as thrombocytopenia, and MAHA may not have sufficient time to manifest.

Neurological manifestations of TTP can be mistaken for acute ischemic stroke, as in the case presented here. Our patient had strong cardiovascular risk factors, tobacco use, dyslipidemia, and history of TIA; hence, CVA was rightly suspected. Moreover, his initial laboratory values showed very mild thrombocytopenia but no schistocytes on the peripheral blood smear, further hindering the early recognition of the disease. Thrombolysis, the treatment of CVA, might have led to severe hemorrhagic complications in the patient; fortunately, he did not have such complications. On the contrary, successful use of thrombolytic therapy in TTP patients with stroke has been described in the literature [6].The patient was transferred to our center because of worsening thrombocytopenia, and we suspected that he might have developed atypical thrombocytopenia even before his arrival to our facility and the examination of his peripheral blood smear. Our higher index for suspicion for atypical TTP was based on our experience with similar cases.

ADAMTS13 activity and autoimmune inhibitors against ADAMTS13 can be measured by lab assays. There are direct and indirect assays for the detection of ADAMTS13 activity, among which the direct FRETS-VWF73 is relatively rapid and simple. ELISA is considered to be more sensitive than an inhibitor assay for detecting ADAMTS13 autoantibodies [14]. Severe acquired ADAMTS13 deficiency is defined as a level less than 10%. Although it is specific for TTP, it is not necessary for diagnosis [2]. The severity of its deficiency in patients with idiopathic TTP corresponds neither to the clinical presentation nor to the response to treatment with plasma exchange. The poor correlation between the severity of disease and the levels of ADAMTS13 still needs to be explained [2, 6, 12, 14]. It may be related to the sensitivity of current assays [2, 7]. A prompt recognition and diagnosis of TTP among the patients presenting with stroke is important, as therapeutic plasma exchange provides immediate improvement but delay in diagnosis, and treatment can be catastrophic.

Although most of the other cases we described from the literature had previous episodes of TTP before an atypical presentation, our patient had an atypical presentation without any earlier history of TTP. Hence, we should have a high index of suspicion for TTP in any patient presenting with stroke and thrombocytopenia. Moreover, empirical plasma exchange should be considered if the patient does not have risk factors for stroke or if thrombocytopenia is persistent or worse without a clear reason. Plasma exchange is the recommended treatment for TTP [2, 12]. The survival rate was 10% before the advent of plasma exchange but is 78% with plasma exchange and 51% with plasma infusion [2]. Corticosteroids and other immunomodulatory drugs should be considered in most patients with acquired TTP to suppress the autoantibodies against ADAMTS13. All patients should be evaluated for possible contributing factors such as underlying infection, autoimmune disease, use of complicating drugs, and familial predisposition. Treatment of underlying condition should be promptly initiated, and any suspected offending drugs should be discontinued. All patients should be on folic acid supplementation. Assessment of baseline B12 levels and iron studies should be considered to ensure that the patient's reserve is adequate to mount a hematopoietic response to anemia. Response to treatment should be assessed by platelet count, and plasma exchange can be performed when platelet count normalizes and remains stable for 2 days, after which the patient can be discharged if clinically stable. After discharge, patients should be evaluated twice weekly for 2 weeks and once a week for another 2 weeks. Estimated risk of relapse for TTP is 41% for 7.5 years and is more common in the first year after occurrence of TTP [2]. The risk of relapse increases when the levels of ADAMTS13 are persistently less than 10% or when the levels continue to decrease during remission. In such a scenario, treatment with rituximab should be considered [11]. Studies indicate that patients with high titers of inhibitors of ADAMTS13 have a delayed response to therapy, high risk of complications, and higher rates of relapse [7]. Many patients have persistent minor cognitive abnormalities even after recovery [14].

In conclusion, TTP should be considered in all patients who develop CVA or TIA and unexplained persistent thrombocytopenia even when they have cardiovascular risk factors. It is imperative to have a high index of suspicion for TTP in this context because delay in diagnosis may lead to death and because early recognition of TTP and proper treatment can lead to rapid improvement of symptoms and can prevent unnecessary therapy resulting in further complications. Empiric therapy with plasma exchange may be appropriate for patients with suspected atypical presentation while awaiting the results of ADAMTS13 tests. Thrombolytic therapy may lead to life-threatening bleeding complications in these patients. TTP can have unusual and atypical presentations that may make the diagnosis extremely difficult, as the patients may lack the expected clinical findings; thus, it is important to be aware of its range of presentations. Atypical presentation of TTP in a patient with cardiovascular risk factors may complicate diagnosis, but a high index of suspicion may save lives.

References

[1] E. L. Amorosi and J. E. Ultmann, "Thrombotic thrombocytopenic purpura," *Medicine*, vol. 45, no. 2, pp. 139–160, 1966.

[2] J. N. George, "How I treat patients with thrombotic thrombocytopenic purpura: 2010," *Blood*, vol. 116, no. 20, pp. 4060–4069, 2010.

[3] R. Sarode, "Atypical presentations of thrombotic thrombocytopenic purpura: a review," *Journal of Clinical Apheresis*, vol. 24, no. 1, pp. 47–52, 2009.

[4] K. A. Downes, R. Yomtovian, H. M. Tsai, B., C. Silver et al., "Relapsed thrombotic thrombocytopenic purpura presenting as an acute cerebrovascular accident," *Journal of Clinical Apheresis*, vol. 19, no. 2, pp. 86–89, 2004.

[5] H.-M. Tsai and K. Shulman, "Rituximab induces remission of cerebral ischemia caused by thrombotic thrombocytopenic purpura," *European Journal of Haematology*, vol. 70, no. 3, pp. 183–185, 2003.

[6] M. Idowu and P. Reddy, "Atypical thrombotic thrombocytopenic purpura in a middle-aged woman who presented with a recurrent stroke," *American Journal of Hematology*, vol. 88, no. 3, pp. 237–239, 2012.

[7] X. L. Zheng, R. M. Kaufman, L. T. Goodnough, and J. E. Sadler, "Effect of plasma exchange on plasma ADAMTS13 metalloprotease activity, inhibitor level, and clinical outcome in patients with idiopathic and nonidiopathic thrombotic thrombocytopenic purpura," *Blood*, vol. 103, no. 11, pp. 4043–4049, 2004.

[8] E. Aksay, S. Kiyan, M. Ersel, and O. Hudaverdi, "Thrombotic thrombocytopenic purpura mimicking acute ischemic stroke," *Emergency Medicine Journal*, vol. 23, no. 9, p. e51, 2006.

[9] M. Furlan, R. Robles, M. Galbusera et al., "von Willebrand factor-cleaving protease in thrombotic thrombocytopenic purpura and the hemolytic-uremic syndrome," *New England Journal of Medicine*, vol. 339, no. 22, pp. 1578–1584, 1998.

[10] Z. Tao, K. Anthony, Y. Peng et al., "Novel ADAMTS-13 mutations in an adult with delayed onset thrombotic thrombocytopenic purpura," *Journal of Thrombosis and Haemostasis*, vol. 4, no. 9, pp. 1931–1935, 2006.

[11] H.-M. Tsai, "Thrombotic thrombocytopenic purpura and the atypical hemolytic uremic syndrome," *Hematology/Oncology Clinics of North America*, vol. 27, no. 3, pp. 565–584, 2013.

[12] S. K. Vesely, J. N. George, B. Lämmle et al., "ADAMTS13 activity in thrombotic thrombocytopenic purpura--hemolytic uremic syndrome: relation to presenting features and clinical outcomes in a prospective cohort of 142 patients," *Blood*, vol. 102, no. 1, pp. 60–68, 2003.

[13] G. A. Rock, K. H. Shumak, N. A. Buskard et al., "Comparison of plasma exchange with plasma infusion in the treatment of thrombotic thrombocytopenic purpura," *New England Journal of Medicine*, vol. 325, no. 6, pp. 393–397, 1991.

[14] J. A. K. Hovinga, S. K. Vesely, D. R. Terrell, B. Lammle, and J. N. George, "Survival and relapse in patients with thrombotic thrombocytopenic purpura," *Blood*, vol. 115, no. 8, pp. 1500–1511, 2009.

34

Chronic Atrophic Gastritis Presenting as Hemolytic Anemia due to Severe Vitamin B12 Deficiency

Amanda M. Woodford,[1] Rabhea Chaudhry,[1] Gabriella A. Conte,[1] Varsha Gupta,[2] and Madhurima Anne[2]

[1]*Department of Medicine, Jersey Shore University Medical Center, Hackensack Meridian Health, Neptune Township, NJ, USA*
[2]*Department of Hematology and Oncology, Jersey Shore University Medical Center, Hackensack Meridian Health, Neptune Township, NJ, USA*

Correspondence should be addressed to Amanda M. Woodford; amandam.woodford@hmhn.org

Academic Editor: Kazunori Nakase

Vitamin B12 is an essential nutrient which plays an important role in neurological function, hematopoiesis, and DNA synthesis. Low levels usually stem from either poor intake or a malabsorptive process. Presently, the most common cause of vitamin B12 deficiency is food-bound cobalamin malabsorption, which occurs when there is impaired release of vitamin B12 from ingested food due to an outstanding factor preventing the release of the nutrient from its transport protein. Such causes include achlorhydria, gastritis, gastrectomy, or the use of PPIs or antacids. A rarer cause is autoimmune chronic atrophic gastritis, resulting in pernicious anemia. In this disease process, there is destruction of parietal cells and thus a reduction in intrinsic factor, which is essential to the absorption of vitamin B12. Deficiency will result in a variety of abnormalities including but not limited to pancytopenia, paresthesias, and neuropsychiatric symptoms. A rare manifestation of vitamin B12 deficiency is hemolytic anemia, which occurs due to intramedullary and extramedullary dysfunction. This case describes a 46-year-old male with no past medical history who presented with chest pain, fatigue, and progressive weakness, found to have hemolytic anemia, ultimately attributed to vitamin B12 deficiency. Antiparietal cell antibodies and intrinsic factor antibodies (IFA) were both negative. Still, the patient underwent an endoscopy with biopsies of the stomach; pathology was consistent with chronic metaplastic atrophic gastritis. The patient improved with intramuscular vitamin B12 supplementation. This case highlights both a rare cause and presentation of vitamin B12 deficiency. Patients with autoimmune chronic atrophic gastritis should have antiparietal cell or intrinsic factor antibodies. Still, seronegative patients have been reported, like this patient. Additionally, hemolytic anemia secondary to vitamin B12 deficiency is uncommon. The presentation will usually mirror that of a thrombotic microangiopathy (TMA), including hemolytic anemia with schistocytes on peripheral blood smear and thrombocytopenia, as it did in this patient. This clinical entity is described as pseudothrombotic microangiopathy and is crucial to identify in order to prevent the initiation of invasive treatment strategies such as plasmapheresis.

1. Introduction

Vitamin B12 (cobalamin) is an essential nutrient that acts as a cofactor for major chemical reactions in the body, including the conversion of methylmalonic acid to succinyl coenzyme A, the conversion of homocysteine to methionine, and the conversion of 5-methyltetrahydrofolate to tetrahydrofolate, which are crucial to proper neurologic function, hematopoiesis, and DNA synthesis [1]. Consequently, deficiency will usually manifest as a compilation of hematologic irregularities (macrocytic anemia, thrombocytopenia, or pancytopenia), neurologic symptoms (paresthesias, loss of proprioception, or autonomic nervous system dysfunction), and/or as neuropsychiatric abnormalities such as depression, dementia, or mania [2]. The prevalence of vitamin B12 deficiency in the United States has been reported to be as high as 3% in those aged 20–39 years old, 4% in those aged 40–59 years old, and 6% in those over 60 years old [3].

A lesser-known complication of vitamin B12 deficiency is hemolytic anemia, sometimes presenting as a pseudo-thrombotic microangiopathy. This can occur due to both intramedullary and extramedullary dysfunction. Deficiency leads to ineffective erythropoiesis, resulting in intramedullary hemolysis and the release of lactate dehydrogenase (LDH), in addition to impaired deformability of the red blood cell membrane, which causes extramedullary fragmentation and hemolysis [2, 4].

Mainly obtained through the ingestion of fish, meat, dairy products, and fortified cereals, vitamin B12 is absorbed in the terminal ileum along with intrinsic factor, which is produced by parietal cells in the stomach [1]. Deficiency usually results from either poor intake or a malabsorptive process. The most common etiology of vitamin B12 deficiency is food-bound cobalamin malabsorption, which occurs when there is impaired release of vitamin B12 from ingested food due to an outstanding factor that prevents the release of the nutrient from its transport protein. Such causes include achlorhydria, gastritis, gastrectomy, or the use of proton-pump inhibitors (PPIs) or antacids [3]. A rarer cause of vitamin B12 deficiency is autoimmune chronic atrophic gastritis, leading to pernicious anemia. In this disease, there is an underlying inflammatory process which leads to the destruction of parietal cells and thus a reduction in intrinsic factor, which is essential to the absorption of vitamin B12. Diagnosis is usually made via positive serologic studies, such as the presence of anti-intrinsic factor antibodies or anti-parietal cell antibodies, or through histological examination [5]. Herein, we present a case of vitamin B12 deficiency manifesting as hemolytic anemia secondary to chronic autoimmune gastritis as observed on histologic examination, although with negative serologic markers.

2. Case Report

A 46-year-old Haitian male with no past medical history presented to the emergency department with chest pain, progressive weakness, and fatigue that had been ongoing for the past month. Prior to these symptoms, the patient was in his usual state of health. He did not routinely follow up with a medical provider. He described the chest pain as an intermittent, substernal burning sensation that occurred mainly at rest. It caused him to have decreased appetite, resulting in an unintentional 30lb weight loss over the preceding several weeks. He denied fevers, chills, cough, night sweats, dysphagia, odynophagia, nausea, or vomiting. He also reported constipation, with bowel movements every 3-4 days associated with occasional rectal pain and bright red blood with wiping. He otherwise denied any rectal bleeding, hematochezia, melena, hematemesis, hematuria, rashes, or bruising. Of note, the patient had no significant family medical history. He took no medications and denied use of over-the-counter agents including NSAIDs, acetaminophen, aspirin, herbs, or supplements. He denied alcohol or tobacco use. He consumed a diet including meat and vegetables with no restrictions. He reported working outside as a landscaper, although denied any known tick or mosquito bites. He denied any recent sick contacts or travel history, with his last trip to Haiti occurring about 1.5 years prior to presentation.

The patient's vital signs on admission were as follows: body temperature 98.1°F, pulse of 84/min, respiratory rate of 18/min, BP 130/67 mmHg, and oxygen saturation of 100% on room air. Physical exam was notable for scleral icterus. There were no oral ulcers or glossitis. The abdomen was soft with no tenderness or hepatosplenomegaly. There was no peripheral edema or rashes. Neurologic examination was unremarkable; muscle strength was 5/5 in the upper and lower extremities, and there was no sensory deficit exhibited. He also had no gait abnormalities.

Initial complete blood count (CBC) revealed pancytopenia with a decreased white blood cell count of 2.4uL (4.5–11.0 10 * 3/uL), hemoglobin level of 4.9 g/dL (13.2–17.5 g/dL), and platelet count of 5710 * 3/uL (140–450 10 * 3/uL). Mean corpuscular volume was 98.7 fL (80.0–100.0 fL). Absolute reticulocyte count was 0.020×10^6/uL ($0.010–0.110 \times 10^6$/uL). Peripheral blood smear was grossly abnormal, demonstrating tear drop cells, few schistocytes, anisopoikilocytosis, left shifted white cells, giant platelets, atypical lymphocytes, and no blasts. Additional blood work revealed normal serum electrolytes and kidney function, an elevation of AST, total bilirubin, direct bilirubin, and LDH, and a decreased haptoglobin level (Table 1). A direct Coombs IgG test was positive. Vitamin B12, folate, and homocysteine levels were also drawn at this time as part of the workup for hemolytic anemia, which demonstrated severe vitamin B12 deficiency (<50 pg/mL), normal folate levels of 22 (>4.0 ng/mL), and elevated homocysteine level of 42.6 (5.0–15.0 umol/L). Urinalysis showed hazy urine, negative for glucose, bilirubin, and ketones, moderate blood, 30–50 RBCs, and 0–2 WBCs. CT scan of the chest/abdomen/pelvis with contrast was significant for mild splenomegaly with the spleen measuring 13.9 cm in length, with no radiographic evidence of splenic infarcts or lesions. There was no hepatomegaly or significant retroperitoneal or mediastinal lymphadenopathy. The stool occult test was positive for occult blood. The patient was transfused 2 units of packed red blood cells and admitted for further workup.

Additional testing was performed to evaluate for hemolytic anemia, including hepatitis panel, HIV, CMV, EBV IgM, ANA, and tick-borne pathogens including malaria/*Babesia* parasite smear, *Lyme* antibodies, *Ehrlichia* antibodies, *Rickettsia rickettsii* antibodies, and ADAMTS13 levels. While the results of these tests were not available on the day of admission, all ultimately came back negative or within normal limits. Peripheral blood flow cytometry showed no immunophenotypic evidence of lymphoproliferative disorder, high-grade myeloid neoplasm/acute leukemia, or plasma cell neoplasm.

Thrombotic thrombocytopenic purpura was initially considered, but less likely given the patient was afebrile, had normal mentation and normal kidney function. ADAMTS13 eventually resulted within normal limits. The leading hypothesis for his pancytopenia and hemolytic anemia was ineffective erythropoiesis and intramedullary hemolysis from severe vitamin B12 deficiency. Antiparietal cell

Table 1: Laboratory data.

Lab	Value	Reference range
WBC	2.4	4.5–11.0 10 * 3/uL
ANC	1.2	1.8–8.0 10 * 3/uL
HGB	4.9	13.2–17.5 g/dL
HCT	14.9	40.0–53.0%
MCV	98.7	80.0–100.0 fL
Platelet	57	140–450 10 * 3/uL
Glucose	93	70–99 mg/dL
Na	138	136–145 mmol/L
K	4.4	3.5–5.2 mmol/L
Chloride	105	96–110 mmol/L
Carbon dioxide	21	24–31 mmol/L
BUN	14	5–25 mg/dL
Cr	1.15	0.61–1.24 mg/dL
AST	105	10–42 U/L
ALT	55	10–60 U/L
ALP	29	38–126 U/L
Total bilirubin	4.2	0.2–1.3 mg/dL
Direct bilirubin	0.5	0.0–0.2 mg/dL
Troponin	0.01	<0.08 ng/mL
LDH	6392	91–200 U/L
Haptoglobin	<6	30–225 mg/dL
Reticulocyte count	1.38	0.40–2.50%
Direct coombs IgG	Positive	Negative
Ferritin	304.3	24–336 ng/mL
Serum iron	81	45–180 ug/dL
TIBC	227	260–480 ug/dL
Vitamin B12	<50	180–914 pg/mL
Folate	22	>4.0 ng/mL
Homocysteine	42.6	5.0–15.0 umol/L
Intrinsic factor antibody	Negative	Negative
Antiparietal cell Antibodies (first test)	20.7	0.0–20.0 units = negative 20.1–24.9 = Equivocal
Antiparietal cell Antibodies (second test)	19.2	0.0–20.0 units = negative 20.1–24.9 = Equivocal

antibodies and intrinsic factor antibodies (IFA) were sent; both ultimately resulted negative. The patient subsequently underwent upper endoscopy (EGD) and colonoscopy. EGD revealed a single, nonbleeding erosion at the gastroesophageal junction and diffuse atrophic appearing mucosa in the gastric body and antrum, which was biopsied. Pathology demonstrated gastric antrum mucosa with chronic gastritis and no intestinal metaplasia or *Helicobacter pylori* identified; gastric mucosa was consistent with chronic gastritis, intestinal metaplasia, and an absence of oxyntic glandular tissues, consistent with metaplastic atrophic gastritis (Figure 1). Colonoscopy showed internal hemorrhoids but was otherwise grossly unremarkable.

The day following admission, the patient's posttransfusion hemoglobin improved to 8.2 g/dL (13.2–17.5 g/dL). He was ultimately treated with 4 days of intravenous dexamethasone 40 mg daily for possible autoimmune hemolytic anemia, given the initial direct positive Coombs test, and was started on daily intramuscular injections of cyanocobalamin 1000 mcq for a total of 10 days. He did not require further blood transfusions. Through the course of his hospitalization, he continued to improve, reporting increased energy and better appetite. On the day of discharge,

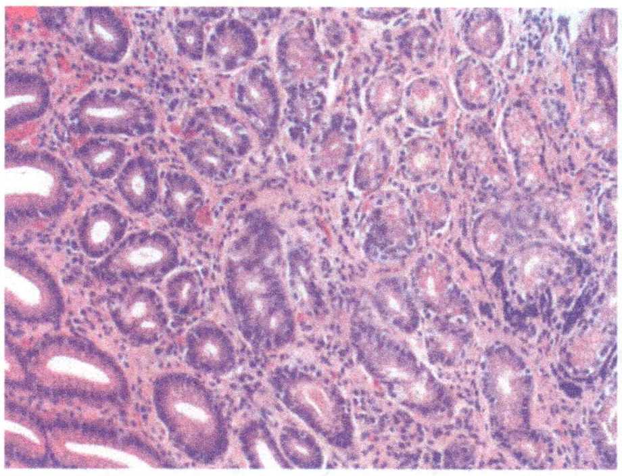

Figure 1: Gastric mucosa demonstrating chronic gastritis, intestinal metaplasia identified by Alcian blue-PAS stain, and absence of oxyntic glandular tissue, consistent with metaplastic atrophic gastritis. No dysplasia identified. No *Helicobacter pylori* identified by Giemsa stain.

the patient's hemoglobin was 9.8 g/dL (13.2–17.5 g/dL). Given that the patient's cell counts showed improvement with vitamin B12 supplementation, bone marrow biopsy was deferred. He was discharged on oral vitamin B12 supplementation and instructions to follow up in the hematology clinic to receive weekly intramuscular vitamin B12 injections for the following month.

3. Discussion

Vitamin B12 deficiency presenting with severe hematologic manifestations is a relatively uncommon occurrence, with only a limited number of reports in the current medical literature. Our case not only serves as an example of this rare clinical entity but also presents a constellation of unique findings of this particular disease process. First, our patient's initial presentation included hemolytic anemia, thrombocytopenia, and dysmorphic red blood cells. These findings are consistent with a thrombotic microangiopathy (TMA). However, because vitamin B12 levels were obtained immediately and were shown to be significantly decreased, the diagnosis of pseudo-TMA, a TMA specifically secondary to vitamin B12 deficiency, was made. Unlike primary TMA syndromes, such as thrombotic thrombocytopenic purpura or hemolytic uremic syndrome, pseudo-TMA does not require invasive interventions like plasmapheresis. It is speculated that the etiology of dysmorphic red blood cells in severe vitamin B12 deficiency stems from both intramedullary and extramedullary dysfunction. From an extramedullary perspective, research has shown that hyperhomocysteinemia, which occurs in vitamin B12 deficiency, may increase the risk of hemolysis in addition to causing endothelial damage, which further leads to intravascular hemolysis and RBC fragmentation [6]. Of note, hyperhomocysteinemia can also be caused by hypothyroidism, obesity, diabetes, hyperlipidemia, medications, and more rarely possessing a methylenetetrahydrofolate reductase gene variant [7]. Testing of this gene variant though is usually only recommended if the cause of the hyperhomocysteinemia is unexplained by another more common cause, thus why our patient did not undergo this form of testing.

Additionally, as more data were accumulated, the suspected cause of our patient's vitamin B12 deficiency was autoimmune atrophic chronic gastritis, given the histologic findings noted on biopsies of his stomach, specifically the intestinal metaplasia and absence of oxyntic glandular tissues in the gastric mucosa, no evidence of *Helicobacter pylori* infection, and lack of metaplasia in the gastric antrum. According to the Updated Sydney System of Classification and Grading of Gastritis, autoimmune gastritis is strongly associated with corpus predominant atrophic gastritis, with little to no atrophy or metaplasia noted in the antrum [8]. This would imply the patient had pernicious anemia, leading to severe vitamin B12 deficiency and thus hemolytic anemia. Although rare, reports of this disease process exist in the literature. However, in a majority of these cases, the diagnosis of pernicious anemia is demonstrated through histological exam in addition to laboratory studies, or evidence of prior gastrectomy or ileum resection [9–11]. Historically, these laboratory studies included surveilling for intrinsic factor deficiency using the Schilling test [12]. However, this method is frequently being replaced by other diagnostics tests such as detecting intrinsic factor antibodies or parietal cell antibodies. Although intrinsic factor or parietal cell antibodies were not detected in our patient, he had histologic evidence of autoimmune gastritis confirming the diagnosis.

At the time of this publication, only a few cases were found which described a patient presenting with hemolytic anemia due to severe vitamin B12 deficiency, likely secondary to seronegative chronic atrophic gastritis. Similar to our patient, this case describes a young male presenting with a macrocytic anemia, elevated LDH, and undetectable vitamin B12 levels, who was discovered to have chronic atrophic gastritis via biopsy. This patient also had negative serologic markers, including parietal cell antibodies and intrinsic factor antibodies [13].

Recently, Conti et al. performed a retrospective, cross-sectional study in Italy examining levels of antiparietal cell antibodies (PCAs) and clinical features of 516 patients diagnosed with autoimmune atrophic gastritis by histology. Of these patients, 21.1% resulted seronegative. The seronegative patients were significantly older than the seropositive patients, with a greater proportion of these patients over the age of 70. It was speculated that the positive correlation between older age and seronegativity could be explained by a seroconversion due to progression of disease, similar to what was observed in other autoimmune conditions, such as autoimmune thyroiditis. However, this study found that seropositivity did not correlate with atrophy severity and that seronegativity was not associated with greater severity of gastric atrophy or clinical symptoms [14]. Interestingly, our case presents a young patient with negative serologic studies.

Lastly, another unique feature of our case was the presence of an initial positive direct antiglobulin test (DAT) in the setting of hemolytic anemia caused by vitamin B12 deficiency. Pernicious anemia associated with a positive DAT has been rarely described in the literature. It has been reported that patients with pernicious anemia may transiently have a positive Coombs test; however, repeat testing will often become negative after that patient is started on vitamin B12 supplementation [15]. Interestingly, in our patient, repeat DAT was negative after the patient had been started on both vitamin B12 supplementation and a course of steroids.

4. Conclusion

This case highlights both a rare cause and manifestation of vitamin B12 deficiency. Deficiency occurs due to poor oral intake or a malabsorptive process of the nutrient. Autoimmune chronic atrophic gastritis is a rare etiology of vitamin B12 deficiency, which results in a destruction of the parietal cells, leading to a reduction in intrinsic factor, which is essential to the absorption of vitamin B12. In this disease process, patients will usual have either antiparietal cell or intrinsic factor antibodies. However, recent studies have demonstrated patients with this disease who are seronegative, making biopsy essential to diagnosis. Additionally, vitamin B12 deficiency usually presents with neurologic and hematologic symptoms. Rarely, it will cause hemolytic anemic and thrombocytopenia, best described as a pseudothrombotic microangiopathy, as demonstrated in this case. It is speculated that the mechanism of hemolysis is due to both intramedullary and extramedullary dysfunction. It is critical to establish this diagnosis early on to prevent unnecessary treatment, such as plasmapheresis.

Consent

The patient described in the case report had given informed consent for the case report to be published.

References

[1] R. C. Langan and A. J. Goodbred, "Vitamin B12 deficiency: recognition and management," *American Family Physician*, vol. 96, no. 6, pp. 384–389, 2017.

[2] S. P. Stabler, "Vitamin B12 deficiency," *The New England Journal of Medicine*, vol. 368, no. 21, pp. 2041-2042, 2013.

[3] M. J. Shipton and J. Thachil, "Vitamin B12 deficiency-A 21st century perspective," *Clinical Medicine*, vol. 15, no. 2, pp. 145–150, 2015.

[4] S. Sasi and M. A. Yassin, "A rare case of acquired hemolytic anemia and pancytopenia secondary to pernicious anemia," *Case Reports in Oncology*, vol. 13, no. 2, pp. 783–788, 2020.

[5] K. I. Rodriguez-Castro, M. Franceschi, A. Noto et al., "Clinical manifestations of chronic atrophic gastritis," *Acta Biomed*, vol. 89, no. 8-S, pp. 88–92, 2018.

[6] Y. Fahmawi, Y. Campos, M. d. Khushman et al., "Vitamin B12 deficiency presenting as pseudo-thrombotic microangiopathy: a case report and literature review," *Clinical Pharmacology: Advances and Applications*, vol. 11, pp. 127–131, 2019.

[7] U.S. Department of Health and Human Services. MTHFR gene variant. Genetic and Rare Diseases Information Center, https://rarediseases.info.nih.gov/diseases/10953/mthfr-gene-variant.

[8] M. F. Dixon, R. M. Genta, J. H. Yardley, and P. Correa, "Classification and grading of gastritis," *The American Journal of Surgical Pathology*, vol. 20, no. 10, pp. 1161–1181, 1996.
[9] K. Veit, "Pseudothrombotic microangiopathy and vitamin B12 deficiency in pernicious anemia," *Baylor University Medical Center Proceedings*, vol. 30, no. 3, pp. 346-347, 2017.
[10] H. Osman, T. A. Alwasaidi, A. Al-Hebshi, N. Almutairi, and H. Eltabbakh, "Vitamin B12 deficiency presenting with microangiopathic hemolytic anemia," *Cureus*, vol. 13, no. 1, p. e12600, 2021.
[11] Y. Harada, I. Komori, K. Morinaga, and T. Shimizu, "Microangiopathic haemolytic anaemia with thrombocytopenia induced by vitamin B12 deficiency long term after gastrectomy," *BMJ Case Reports*, vol. 2018, 2018.
[12] N. M. Rodriguez and K. Shackelford, "Pernicious anemia," in *StatPearls*StatPearls Publishing, Treasure Island, FL, USA, 2021, https://www.ncbi.nlm.nih.gov/books/NBK540989/.
[13] G. F. Cittolin-Santos, S. Khalil, J. K. Bakos, and K. Baker, "Chronic atrophic gastritis with negative intrinsic factor and parietal cell antibody presenting as a severe hemolytic anemia," *Case Reports in Hematology*, vol. 2020, Article ID 8697493, 4 pages, 2020.
[14] L. Conti, M. V. Lenti, A. Di Sabatino et al., "Seronegative autoimmune atrophic gastritis is more common in elderly patients," *Digestive and Liver Disease*, vol. 52, no. 11, pp. 1310–1314, 2020.
[15] S. L. H. Yeruva, R. P. Manchandani, and P. Oneal, "Pernicious anemia with autoimmune hemolytic anemia: a case report and literature review," *Case Reports in Hematology*, vol. 2016, Article ID 7231503, 4 pages, 2016.

35

Persistent Increase in Serum Alkaline Phosphatase in a Patient with Monoclonal Gammopathy of Undefined Significance

I. Ramasamy

Worcester Royal Hospital, Charles Hastings Way, Worcester WR41DD, UK

Correspondence should be addressed to I. Ramasamy; indrar@ozemail.com.au

Academic Editor: Sylvain Choquet

We report the finding of alkaline phosphatase-immunoglobulin complex (macro-alkaline phosphatase (macro-ALP)) in a patient with persistently increased ALP activity. The identification of macro-ALP is important to rule out pathological causes of increased ALP activity and to avoid unnecessary diagnostic investigation. The patient was subsequently diagnosed with vitamin D deficiency, gallstone pancreatitis, and monoclonal gammopathy of undefined significance (MGUS). Macro-ALP can coexist with disease that can increase serum ALP activity. We report, for the first time, a case of macro-ALP in a patient with a monoclonal protein (M-protein).

1. Introduction

The tissue-nonspecific alkaline phosphatase (ALP) is the major fraction found in the serum and is coded by a single gene expressed in the liver, bone, and kidney. Intestinal alkaline phosphatase, which is about 25% of normal sera, is coded by a separate gene which is separate from the gene that codes for placental alkaline phosphatase and the placental-like isoenzyme (which is an oncofetal form the enzyme). Raised serum ALP may be due to the liver ALP isoenzyme as a result of hepatic damage or cholestatasis. Increased bone-specific ALP can be caused by a number of pathologies affecting the bone: fracture, Paget's disease, osteomalacia, and bone metastases. Raised intestinal ALP has been reported in liver cirrhosis, diabetes, chronic kidney disease, and bowel ischemia and infarction. Alkaline phosphatase isoenzyme analysis is used to understand the changes in serum values of ALP and has many diagnostic advantages in identifying underlying pathology [1, 2].

Rarely increased serum ALP activity will be due to an immunoglobulin-bound form of ALP (macro-ALP). Macro-ALP has reduced renal clearance usually due to a high molecular weight form of the enzyme. The importance for the diagnosis of macro-ALP lies in their ability to cause diagnostic confusion when plasma ALP activities are elevated, leading to unnecessary and potentially harmful investigations [3]. We report here, to our knowledge for the first time, the finding of macro-ALP in a patient with monoclonal gammopathy of undefined significance (MGUS).

2. Case Presentation

A 73-year-old man with a total ALP of 70 IU/L (reference range (RR) 30–130, using p-nitrophenyl phosphate as a substrate, Roche UK) was found to have a minor IgG kappa monoclonal band (M-band) of 2.8 g/L in 2009. His total ALP increased to 142 IU/Lin 2012 and to 178 IU/L in 2013 (Figure 1). His gamma-glutamyl transferase (gamma-GT, RR 10–70 IU/L), alanine aminotransaminase, and total bilirubin remained within the reference range. His 25-hydroxy vitamin D level was found to be 28.2 nmol/L (RR > 50 nmol/L for adequate vitamin D status). He was treated with vitamin D. Vitamin D status was assessed as adequate in Feb 2014 at 66.5 nmol/L. His 25-hydroxy vitamin D concentration remained at 76.2 nmol/L in 2018, with a parathyroid hormone level of 29 ng/L (RR 15–65), and his

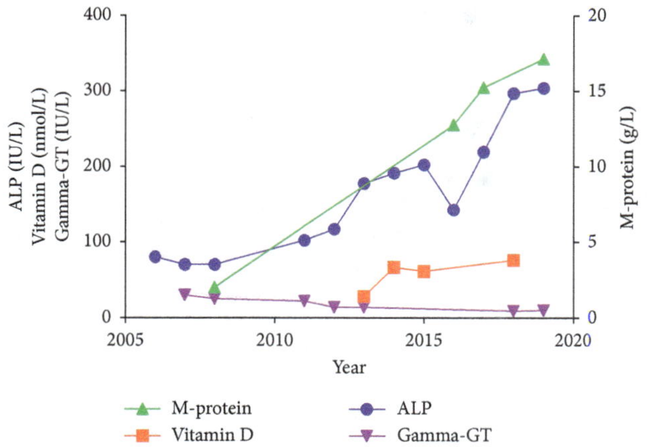

Figure 1: Changes in ALP, M-protein, vitamin D, and gamma-GT in the patient's sera with time.

unadjusted calcium was 2.3 mmol/L (RR 2.2–2.6). His full blood count profile and renal function remained within the reference limit. The ALP remained persistently high at 192 IU/L and remained high during 2015 at 174 IU/L. In March 2016, his M-band was 15.3 g/L, kappa light chain was 56.6 mg/L (RR 3.3–19.4 mg/L), lambda light chain was 31.1 mg/L (RR 5.7–26.3 mg/L), and the ratio was 1.821 (RR 0.26–1.65). Progression in his M-protein is shown in Figure 1. He presented with acute pancreatitis in 2017. Radiological investigation identified multiple gallstones within the gallbladder leading to a diagnosis of gallstone pancreatitis. He was admitted for laparoscopic cholecystectomy and remained well following surgery. He had an extensive past medical history which included hypertension, chronic obstructive pulmonary disease, diabetes, and total knee replacement. His treatment included amlodipine, vitamin D, clopidogrel, omeprazole, pravastatin, and lisinopril.

Following cholecystectomy, his ALP remained raised, and alanine aminotransaminase, bilirubin, gamma-GT, serum calcium, and renal function were within the reference limit. Liver screening for antinuclear antibody, mitochondrial antibody, smooth muscle antibody, and anti-liver-kidney microsomal antibody was negative. Referral to a hospital gastroenterologist and an abdominal ultrasound detected a post inflammatory pancreatic cyst but did not report liver disease.

3. Investigations

ALP isoenzyme analysis was carried out by the Sebia (UK) serum enzyme electrophoresis method. The SEBIA system utilizes the different degrees of sialylation of liver and bone isoenzymes to separate them. Wheat germ lectin presents a strong affinity for the sialic acid residues and consequently binds preferentially to the bone isoenzyme that is sialated to a higher degree. The separated ALP isoenzymes are visualized at 37°C and 50°C using an ALP-specific chromogenic substrate, 5-bromo-4-chloro-3-indolyl phosphate/nitro blue tetrazolium in aminomethyl propanol (AMP) buffer, with pH 10.1. Isoenzyme analysis of the patient's sera in 2018 identified an unusual form of ALP (Figure 2(a)).

Further investigation showed that the electrophoretic mobility of the unusual alkaline phosphatase isoform was not affected by lectin. Equal volumes of the patient's sera and poly ethylene glycol (PEG) 6000 (240 g/L in 9 g/L of saline) were mixed, and the residual activity was measured. Fifteen patient sera with liver, bone, and intestinal alkaline phosphatase isoenzymes were used as controls. The average measured residual activity was 95.4% in controls (range 84.8–108.5), compared to 25.2% ($n = 3$) in the patient. Isoenzyme electrophoresis of the patient's sera before and after PEG precipitation showed that the unusual form was precipitated by PEG and identified an immunoglobulin-alkaline phosphatase macroenzyme complex (Figure 2(b)).

The Sebia (UK) immunofixation method allows the separation and characterization of M-protein heavy and light chains using specific antisera. Following agarose gel electrophoresis, the gel is incubated with antisera to IgG, IgA, and IgM heavy chains and kappa and lambda light chains. The excess antisera are removed, the precipitated (immunofixed) immunoglobulin is visualised, and the M-protein is identified by staining. The patient's sera and three controls with total alkaline phosphatase in the range 200–300 IU/L were electrophoresed on the immunofixation gel (Sebia, UK). Following electrophoresis serum, ALP was visualised using the specific substrate for ALP. Visualisation was performed by a manual technique in which the gel was overlaid with the substrate and incubated at 37°C. A discrete band that was visualised by the ALP chromogenic substrate was identified in the patient's sera but not in controls (Figure 3(a)). Comparison with the gel visualised with antisera to immunoglobulin heavy and light chains showed that the band had a slightly higher mobility than the IgG kappa M-band found in the patient's sera (Figure 3(b)).

The discrete band found using specific substrate staining following electrophoresis on the immunofixation gel suggested a monoclonal (M) component to the ALP-immunoglobulin complex. The molecular weight of IgG is 150,000 and of the non-tissue-specific form of ALP is 186,000 [4]. It is likely that the electrophoretic mobility of the immunoglobulin-ALP complex differs from the IgG M-protein. It is probable at the activity of 180 IU/L, and the concentration of the macro-ALP in mg/L is below the detection limit of the immunofixation technique (manufacturer detection limit: 150 mg/L by precipitation using the anti-IgG sera) [5].

4. Discussion

There have been several reports of macro-ALP in the literature. Reported macro-ALP were bound to IgG [6, 7] and to a lesser extent IgA [8, 9]. The ALP is usually of liver and bone origin or both [10]. Gel filtration analysis of the macro-ALP suggested that the results will be consistent with equimolar complexes of IgG-ALP or a complex made up of two molecules of IgG with one of ALP or one molecule of IgG and two molecules of ALP [6]. Wenham et al. [9] reported two peaks on gel chromatography and suggested different molar ratios of ALP and IgA immunoglobulin complexes as well as lipid forms within the macro-ALP complex. Maekawa et al. [8] suggested that ALP was attached

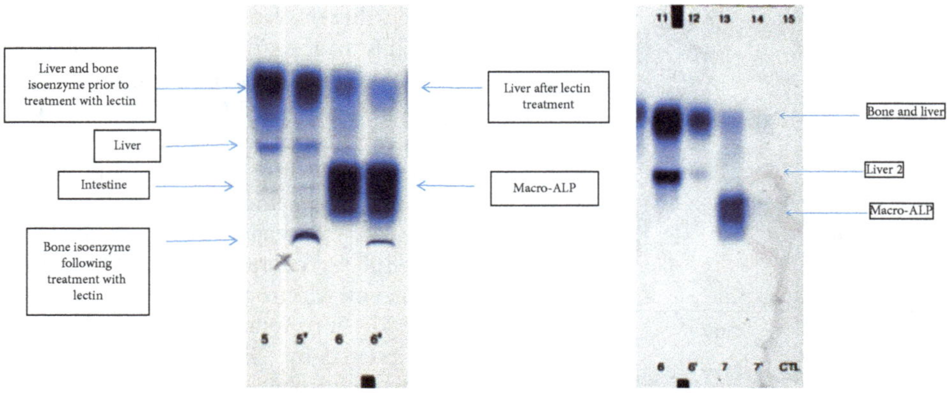

(a) (b)

FIGURE 2: (a) ALP isoenzyme analysis following lectin treatment. Lane 5: Control sera with liver, bone, and intestinal isoenzyme. Lane 5′: control sera following lectin treatment. Lane 6: the patient's sera. Lane 6′: the patient's sera following treatment with lectin. Lectin precipitates the bone isoenzyme, allowing the liver isoenzyme to be quantitated. Electrophoretic mobility of the macro-ALP is not affected by lectin. (b) ALP isoenzyme analysis following PEG precipitation. Lane 6: control with liver ALP isoenzyme. Lane 6′: control following treatment with PEG. Lane 7: the patient's sera. Lane 7′: the patient's sera following treatment with PEG. PEG treatment precipitates the macroenzyme in the patient's sera.

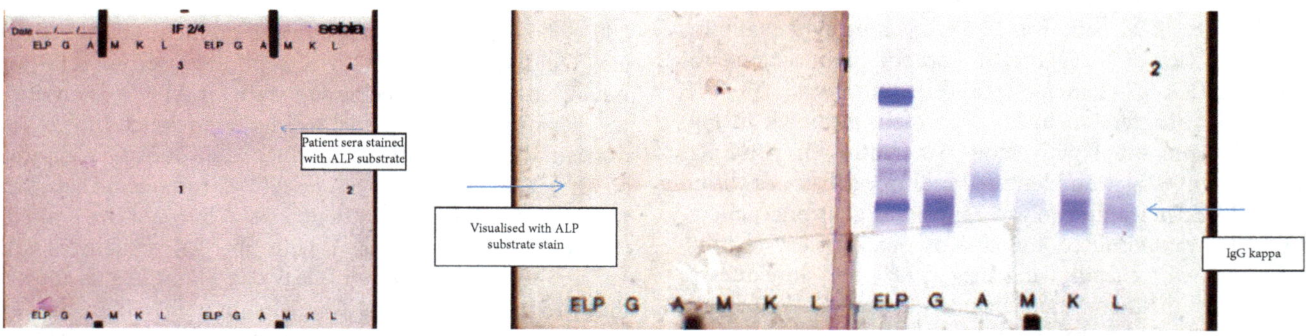

(a) (b)

FIGURE 3: (a) Immunofixation gels stained with alkaline phosphatase substrate. Three control sera and the patient's sera were electrophoresed using the Sebia immunofixation gel and stained with ALP substrate. Gel 1–3: three control sera on all lanes. Gel 4: lanes 1 and 2: the patient's sera. (b) Comparative stain of the immunofixation gel with alkaline phosphatase substrate and anti-IgG/A/M heavy chain and kappa/lambda light chain. Gel 1: lanes 1–6: the patient's sera stained with alkaline phosphatase substrate. Gel 2: lanes 1–6: the patient's sera stained with antisera to immunoglobulin heavy chain and light chains.

through the F (ab′) 2 fragment of IgA and that the molecular weight of the complexes suggested that 2 molecules of ALP was associated with one molecule of divalent IgA.

Characterisation of the macro-ALP was performed by gel filtration [7], immunoelectrophoresis [7], PEG precipitation [11], and proteolytic digestion [9]. Protein A/G agarose affinity chromatography was used to demonstrate the presence of macro-ALP [12]. This method will not detect complexes to immunoglobulins other than IgG so has limitations [10]. In a further case study, Nagakawa et al. [13] reported an intestinal ALP-IgG complex in which the IgG had the ability to inhibit ALP in a patient's serum. The electrophoretic mobility of the unusual form of ALP found in this patient coincided with that of the intestinal enzyme. However, we confirmed the presence of the immunoglobulin-ALP complex by PEG precipitation. The presence of a discrete band detected by specific ALP substrate stain in the gamma region following protein electrophoresis was further supportive of an immunoglobulin-ALP complex.

Macro-ALP has been reported in patients with ulcerative colitis [11], carcinoma of prostate [10], bronchopneumonia and recurrent infections [9], and liver cirrhosis and cholestasis [6]. Atypical ALP with posttranslational modification has been described in a patient with Hodgkin's disease [14]. There was no observed correlation with the presence of the macro-ALP and clinical abnormalities. The question as to why autoantibodies to ALP occur in sera is not fully understood at present.

Isolated increase in ALP is associated with a variety of medical illnesses. In the first instance, a reasonable approach would be a careful medical and drug history and physical examination. The within-subject variation for ALP was reported as 6.4% [15], suggesting minor increases in ALP can be within biological variation. Raised ALP of unknown cause requires further tests to define associated pathology.

The finding of an isolated increase in ALP triggered several investigations in this patient. The increase was at first attributed to vitamin D deficiency. The persistent increase following repletion with vitamin D resulted in carrying out further investigations for liver disease and a referral to a hospital based specialist gastroenterologist. Conditions that favour the presence of a macro-ALP are the absence of symptoms, an isolated and persistently increased ALP, symptoms atypical for the abnormal level of the enzyme. However, as in this patient, the presence of macro-ALP can coexist with disease that can cause an increase in ALP, vitamin D deficiency, gallstone pancreatitis, and MGUS. Identification of macro-ALP in this context becomes of relevance in the correct interpretation of increased total ALP. Interestingly, macro-ALP in this patient raises the possibility of ALP bound to the M-protein as a cause of the immunoglobulin-ALP complex.

Recent studies have indicated an increased fracture risk in multiple myeloma around the time of presentation [16]. MGUS usually precedes multiple myeloma, and the risk of fractures is increased in MGUS patients [17]. The consequences of skeletal involvement are severe pain, spinal cord compressions, and bone fractures which have a dramatic impact on a patient's quality of life. In serial monitoring of patients with skeletal metastases bone, ALP correlated with progression or regression of metastatic spread [18]. In multiple myeloma, the bone remodelling balance is disrupted and osteolytic lesions develop. In multiple myeloma, the effects of upregulated osteoclastogenesis is amplified by the inhibition of osteoblast activity [19]. Changes in bone remodelling may be monitored by the detection of specific serum markers, including carboxy-terminal telopeptide of type 1 collagen, β-crosslaps, and deoxypyridinoline characteristic of bone degradation as well as bone-specific alkaline phosphatase, osteocalcin, amino-terminal propeptide of type I collagen, and carboxy-terminal propeptide of type I collagen characteristic of bone formation [20]. In a goal in which state-of-the-art treatment strategies are used to restore balanced bone remodelling, biochemical markers of bone remodelling may play a role in slowing down bone damage. In this clinical scenario, identification of a macro-ALP becomes important to prevent unnecessary investigation and incorrect interpretation of increased total ALP.

In summary, we report a case of macro-ALP in a patient with IgG kappa MGUS. Diagnostic use of ALP isoenzyme characterisation is of value and can provide useful information on underlying pathology. The presence of macro-ALP can confuse the interpretation of increased total ALP and can lead to unnecessary investigation. This is particularly true in disease states, such as MGUS and multiple myeloma which can lead to pathology that can result in increased total ALP.

5. Learning Points

(1) Differential diagnosis of an isolated increased ALP can be a challenge and can trigger several investigations

(2) We report for the first time, macro-ALP in a patient with M-protein

(3) Macro-ALP can coexist with several pathologies which can increase ALP

(4) It is important to detect the presence of macro-ALP as they can cause diagnostic confusion leading to several unnecessary investigations

References

[1] D. Lowe and S. John, *Alkaline Phosphatase. StatPearls*, StatPearls Publishing, Treasure Island, FL, USA, 2019.

[2] D. W. Moss, "Alkaline phosphatase isoenzymes," *Clinical Chemistry*, vol. 28, no. 10, pp. 2007–2016, 1982.

[3] P. J. Galasso, S. C. Litin, and J. F. O'Brien, "The macroenzymes: a clinical review," *Mayo Clinic Proceedings*, vol. 68, no. 4, pp. 349–354, 1993.

[4] R. A. Stinson, "Size and stability to sodium dodecyl sulfate of alkaline phosphatases from their three established human genes," *Biochimica et Biophysica Acta (BBA)—Protein Structure and Molecular Enzymology*, vol. 790, no. 3, pp. 268–274, 1984.

[5] H. H. Sussman, P. A. Small Jr., and E. Cotlove, "Human alkaline phosphatase. Immunochemical identification of organ-specific isoenzymes," *Journal of Biological Chemistry*, vol. 243, no. 1, pp. 160–166, 1968.

[6] M. Owen, L. Pike, P. George, M. Barclay, and C. Florkowski, "Macro-alkaline phosphatase due to IgG complex: demonstration with polyethylene glycol precipitation and immunofixation," *Annals of Clinical Biochemistry*, vol. 39, no. 5, pp. 523–525, 2002.

[7] M. E. De Broe, T. E. Mets, G. G. Leroux-Roels, and R. J. Wieme, "Occurrence of immunoglobulin G-alkaline phosphatase complexes in human serum," *Annals of Internal Medicine*, vol. 90, no. 1, pp. 30–35, 1979.

[8] M. Maekawa, K. Sudo, and T. Kanno, "Characteristics of the complex between alkaline phosphatase and immunoglobulin A in human serum," *Clinica Chimica Acta*, vol. 150, no. 3, pp. 185–195, 1985.

[9] P. R. Wenham, B. Chapman, and A. F. Smith, "Two macromolecular complexes between alkaline phosphatase and immunoglobulin A in a patient's serum," *Clinical Chemistry*, vol. 29, no. 10, pp. 1845–1849, 1983.

[10] J. E. Buttery, C. R. Milner, P. Nenadovic, and P. R. Pannall, "Detection of alkaline phosphatase/immunoglobulin complexes," *Clinical Chemistry*, vol. 26, no. 11, pp. 1620-1621, 1980.

[11] M. P. McTaggart, C. Rawson, D. Lawrence et al., "Identification of a macro-alkaline phosphatase complex in a patient with inflammatory bowel disease," *Annals of Clinical Biochemistry*, vol. 49, no. 4, pp. 405–407, 2012.

[12] M. A. Cervinski, H. K. Lee, I. W. Martin, and D. K. Gavrilov, "A macro-enzyme cause of an isolated increase of alkaline phosphatase," *Clinica Chimica Acta*, vol. 440, pp. 169–171, 2015.

[13] H. Nakagawa, K. Umeki, K. Yamanaka, N. Kida, and S. Ohtaki, "Macromolecular alkaline phosphatase and an immunoglobulin G that inhibited alkaline phosphatase in a patient's serum," *Clinical Chemistry*, vol. 29, no. 2, pp. 375–378, 1983.

[14] J. P. Beilby, P. Garcia-Webb, C. I. Bhagat, and A. Prins, "Atypical alkaline phosphatase isoenzyme in serum from a patient with Hodgkin's disease," *Clinical Chemistry*, vol. 30, no. 5, pp. 800–802, 1984.

[15] C. Ricós, N. Iglesias, J.-V. García-Lario et al., "Within-subject biological variation in disease: collated data and clinical consequences," *Annals of Clinical Biochemistry*, vol. 44, no. 4, pp. 343–352, 2007.

[16] L. J. Melton III, R. A. Kyle, S. J. Achenbach, A. L. Oberg, and S. V. Rajkumar, "Fracture risk with multiple myeloma: a population-based study," *Journal of Bone and Mineral Research*, vol. 20, pp. 487–493, 2005.

[17] L. J. Melton III, S. V. Rajkumar, S. Khosla, S. J. Achenbach, A. L. Oberg, and R. A. Kyle, "Fracture risk in monoclonal gammopathy of undetermined significance," *Journal of Bone and Mineral Research*, vol. 19, pp. 25–30, 2004.

[18] A. Burlina, D. Rubin, S. Secchiero, L. Sciacovelli, M. Zaninotto, and M. Plebani, "Monitoring skeletal cancer metastases with the bone isoenzyme of tissue unspecific alkaline phosphatase," *Clinica Chimica Acta*, vol. 226, no. 2, pp. 151–158, 1994.

[19] S. Vallet, J.-M. Filzmoser, M. Pecherstorfer, and K. Podar, "Myeloma bone disease: update on pathogenesis and novel treatment strategies," *Pharmaceutics*, vol. 10, no. 4, p. 202, 2018.

[20] R. H. Christenson, "Biochemical markers of bone metabolism: an overview," *Clinical Biochemistry*, vol. 30, no. 8, pp. 573–593, 1997.

36

Essential Thrombocythemia Complicated by Occlusive Thrombosis of the Abdominal Aorta

Jamie Geringer, Joshua Fenderson, and Michael Osswald

San Antonio Uniformed Services Health Education Consortium, 3551 Roger Brooke Drive JBSA, Fort Sam Houston, San Antonio, TX 78234, USA

Correspondence should be addressed to Jamie Geringer; jlgordon410@gmail.com

Academic Editor: Gergely Feher

Introduction. Essential thrombocythemia (ET) is a myeloproliferative neoplasm of excessive platelet production complicated by thrombohemorrhagic events. Thrombosis typically occurs in small to medium vessels; thrombosis of large vessels is rare. *Case Presentation.* A 75-year-old woman with ET complicated by bilateral retinal vein occlusion was evaluated for fatigue, early satiety, and unintentional weight loss. Her hypertension was well controlled, and her chronic lower extremity claudication from peripheral artery disease was stable. She reported adherence to aspirin 81 mg and hydroxyurea 1000 mg daily, and her platelets (375×10^9/L) were at goal. Bone marrow biopsy was consistent with ET without progression to myelofibrosis or leukemia. CT abdomen demonstrated complete occlusion of the infrarenal aorta, extending into the common iliac arteries, with reconstitution of flow distally via collaterals. The addition of clopidogrel, for platelet inhibition, and cilostazol, for claudication, caused symptom improvement without further thrombosis or bleeding. *Discussion.* There are few published reports of ET complicated by aortic thrombosis. To our knowledge, this is the first report of aortic thrombosis occurring in an ET patient with normal platelet count on antiplatelet and cytoreductive therapies. There is limited evidence to guide treatment, but medical management with triple antiplatelet therapy may be effective in selected patients.

1. Introduction

Essential thrombocythemia (ET) is a myeloproliferative neoplasm characterized by increased platelet counts and excessive large and morphologically mature megakaryocytes in the bone marrow [1]. ET may be complicated by thrombotic and/or hemorrhagic events. Small and medium vessel thrombosis is most common and may manifest as erythromelalgia, transient ischemic attack, myocardial infarction, deep vein thrombosis, or pulmonary embolism [2]. Thrombosis of the large vessels rarely occurs, and there is limited evidence to guide management, particularly in cases without acute tissue ischemia. A small number of case reports suggest pharmacologic management alone can be successful in patients with minimally symptomatic ET-associated aortic thrombosis; however, the agents chosen and treatment rationale are quite varied [3–7].

2. Case Presentation

A 75-year-old African American female with a history of hypertension, hyperlipidemia, peripheral artery disease, and essential thrombocythemia, complicated by sequential bilateral central retinal vein occlusion, was seen for follow-up. She first presented to hematology in March 2015 with a history of left central retinal vein occlusion, stable claudication from peripheral arterial disease, and progressive thrombocytosis. She had quit smoking three months prior. Laboratory review revealed persistent increased platelet counts ($>800 \times 10^9$/L) over the previous six months. Blood smear was notable for increased large mature megakaryocytes relative to red blood cells; no left shift, leukoerythroblastosis, or dysplasia was observed. Iron studies, lactate dehydrogenase, BCR-ABL translocation, and JAK2 V617F mutation studies were unremarkable. The patient refused bone marrow biopsy, and a presumptive diagnosis of ET was given, supported by calreticulin (CALR) mutation detected. Low-dose aspirin and hydroxyurea were initiated, and platelets were at goal ($<400 \times 10^9$/L) two months later. Her history was further complicated by right central retinal vein occlusion in December 2016 during a period of poor compliance with cytoreductive therapy.

In May 2018, she reported progressive fatigue and 15 lb unintentional weight loss over the preceding three months. Laboratory evaluation was notable for a macrocytic anemia and platelets at goal (WBC 6×10^9/L; Hb 10 g/dL; MCV 101.7 fL; Plt 375×10^9/L). She agreed to bone marrow evaluation which revealed a normocellular marrow with an increased number of enlarged and hyperlobated megakaryocytes and variable mild reticulin fibrosis (less than MF-1); blasts were not increased. Fluorescent in situ hybridization analysis for BCR/ABL, PDGFRA, PDGFRB, and FGFR1 was negative. Peripheral blood molecular analysis revealed a mutation in the calreticulin (CALR) gene; JAK2 V617F, JAK2 exon 12, and myeloproliferative leukemia virus (MPL) oncogene mutations were not identified. These findings confirmed a diagnosis of essential thrombocythemia and excluded myelofibrosis as the cause of her fatigue and weight loss. Further evaluation with CT scan of the chest, abdomen, and pelvis demonstrated atherosclerosis and completely occlusive thrombosis of the infrarenal aorta, extending bilaterally into the common iliac arteries, with reconstitution of flow distally via collaterals (Figure 1). There was no splenomegaly. Subsequent CT angiogram of the abdomen showed redemonstration of the aortic thrombus without occlusion of the mesenteric arteries, the celiac trunk, or the hepatic, splenic, and renal arteries.

The patient's only symptom was mild chronic claudication which had not changed in quality; she denied lower extremity swelling or skin mottling. She reported compliance with her prescribed medications for hypertension, hyperlipidemia, and ET. Lower extremity ultrasound and ankle brachial index were not significantly changed from prior studies. An evaluation for inflammatory disorders and thrombophilia, including erythrocyte sedimentation rate, C-reactive protein, anti-nuclear antibodies, anti-neutrophil cytoplasmic antibodies, lupus anticoagulant, anti-phospholipid antibodies, factor V Leiden mutation, prothrombin gene mutation, and protein C and protein S, was unremarkable.

In light of her very mild symptoms and good collateralization on imaging, she was offered medical management with surgical intervention reserved for treatment refractoriness or acute ischemia. Clopidogrel 75 mg daily was added to the aspirin 81 mg and hydroxyurea 1000 mg she was already taking. Additionally, she was started on cilostazol 100 mg twice daily by her vascular surgeon to treat her claudication. She reported initial improvement in her symptoms one month after starting therapy. She did not return for follow-up until February 2019 due to temporarily relocating out of the state. She had been noncompliant with therapy for ET. Her platelet count was 948×10^9/L, and a CT scan showed no significant interval change in the occlusive thrombus of the infrarenal abdominal aorta and proximal common iliac arteries. She refused surgical intervention and was restarted on previous medical therapy.

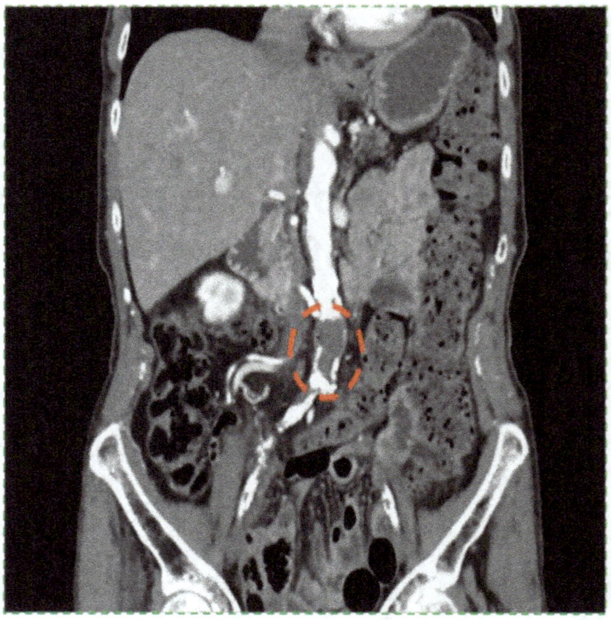

FIGURE 1: Computed tomography (CT) abdomen and pelvis demonstrating an occlusive thrombus in the abdominal aorta distal to the mesenteric artery. There is thrombus extension into the common iliac arteries with reconstitution of flow distally via collaterals.

3. Discussion

According to the 2016 World Health Organization, the diagnosis of ET can be made if the following major criteria are met: (1) platelet count $\geq 450 \times 10^9$/L; (2) increased numbers of enlarged and hyperlobated mature megakaryocytes in the bone marrow without left shift and no more than grade 1 reticulin fibrosis; (3) not meeting criteria for other myeloproliferative neoplasms, myelodysplastic syndrome, leukemia, or other myeloid disorders; (4) presence of JAK2, CALR, or MPL mutation. Alternatively, ET may be diagnosed if the first three major criteria are met, and another clonal marker is identified or reactive thrombocytosis is excluded [1].

In this case, a clinical diagnosis of ET was originally given based on progressive thrombocytosis, increased large platelets on peripheral blood smear, and history of retinal vein thrombosis. The characteristic morphology on bone marrow evaluation three years later, negative evaluation for iron deficiency, infection, or inflammatory disorder, and CALR mutation detected confirmed the diagnosis of essential thrombocythemia. CALR is mutated in approximately 70% of patients with JAK2-negative essential thrombocythemia. The detection of a CALR gene mutation helps distinguish this clonal disease from a benign reactive process [8, 9].

Occlusive thrombosis of the aorta is rare and typically associated with aneurysm, dissection, or severe atherosclerosis. Hypercoagulable disorders, malignancy, and myeloproliferative disorders are less frequently described causative or contributing etiologies [10]. While small and medium vessel thromboses frequently complicate ET, only a small number of case reports have described thrombosis of the aorta. As such, there is no evidence-based consensus on how to treat these patients.

Thrombosis in ET is a result of spontaneous activation and aggregation of hypersensitive platelets [11]. Histopathologic evaluations of arterial thrombi in ET have revealed platelet-rich clots with abundant von Willebrand factor (VWF) and very little fibrin [12]. This pathophysiology supports the efficacy of antiplatelet and cytoreductive therapies in preventing and treating thrombosis and microvascular circulation disturbances in ET. Thrombosis while the platelet count is normal supports the view that platelet count is not the sole factor responsible for the thrombosis and thus, medical therapy targeted at thrombin generation may be less effective, given the limited fibrin in these platelet-rich thrombi [13].

The goal of medical therapy in ET is to prevent thrombohemorrhagic events in high-risk patients or prevent growth and embolization in patients with an existing thrombus. This is commonly accomplished with low-dose aspirin, which inhibits platelet activation, and hydroxyurea, which decreases the clonal production of hypersensitive platelets. Of the few cases of ET-related aortic thrombosis that have been published, most were managed with a combination of surgical and pharmacologic therapies; however, successful medical management alone has been reported [3–7, 14].

Fang et al. reported complete resolution of an intra-aortic thrombus, confirmed by CT scan, in an ET patient three weeks after starting aspirin and hydroxyurea [5]. Additionally, Lorelli and Shepard reported resolution of abdominal pain in an elderly patient with ET-related thrombosis of the aorta, splenic infarction, and portal vein thrombosis treated with anegralide and systemic anticoagulation with warfarin [3]. In a patient with myelodysplastic syndrome and/or myeloproliferative disorder unclassifiable (MDS/MPD-U) complicated by myeloproliferative thrombocytosis and aortic thrombosis, treatment with low-dose aspirin, hydroxyurea, and ticlopidine, a platelet adenosine diphosphate (ADP) receptor $P2Y_{12}$ inhibitor, resulted in complete resolution of the thrombus on CT scan after one week of therapy [15].

In our patient, we hypothesize that atherosclerotic narrowing of the aorta and iliac vessels created a high shear environment whereby hypersensitive platelets, characteristic of ET, were activated and formed a platelet-rich thrombus despite a normal platelet count and reported compliance with antiplatelet and cytoreductive therapies. Noncompliance with antiplatelet therapy, though, cannot be ruled out, and unfortunately, platelet function testing was unavailable at our institution at that time. Our patient was minimally symptomatic, and so, the chronicity of her aortic thrombosis is unclear. She had numerous collateral vessels identified on imaging which likely developed as a result of her longstanding peripheral arterial disease. These collaterals may have protected her from experiencing acute symptoms when the occlusive thrombosis occurred. There was no acute indication for surgery at her initial presentations, so we aimed to intensify her medical therapy.

Taking into account the pathophysiology of arterial thrombosis in ET, additional platelet directed therapies were chosen over systemic anticoagulation. Clopidogrel, an irreversible adenosine diphosphate (ADP) receptor $P2Y_{12}$ inhibitor, was added to aspirin and hydroxyurea to increase platelet inhibition. The patient was also started on a third antiplatelet agent: cilostazol, a phosphodiesterase type 3 inhibitor (PDE_3), by her vascular surgeon to improve claudication. PDE_3 inhibition leads to a cyclic AMP-dependent increase in protein kinase A (PKA) which prevents smooth muscle contraction resulting in vasodilation [16]. PKA also directly inhibits platelet activation and aggregation by a mechanism that remains poorly understood [17]. Though it has not been studied in ET, the safety and efficacy of this triple antiplatelet combination is supported by studies in other vascular diseases [18, 19]. Unfortunately, we could not assess the efficacy of this therapy in our patient due to poor compliance.

In conclusion, aortic thrombosis is a rare complication of ET and pharmacologic therapy alone may be appropriate in patients without acute surgical indications or who are poor surgical candidates. In patients who develop large vessel thrombosis on first-line therapies, additional platelet-directed therapies may be effective. This case also underscores the importance of managing cardiovascular comorbidities which increase thrombosis risk in patients with ET.

Disclosure

The view(s) expressed herein are those of the authors and do not reflect the official policy or position of Brooke Army Medical Center, the U.S. Army Medical Department, the U.S. Army Office of the Surgeon General, the Department of the Army, the Department of the Air Force, or the Department of Defense or the U.S. Government.

References

[1] D. A. Arber, A. Orazi, R. Hasserjian et al., "The 2016 revision to the World Health Organization classification of myeloid neoplasms and acute leukemia," *Blood*, vol. 127, no. 20, pp. 2391–2405, 2016.

[2] J. Loscalzo, "Resolution of platelet-rich thrombi in essential thrombocythemia: mechanisms, risks, and benefits of antiplatelet therapy," *Mayo Clinic Proceedings*, vol. 76, no. 4, pp. 356-357, 2001.

[3] D. R. Lorelli and A. D. Shepard, "Aortic mural thrombus embolization: an unusual presentation of essential thrombocytosis," *Annals of Vascular Surgery*, vol. 16, no. 3, pp. 375–379, 2002.

[4] M. Johnson, T. Gernsheimer, and K. Johansen, "Essential thrombocytosis: underemphasized cause of large-vessel thrombosis," *Journal of Vascular Surgery*, vol. 22, no. 4, pp. 443–449, 1995.

[5] M. Fang, S. Agha, L. Lockridge, R. Lee, J. P. Cleary, and E. M. Mazur, "Medical management of a large aortic thrombus in a young woman with essential thrombocythemia," *Mayo Clinic Proceedings*, vol. 76, no. 4, pp. 427–431, 2001.

[6] B. K. Chong, D. Mun, C. H. Kang, C.-b. Park, and W. C. Cho, "Essential thrombocytosis-associated thromboembolism in the abdominal aorta," *Korean Journal of Thoracic and Cardiovascular Surgery*, vol. 49, no. 5, pp. 397–400, 2016.

[7] M. Oki, M. Moriuchi, H. Kawada, Y. Ogawa, and K. Ando, "A case of essential thrombo-cythemia presenting with aortic thrombosis," *Tokai Journal of Experimental and Clinical Medicine*, vol. 33, no. 4, pp. 135–137, 2008.

[8] T. Klampfel, H. Gisslinger, A.S. Harutyunyan et al., "Somatic mutations of calreticulin in myeloproliferative neoplasms," *New England Journal of Medicine*, vol. 369, pp. 2379–2390, 2013.

[9] J. Nangalia, C. E Massie, E. J Baxter et al., "Somatic CALR mutations in myeloproliferative neoplasms with nonmutated JAK2," *New England Journal of Medicine*, vol. 369, no. 25, pp. 2391–2405, 2013.

[10] Z. Y. Fayad, E. Semaan, B. Fahoum, M. Briggs, A. Tortolani, and M. D'Ayala, "Aortic mural thrombus in the normal or minimally atherosclerotic aorta," *Annals of Vascular Surgery*, vol. 27, no. 3, pp. 282–290, 2013.

[11] S. Bellucci and J. J. Michiels, "Spontaneous proliferative megakaryocytopoiesis and platelet hyperreactivity in essential thrombocythemia: is thrombopoietin the link?," *Annals of Hematology*, vol. 79, no. 2, pp. 51–58, 2000.

[12] P. V. Genderen, I. Lucas, R. V. Strik et al., "Erythromelalgia in essential thrombocythemia is characterized by platelet activation and endothelial cell damage but not by thrombin generation," *Thrombosis and Haemostasis*, vol. 76, no. 3, pp. 333–338, 1996.

[13] J. J. Michiels, Z. N. Berneman, W. Schroyens, and H. H. D. M. Van Vliet, "Review," *Platelets*, vol. 15, no. 2, pp. 67–84, 2004.

[14] V. Sohn, Z. Arthurs, C. Andersen, and B. Starnes, "Aortic thrombus due to essential thrombocytosis: strategies for medical and surgical management," *Annals of Vascular Surgery*, vol. 22, no. 5, pp. 676–680, 2008.

[15] H. Yamamoto, H. Nishimaki, N. Imai, M. Nitta, and O. Daimaru, "Aortic thrombus in a patient with myeloproliferative thrombocytosis, successfully treated by pharmaceutical therapy: a case report," *Journal of Medical Case Reports*, vol. 4, no. 1, p. 219, 2010.

[16] F. Biscetti, G. Ferraccioli, and A. Flex, "New therapeutic effects of cilostazol in patients with ischemic disorders," *Current Vascular Pharmacology*, vol. 13, no. 3, pp. 399–404, 2015.

[17] A. Smolenski, "Novel roles of cAMP/cGMP-dependent signaling in platelets," *Journal of Thrombosis and Haemostasis*, vol. 10, no. 2, pp. 167–176, 2012.

[18] Y. Han, Y. Li, S. Wang et al., "Cilostazol in addition to aspirin and clopidogrel improves long-term outcomes after percutaneous coronary intervention in patients with acute coronary syndromes: a randomized, controlled study," *American Heart Journal*, vol. 157, no. 4, pp. 733–739, 2009.

[19] D.-F. Geng, M. Liu, D.-M. Jin, W. Wu, J. Deng, and J.-F. Wang, "Cilostazol-based triple antiplatelet therapy compared to dual antiplatelet therapy in patients with coronary stent implantation: a meta-analysis of 5,821 patients," *Cardiology*, vol. 122, no. 3, pp. 148–157, 2012.

Two Rare Complications in One Patient: Acquired von Willebrand Syndrome Associated with Intracranial Plasmacytoma

H. Auge,[1] C. Yguel,[2] E. Schmitt,[3] B. Frotscher,[4] H. Busby-Venner,[2] R. Morizot,[1] C. Moulin,[1] P. Feugier,[1] A. Perrot,[1] and L. Filliatre-Clement[1]

[1]*Hematology Department, University Hospital of Nancy, 5 Rue du Morvan, 54500 Vandoeuvre les Nancy, France*
[2]*Histopathology Department, University Hospital of Nancy, 5 Rue du Morvan, 54500 Vandoeuvre les Nancy, France*
[3]*Neuroradiology Department, University Hospital of Nancy, 29 Avenue du Maréchal de Lattre de Tassigny, 54035 Nancy, France*
[4]*Hemostasis Department, University Hospital of Nancy, 5 Rue du Morvan, 54500 Vandoeuvre les Nancy, France*

Correspondence should be addressed to H. Auge; h.auge@chru-nancy.fr

Academic Editor: Sudhir Tauro

Here, we describe a rare case of acquired von Willebrand syndrome (VWS) associated with intracranial plasmacytoma. The literature includes reports of a few cases of plasmacytoma with central nervous involvement, but none of them with acquired VWS. Diagnosis was made based on a stereotaxic intracerebral biopsy. During this biopsy, a ventriculoperitoneal shunt was established, which was complicated with abnormal bleeding. Subsequent hemostasis assessment related to hemopathy revealed acquired von Willebrand disease. The patient received induction therapy with bortezomib, thalidomide, and dexamethasone (VTD), followed by high-dose melphalan chemotherapy and autologous stem cell transplantation, and then VTD consolidation, and finally maintenance with lenalidomide. Our patient currently remains in very good partial response without neurological symptoms after 4 months of maintenance. The patient is free of progression 14 months after their original presentation.

1. Introduction

Multiple myeloma (MM) is a rare hematological malignant pathology, but its incidence has increased over recent years (5-6 cases per 100,000 population). Therapeutic advances have increased the 5-year survival rate to around 70% [1]. Patients rarely present with central nervous system (dural or extradural) involvement at diagnosis, with only a few such cases described in the literature [2]. MM can also be complicated with an acquired von Willebrand syndrome (VWS). Although von Willebrand disease is the most common hereditary hemorrhagic pathology (affecting up to 1% of the general population), the acquired form of VWS is an unusual complication of certain lymphoproliferative disorders, particularly MM [3].

2. Case Presentation

Here, we report the case of a 48-year-old Caucasian male with no previous relevant medical/surgical history, who was admitted to neurology services due to intermittent headaches, dysgeusia, and persistent dizziness for two months. His symptoms also included spontaneously resolving gum bleeding. An MRI was performed (Figure 1(a)), revealing a voluminous left extraparenchymal posterior fossa tumor, complicated by occipital osteolysis and hydrocephalus, without distant metastatic lesions. Computerized tomography (CT) scanning revealed no other suspicious lesion (Figure 1(b)).

A stereotaxic intracerebral biopsy was performed, and at the same time, a ventriculoperitoneal shunt was established to control intracranial hypertension. These procedures were complicated by a voluminous right parietal hematoma with mass effect and falcorial and temporal commitment, resulting in a secondary epileptic seizure. No hemostasis report was available before this intervention.

To explore this major bleeding, a hemostasis assessment was performed. This revealed a prolonged activated partial thromboplastin time (APTT) of 44 s (normal value (NV):

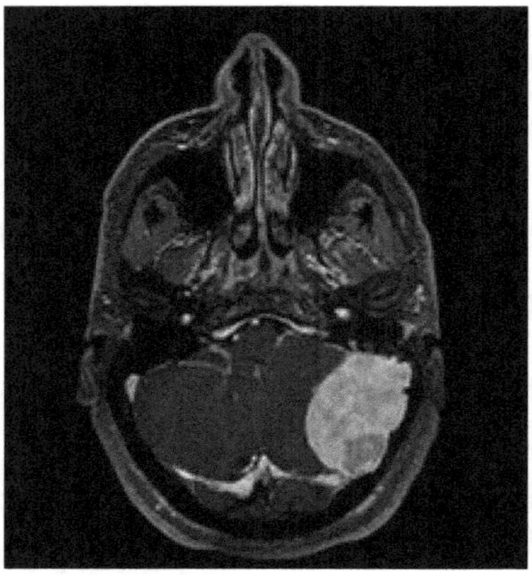

MRI at diagnosis:
Axial 3DT1 sequence with gadolinium injection. Well-limited mass, relatively homogeneous, with intense enhancement of extraparenchymal localization, pushing the left cerebellar hemisphere and compressing the 4th ventricle.

(a)

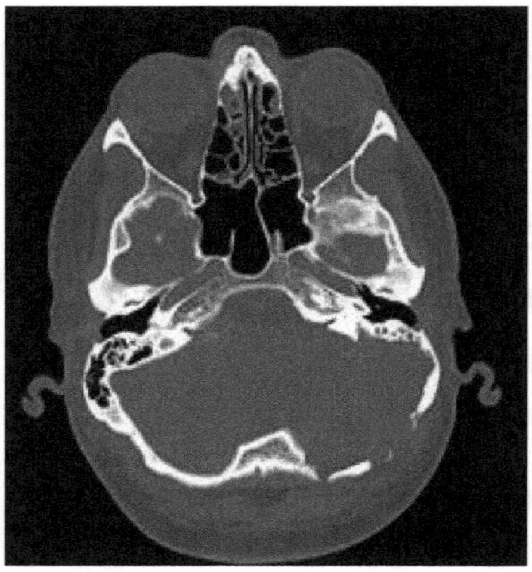

CT scan at diagnosis:
Osteomeningeal mass syndrome, lytic, centered on occipital bone and left mastoid

(b)

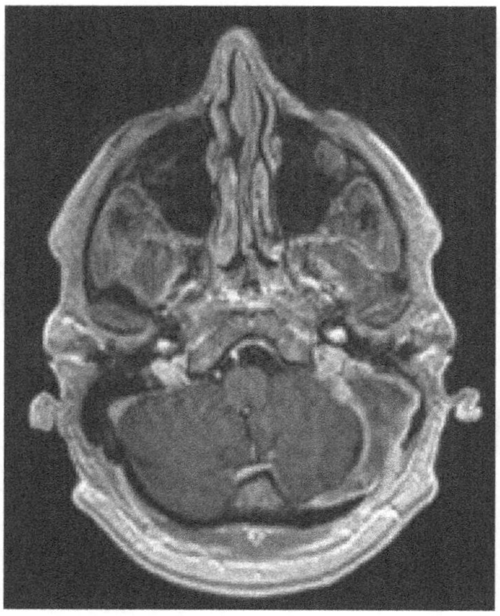

Axial 3DT1 sequence with gadolinium injection. Strong regression of left osteomeningeal mass syndrome with more necrotic appearance. Regression of the mass effect on the cerebellum

(c)

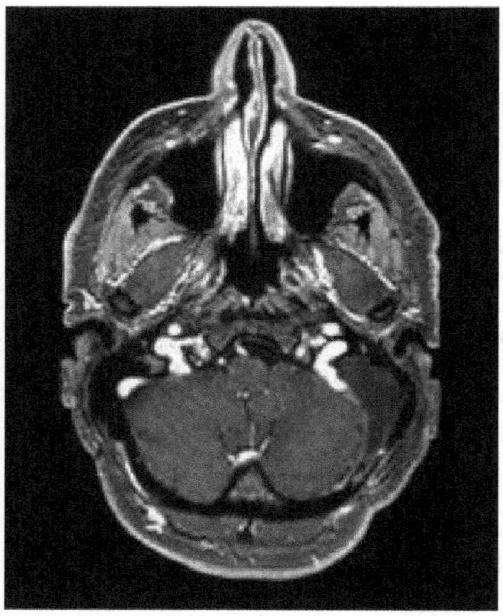

Axial 3DT1 sequence with gadolinium injection. Persistant regression of mass syndrome with disappearance of contrast enhancement. Disappearance of the mass effect on the cerebellum

(d)

FIGURE 1: (a) MRI at diagnosis. (b) CT scan at diagnosis. (c) Follow-up MRI after two courses of bortezomib, thalidomide, and dexamethasone. (d) Follow-up MRI after two courses of lenalidomide maintenance.

23–35 s) and a decreased factor VIII level (FVIII: 10%; NV: 60–150%). In addition, the level of von Willebrand factor antigen was low (vWF : Ag < 10%; NV > 60%), and the activity of vWF ristocetin cofactor was severely decreased (vWF : RCo < 4%, undetectable; NV > 60%), indicating an acquired von Willebrand syndrome (VWS).

Biological evaluation, including serum protein electrophoresis, revealed a monoclonal gammopathy IgG kappa of 16 g/L, associated with high kappa-free light chain of 109 mg/L (NV, 3.3–19.4 mg/L). The lambda-free light chain level was 37.2 mg/L (NV, 5.7–26.3 mg/L), and the kappa/lamba ratio was 2.94 (NV, 0.26–1. 65). Complete blood count (CBC), renal function, and corrected serum calcium were normal. We detected a Bence-Jones proteinuria, with global proteinuria of 1.73 g/L, and B2 microglobulin of 1.88 mg/L (NV, 0.9–2 mg/L). The albumin level was 12.3 g/L

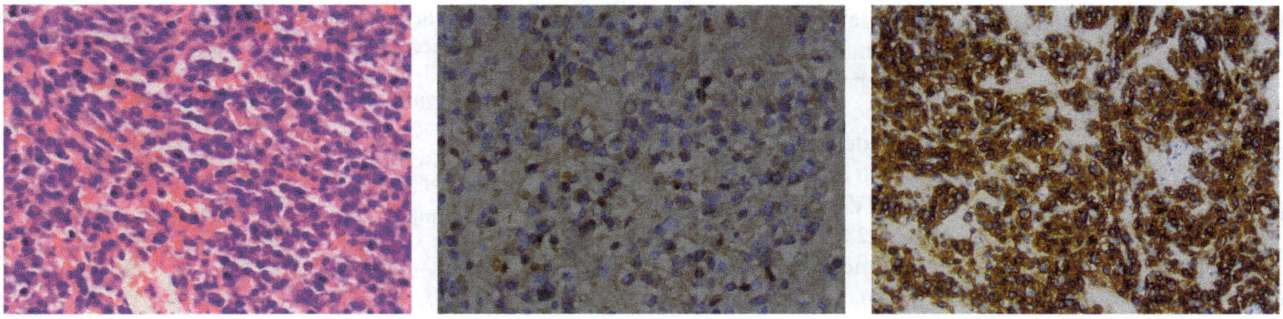

(a) (b) (c)

FIGURE 2: (a) Neoplastic plasma cell proliferation. Hematoxylin-eosin-saffron (HES) coloration, ×400 magnification. (b) Monotypic plasma cell proliferation. Anti-kappa antibody, ×400 magnification. (c) CD138 expression by plasma cells. Anti-CD138 antibody, ×400 magnification.

(NV, 35–52 mg/L), and the LDH level was 265 U/L (NV, <248 U/L).

Histological examination of the biopsy supported a diagnosis of plasmacytoma (Figures 2(a)–2(c)), revealing the following atypical plasma cells proliferation markers: $CD38^+$, MUM–$IRF4^+$, positive expression of kappa-free light chain (KP-53 clone) without expression of lambda-free light chain (K22-Y clone), $CD20^-$, $CD3^-$, and proliferation index ki67 of 5%. Bone marrow aspiration showed 5% atypical plasma cells. Serum and bone marrow immunophenotyping were not performed. Cytogenetic analysis supported the conclusion of a standard risk, without *t*(4;14) or del(17p). The revised prognostic score R-ISS was evaluated to be 2.

Prior to myeloma confirmation, the initial case management comprised symptomatic treatment, including evacuation of intraparenchymal hematoma, and establishment of an external ventricular bypass. Immediately before this surgical intervention, FVIII was administered in association with VWF (KOVALTRY® 70 UI/kg + WILFACTIN® 52 UI/kg UI). Immediately after surgical intervention, FVIII (KOVALTRY® 70 UI/kg) was administered without VWF. During the night, this treatment was switched to recombinant factor VII (NOVOSEVEN® 86 μg/kg). FVIII treatment increased the circulating FVIII level to 59% with persisting low levels of vWF : Ag (11%) and vWF : Rco (4%). Administration of high-dose intravenous immunoglobulins (CLAYRIG® 0.8 mg/kg) allowed the FVIII level to increase to >200%, with a vWF : Ag level of 68% and vWF : Rco level of 70%, causing the bleeding to stop. The patient's FVIII and VWF levels remained normal for 3 weeks. At 3 weeks after the first infusion, VWF activity decreased to 55%, with a vWF : Ag level of 120% and normal FVIII at 135%, without bleeding event, necessitating another treatment with intravenous immunoglobulins before a new surgical intervention (laparoscopy) was required to eliminate peritonitis by infection of the external ventricular bypass valve. Subsequently, we observed normalization of hemostasis (FVIII > 150%; VWF activity > 60%; vWF : RCo > 60%).

For symptomatic myeloma with extraparenchymal plasmacytoma developed at the expense of the occipital bone, the specific treatment started with 4 days of administration of 40 mg of dexamethasone treatment alone. This was followed by the induction of four 28-day cycles of VTD plus bortezomib 1.3 mg/m^2 on D1, D4, D8, and D11; thalidomide 100 mg continuously; and dexamethasone 40 mg on D1-D2, D8-D9, D15-D16, and D22-D23. After one cycle of VTD, the ventriculoperitoneal shunt could be removed. After two cycles, MRI showed regression of the plasmacytoma, which was considered complete (Figure 1(b)). After the third cycle, we observed a very good partial response, with non-measurable serum and urine M-proteins and normalization of the light chain ratio, as well as complete normalization of the hemostasis balance parameters.

The patient then received high-dose melphalan chemotherapy and autologous stem cell transplantation, followed by two VTD consolidation courses, and then maintenance with lenalidomide. After two courses of maintenance, MRI revealed a net decrease of the extraparenchymal posterior fossa tumor, with a greater necrotic aspect and less enhancement (Figure 1(c)). To date, our patient remains in VGPR without neurological symptoms after 4 months of maintenance. The patient is free of progression 14 months after their original presentation.

3. Discussion

To our knowledge, this is the first reported case of extraparenchymal intracranial plasmacytoma associated with acquired VWS. Kumar et al. [4] suggested that physiopathological mechanisms of acquired VWS are poorly understood, but its occurrence with malignant hematologic disorders, especially dysproteinemias, has been described. [5–11]. Acquired VWS is usually similar to the "2A" type inherited disease, in that it involves decreases of both the activity and concentration of vWF (vWF : RCo and vWF : Ag) [12]. In addition, type 1 or type 3 VWD can also be detected in individuals in whom acquired VWS is associated with abnormal synthesis of vWF (e.g., hypothyroidism) [12], and optimally, a multimeric analysis completes the diagnosis of acquired VWS. Acquired VWD in MM is based on several mechanisms: antibodies specifically directed against functional domains of VWF [11, 13], the monoclonal protein can also accelerate immunologic clearance of VWF [14], adsorption of VWF by malignant cells [15], and finally a GpIb-mediated selective adsorption of VWF on malignant cells [16].

Intravenous immunoglobulin (IVIg) has shown efficacy for treatment of acquired VWS with type immunoglobulin (Ig) G monoclonal gammopathies of undetermined significance (MGUS) [17, 18]. Such treatment can reportedly induce a prompt and sustained increase of FVIII/VWF activities and shorten the bleeding time for at least 15–20 days for all IgG-MGUS with a correction of VWF multimeric structure [6]. Data from the International Society on Thrombosis and Hemostasis (ISTH) registry indicate that patients exhibiting acquired VWS along with lymphoproliferative disease (48% of patients with acquired VWS) may also benefit from IVIg therapy [6, 18]. Normalization of plasma vWF activity is usually observed no earlier than 24–48 h after IVIg administration. Thus, it was surprising and unusual that vWF : Ag and vWF : Rco increased immediately (<8 h) after IVIg administration in our present case.

With regard to intracranial extramedullary involvement, a recently reported series of 50 patients included 14 patients with dural or extradural involvement at diagnosis [2]. Of these patients, 78% exhibited spinal osteolytic abnormalities, which were not observed in our present patient. Of the 50 patients, 10 were able to benefit from an autotransplant, including 7 who exhibited complete remission/very good partial response. Multivariate analysis in that study revealed that survival was associated with B2 microglobulin levels and complete response or very good partial response. The median survival was 25 months among patients with plasmacytoma exhibiting dural or extradural involvement and was 46 months among MM patients without CNS involvement.

In conclusion, the survival of patients with multiple myeloma and extradural disease remains lower than that of other MM patients. However, new therapeutic options and reinforcement with autotransplant have yielded encouraging results. Our currently described patient presented with a serious initial disease associated with acquired VWS, but highly effective treatment led to regression of the symptoms without sequelae.

Consent

The patient gave consent for his case to be reported in a scientific manuscript.

References

[1] I. Turesson, M. Bjorkholm, C. H. Blimark, S. Kristinsson, R. Velez, and O. Landgren, "Rapidly changing myeloma epidemiology in the general population: increased incidence, older patients, and longer survival," *European Journal of Haematology*, vol. 101, no. 2, pp. 237–244, 2018.

[2] A. Gozzetti, A. Cerase, F. Lotti et al., "Extramedullary intracranial localization of multiple myeloma and treatment with novel agents: a retrospective survey of 50 patients," *Cancer*, vol. 118, no. 6, pp. 1574–1584, 2012.

[3] C. Dicke, S. Schneppenheim, K. Holstein et al., "Distinct mechanisms account for acquired von Willebrand syndrome in plasma cell dyscrasias," *Annals of Hematology*, vol. 95, no. 6, pp. 945–957, 2016.

[4] S. Kumar, R. K. Pruthi, and W. L. Nichols, "Acquired von Willebrand disease," *Mayo Clinic Proceedings*, vol. 77, no. 2, pp. 181–187, 2002.

[5] G. I. C. Ingram, P. J. Kingston, J. Leslie, and E. J. W. Bowie, "Four cases of acquired von Willebrand's syndrome," *British Journal of Haematology*, vol. 21, no. 2, pp. 189–199, 1971.

[6] A. B. Federici, F. Stabile, G. Castaman, M. T. Canciani, and P. M. Mannucci, "Treatment of acquired von Willebrand syndrome in patients with monoclonal gammopathy of uncertain significance: comparison of three different therapeutic approaches," *Blood*, vol. 92, no. 8, pp. 2707–2711, 1998.

[7] N. Jin, F. F. Salahuddin, and J. A. Nesbitt, "Acquired von Willebrand disease and multiple myeloma," *Blood Coagulation and Fibrinolysis*, vol. 25, no. 8, pp. 890–893, 2014.

[8] S. Katagiri, D. Akahane, K. Amano, and K. Ohyashiki, "Long-term remission of acquired von Willebrand syndrome associated with multiple myeloma using bortezomib and dexamethasone therapy," *Haemophilia*, vol. 22, no. 6, pp. e557–e559, 2016.

[9] B. M. Sampson, M. Greaves, R. G. Malia, and F. E. Preston, "Acquired von Willebrand's disease: demonstration of a circulating inhibitor to the factor VIII complex in four cases," *British Journal of Haematology*, vol. 54, no. 2, pp. 233–244, 1983.

[10] E. G. Bovill, W. B. Ershler, E. A. Golden, B. H. Tindle, and J. R. Edson, "A human myeloma-produced monoclonal protein directed against the active subpopulation of von Willebrand factor," *American Journal of Clinical Pathology*, vol. 85, no. 1, pp. 115–123, 1986.

[11] H. Mohri, J. Tanabe, M. Ohtsuka et al., "Acquired von Willebrand disease associated with multiple myeloma; characterization of an inhibitor to von Willebrand factor," *Blood Coagulation and Fibrinolysis*, vol. 6, no. 6, pp. 561–566, 1995.

[12] A. Mital, "Acquired von Willebrand syndrome," *Advances in Clinical and Experimental Medicine*, vol. 25, no. 6, pp. 1337–1344, 2016.

[13] H. Mohri, T. Noguchi, F. Kodama, A. Itoh, and T. Ohkubo, "Acquired von Willebrand disease due to inhibitor of human myeloma protein specific for von Willebrand factor," *American Journal of Clinical Pathology*, vol. 87, no. 5, pp. 663–668, 1987.

[14] O. Zettervall and I. M. Nilsson, "Acquired von Willebrand's disease caused by a monoclonal antibody," *Acta Medica Scandinavica*, vol. 204, no. 1–6, pp. 521–528, 2009.

[15] C. Richard, M. A. Cuadrado, M. Prieto et al., "Acquired von Willebrand disease in multiple myeloma secondary to absorption of von Willebrand factor by plasma cells," *American Journal of Hematology*, vol. 35, no. 2, pp. 114–117, 1990.

[16] M.-L. Scrobohaci, M.-T. Daniel, Y. Levy, J.-P. Marolleau, and J.-C. Brouet, "Expression of GpIb on plasma cells in a patient with monoclonal IgG and acquired von Willebrand disease," *British Journal of Haematology*, vol. 84, no. 3, pp. 471–475, 1993.

[17] A. Tiede, J. H. Rand, U. Budde, A. Ganser, and A. B. Federici, "How I treat the acquired von Willebrand syndrome," *Blood*, vol. 117, no. 25, pp. 6777–6785, 2011.

[18] A. B. Federici, "Use of intravenous immunoglobulin in patients with acquired von Willebrand syndrome," *Human Immunology*, vol. 66, no. 4, pp. 422–430, 2005.

38

Rivaroxaban Treatment for Heparin-Induced Thrombocytopenia: A Case Report and a Review of the Current Experience

Mohamed Aon[1,2] **and Omar Al-Shammari**[1]

[1]*Department of Medicine, Jahra Hospital, Ministry of Health (HOM), Jahra city, Kuwait*
[2]*Department of Medicine, Faculty of Medicine, Cairo University, Giza, Egypt*

Correspondence should be addressed to Mohamed Aon; maon2004@cu.edu.eg

Academic Editor: Gergely Feher

Heparin-induced thrombocytopenia is a life-threatening complication of exposure to heparin. Heparin-induced thrombocytopenia results from an autoantibody directed against platelet factor 4 in complex with heparin. Heparin-induced thrombocytopenia is traditionally treated with bivalirudin, argatroban, danaparoid, or fondaparinux. Recently, direct oral anticoagulants administration to treat heparin-induced thrombocytopenia has been reported. Direct oral anticoagulants do not cause platelet activation in the presence of heparin-platelet factor 4 antibodies, nor do they provoke autoantibody production. Direct oral anticoagulants offer advantages such as consistent and predictable anticoagulation, oral administration with good patient compliance, and a good safety profile. We report a case of heparin-induced thrombocytopenia with deep venous thrombosis successfully treated with rivaroxaban and review the current experience with rivaroxaban for the treatment of heparin-induced thrombocytopenia.

1. Introduction

Heparin-induced thrombocytopenia (HIT) is a clinical syndrome complicating exposure to heparin that occurs in a small percentage of patients. HIT is caused by antibodies to complexes of platelet factor 4 (PF4) and heparin that can cause thrombosis along with thrombocytopenia. HIT diagnosis rests on the presence of thrombocytopenia and/or thrombosis after heparin exposure while excluding other possible causes of thrombocytopenia [1]. HIT requires immediate treatment to reduce the risk of serious thrombosis. There are several nonheparin anticoagulants that can be used in the treatment of HIT, e.g., argatroban, bivalirudin, danaparoid, and fondaparinux. Accumulating evidence suggests that direct oral anticoagulants (DOACs) are effective in treating HIT [2].

In this article, we report a case of HIT complicated with deep venous thrombosis (DVT) successfully treated with rivaroxaban and review the accumulating experience with rivaroxaban for the treatment of HIT.

2. Case Presentation

A 25-years-old male presented to Jahra Hospital, Kuwait, with confusion after the ingestion of methanol. In the emergency room, he had high anion gap metabolic acidosis (pH 6.8, HCO_3 8 mmol/L, anion gap 31 mmol/L), elevated serum lactate (16.6 mmol/L), and hypoglycemia. Treatment was started with intravenous dextrose, thiamine, and sodium bicarbonate infusion. Due to persistent acidosis, dialysis was started through a right femoral catheter. After dialysis, his metabolic parameters improved, and the catheter was removed. His medication included enoxaparin 40 mg once daily for DVT prophylaxis, omeprazole, folic acid, and thiamine. On the 5th day of hospital stay, the patient's platelet count decreased (Figure 1), with normal white blood cells, hemoglobin, and coagulation profile, so his enoxaparin prophylaxis was substituted with fondaparinux 2.5 mg once daily. On the 6th day of hospital stay, he started to develop right-sided thigh pain and swelling. Urgent ultrasound examination of the deep venous system revealed right

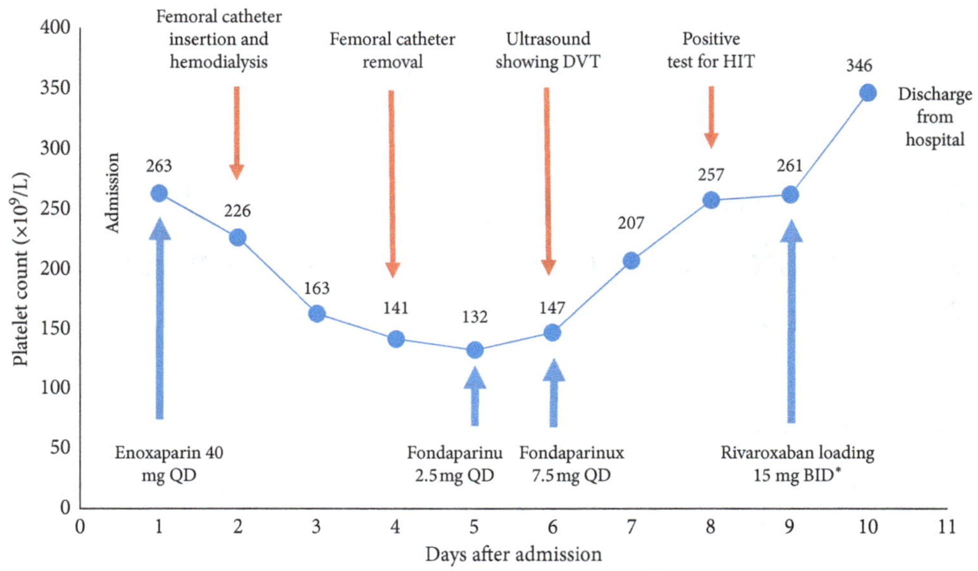

Figure 1: Platelet count charted against time and timeline of clinical events and medications used until day of discharge. QD, once daily; BID, twice per day; DVT, deep venous thrombosis; HIT, heparin-induced thrombocytopenia. *Loading for 21 days and then 20 mg QD to complete a total of three months.

external iliac, femoral, and popliteal vein recent thrombosis. Fondaparinux was increased to a therapeutic dose according to his body weight (7.5 mg once daily) and HIT serology was sent. Over the next days, the patient's condition was improving, and blood examination showed recovery of platelet count (Figure 1). Heparin-induced anti-platelet antibodies were detected at 0.846 optical density (OD) units, and the confirmatory functional assay was positive. Given his clinical and laboratory improvement, we decided to start him on rivaroxaban. Loading dose 15 mg twice daily for 21 days was started and the patient was released to outpatient care. Follow-up in outpatient revealed continued clinical improvement. The treatment was well tolerated with no adverse effects and the dosing was switched to 20 mg once daily to complete a total of three months of treatment. Three months after the hospital discharge, the patient underwent outpatient examination that revealed a good overall condition with a normal platelet count and recanalization of the deep venous system on ultrasound examination. Rivaroxaban was stopped and the patient was instructed to avoid heparin for life.

3. Discussion

HIT is a clinical syndrome caused by antibodies to complexes of PF4 and heparin. This syndrome has also been called heparin-induced thrombocytopenia and thrombosis (HITT) because antibodies can cause thrombosis along with thrombocytopenia [1]. Antibody-coated platelets are removed by the reticuloendothelial system causing thrombocytopenia. Consumption of platelets at sites of thrombosis is another mechanism of thrombocytopenia in HIT [3]. HIT is a prothrombotic disorder and the primary mechanism of thrombosis is due to the binding of HIT antibodies to the platelet which elicits platelet activation and release of procoagulant microparticles. Platelet activation in HIT is also accompanied by endothelial cell activation and injury leading to increased tissue factor expression and thrombin generation [4]. Affected individuals have a 50% risk of developing new thromboembolic events which can involve both the arterial and the venous systems. The mortality rate is approximately 15%, and 10% of patients require amputations or suffer another major morbidity [5]. HIT is more common in surgical patients compared with medical patients and more common among females. Absolute risks of developing HIT after exposure to prophylactic unfractionated heparin is 2.6% versus 0.2% after low molecular weight heparin (LMWH) exposure [6]. HIT diagnosis rests on the presence of thrombocytopenia and/or thrombosis in temporal association with heparin exposure while excluding other causes of thrombocytopenia. If HIT is suspected, it is recommended to use the 4Ts score to estimate the probability of HIT [7]. If there is an intermediate to high probability of HIT (4Ts score ≥4), heparin should be discontinued and an immunoassay for HIT antibodies is obtained. If the immunoassay is positive, a functional assay is used to confirm the results. A functional assay may not be necessary for patients with a high probability score and a strongly positive immunoassay >2.0 OD units [8].

Given that platelet drop is 50% on the 5th day after LMWH exposure, associated with a new DVT, and no other causes for thrombocytopenia are present, our patient's 4Ts score is 7 points, i.e., a high probability of HIT. His immunoassay is positive (OD 0.846; OD values ≥0.400 are considered positive in our reference laboratory and the confirmatory test is positive).

Once HIT is diagnosed, heparin must be discontinued, and a nonheparin anticoagulant is used instead. The latest American Society of Hematology (ASH) HIT treatment guidelines endorse the use of either argatroban, bivalirudin, danaparoid, or fondaparinux. Because of their short

Table 1: Cohort studies and case reports of rivaroxaban for the treatment of HIT.

Study reference	Number of patients	HITT*	Rivaroxaban treatment for acute or subacute HIT*	Primary or secondary treatment*	Extension of thrombosis or major bleeding	Dose*
[2, 9]	28	12/28	19/28 acute 9/28 subacute	13/28 primary 15/28 secondary	Yes[a,b]	20/28 standard dose 4/28 20 mg once daily 4/28 10 mg once daily
[10, 11][c]	9	9/9	9/9 acute	9/9 primary	No	4/9 standard dose 5/9 10 mg once daily
[12]	9[d]	4/9	9/9 acute	9/9 secondary	No	9/9 20 mg once daily
[13]	3	2/3	3/3 acute	3/3 secondary	No	3/3 15 mg twice daily
[14]	2	2/2	2/2 acute	2/2 secondary	Yes[e]	2/2 Standard dose
[15]	1	No	Acute	Secondary	No	Not specified
[16]	1	Yes	Acute	Secondary	No	Standard dose
[17]	1	Yes	Acute	Primary	No	20 mg twice daily
[18]	1	No	Acute	Primary	No	10 mg once daily
[19]	1	Yes	Acute	Primary	No	Standard dose
[20]	1	Yes	Acute	Secondary	No	Standard dose
[21]	1	Yes	Acute[f]	Secondary	No	20 mg once daily
[22]	1	No	Acute	Primary	No	15 mg twice daily
[23]	1	Yes	Acute	Secondary	No	Not specified
[24, 25][g]	1	Yes	Acute	Primary	No	Standard dose
[26]	1	Yes	Subacute	Primary	No	10 mg once daily
[27]	1	Yes	Acute	Primary	No	Not specified
[28]	1	Yes	Acute	Secondary	No	Standard dose
[29]	1	Yes	Acute	Secondary	No	Not specified
Total (%)	65	40/65 (61.5%)	55/65 acute (84.6%) 10/65 subacute (15.4%)	29/65 primary (44.6%) 36/65 secondary (55.4%)	1/65 extension of thrombosis (1.5%) 1/65 major bleeding (1.5%)	33/65 standard dose (51%) 28/65 other doses (43%) 4/65 not specified (6%)
Our case	1	Yes	Subacute	Secondary	No	Standard dose

*See text for details. [a]Possible extension of a catheter-related arm DVT with full recovery after catheter removal and despite the continuation of rivaroxaban. [b]One rectal bleeding episode with a known gastric cancer occurred 9 days after discontinuing rivaroxaban and while receiving fondaparinux, so not included. [c]The articles are combined because the 3 patients first reported by Ng et al. are also included among the 9 patients reported by Ong et al. [d]Out of the 11 patients who received rivaroxaban, 2 tested negative for HIT antibodies and thus are excluded in this table. [e]Moderate hemoptysis secondary to known squamous cell lung cancer. [f]Platelets dropped <50% but did not drop below 150×10^9/L. [g]Articles in Spanish but data from Barlow et al.

duration of action, argatroban and bivalirudin are preferred in critically ill patients, patients with high bleeding risk, or patients who may need urgent procedures. However, they are expensive and require a hospital stay for parenteral administration and frequent monitoring. Fondaparinux is being increasingly used in clinically stable patients at average risk of bleeding. Danaparoid is no longer available in the United States and parts of Europe [8]. In our case, the patient's stable condition and the average risk of bleeding is the reason to choose fondaparinux as a nonheparin anticoagulant initially.

Accumulating evidence suggests that DOACs are effective in treating HIT, without stimulating HIT antibodies. DOACs are an attractive treatment option for HIT as they offer many potential benefits, including ease of administration, rapid onset of action, no required monitoring, the competitive cost to other anticoagulants, and efficacy during longer-term anticoagulation. However, the evidence for the efficacy of DOACs for HIT is only based on prospective cohort studies or retrospective case series while an RCT is lacking [2]. Ideally, an RCT demonstrating the efficacy of a DOAC in HIT is preferred before it becomes an approved treatment. However, the rarity of HIT and the challenges in diagnosis delay any trial recruitment.

With respect to the choice of a DOAC, most of the published experience in HIT is with rivaroxaban which is an oral direct factor Xa inhibitor. After carrying out a search on PubMed and MEDLINE database using the words "heparin-induced thrombocytopenia," and "rivaroxaban," 59 references were identified, dating from 2008 to 2020. Until February 2020, twenty-one articles in English contained reports of HIT cases treated with rivaroxaban: 1 prospective study, 5 retrospective cohort studies, and 14 case reports, totaling 65 patients. In the previously discussed literature, 61.5% of cases had HIT-related thrombosis, treatment with rivaroxaban was started while the patient was still thrombocytopenic (i.e., acute HIT) in 84.6% of cases, while it was initiated after platelet recovery (i.e., subacute HIT) in 15.4%. Out of the 65 cases, one (1.5%) had recurrent venous thromboembolism and one case (1.5%) experienced a moderate bleeding episode while receiving rivaroxaban (Table 1).

Rivaroxaban was the initial nonheparin anticoagulant selected to treat HIT (i.e., primary therapy of HIT) in 44.6% of HIT cases. Switch from another parenteral nonheparin anticoagulant to rivaroxaban therapy (i.e., secondary therapy of HIT) was noticed in 55.4% of cases. Half of the published cases used the standard dose regimen for venous thromboembolism: 15 mg twice daily for the initial 21 days followed by 20 mg once daily, while others used different dosing regimens (Table 1).

Of all the DOACs, rivaroxaban has the largest body of literature for its use in HIT and is the only DOAC that has been evaluated in a prospective study. While the current experience remains limited, it is suggestive of the potential role of rivaroxaban in HIT, which has led to its integration into the 2018 ASH guidelines with a conditional recommendation [8].

In our case, after the initial use of fondaparinux for 3 days, platelets recovered, and rivaroxaban was started before discharging the patient. We used the standard dose of rivaroxaban: 15 mg twice daily for the initial 21 days followed by 20 mg once daily for 3 months. After 3 months of treatment, rivaroxaban was stopped.

In conclusion, this case report demonstrates the effectiveness and safety of rivaroxaban in the treatment of HIT. Given the rarity of HIT itself, there are no consensus management guidelines for the treatment of HIT with rivaroxaban. More research is needed including encouraging physicians to present outcome data when using rivaroxaban, creating registries of HIT treatment with rivaroxaban and conducting studies that compare rivaroxaban and other nonheparin anticoagulants.

References

[1] G. M. Arepally, "Heparin-induced thrombocytopenia," *Blood*, vol. 129, no. 21, pp. 2864–2872, 2017.

[2] T. E. Warkentin, M. Pai, and L.-A. Linkins, "Direct oral anticoagulants for treatment of HIT: update of Hamilton experience and literature review," *Blood*, vol. 130, no. 9, pp. 1104–1113, 2017.

[3] B. H. Chong, "Heparin-induced thrombocytopenia," *Journal of Thrombosis and Haemostasis*, vol. 1, no. 7, pp. 1471–1478, 2003.

[4] T. Warkentin, C. Hayward, L. Boshkov et al., "Sera from patients with heparin-induced thrombocytopenia generate platelet-derived microparticles with procoagulant activity: an explanation for the thrombotic complications of heparin-induced thrombocytopenia," *Blood*, vol. 84, no. 11, pp. 3691–3699, 1994.

[5] C. Kearon, E. A. Akl, A. J. Comerota et al., "Antithrombotic therapy for VTE disease: antithrombotic therapy and prevention of thrombosis, 9th ed: American College of Chest Physicians evidence-based clinical practice guidelines [published correction appears in chest. 2012 Dec; 142 (6): 1698–1704]," *Chest*, vol. 141, no. 2, pp. e419S–e496S, 2012.

[6] N. Martel, J. Lee, and P. S. Wells, "Risk for heparin-induced thrombocytopenia with unfractionated and low-molecular-weight heparin thromboprophylaxis: a meta-analysis," *Blood*, vol. 106, no. 8, pp. 2710–2715, 2005.

[7] G. K. Lo, D. Juhl, T. E. Warkentin, C. S. Sigouin, P. Eichler, and A. Greinacher, "Evaluation of pretest clinical score (4 T's) for the diagnosis of heparin-induced thrombocytopenia in two clinical settings," *Journal of Thrombosis and Haemostasis*, vol. 4, no. 4, pp. 759–765, 2006.

[8] A. Cuker, G. M. Arepally, B. H. Chong et al., "American Society of Hematology 2018 guidelines for management of venous thromboembolism: heparin-induced thrombocytopenia," *Blood Advances*, vol. 2, no. 22, pp. 3360–3392, 2018.

[9] L. A. Linkins, T. E. Warkentin, M. Pai et al., "Rivaroxaban for treatment of suspected or confirmed heparin-induced thrombocytopenia study," *Journal of Thrombosis and Haemostasis*, vol. 14, no. 6, pp. 1206–1210, 2016.

[10] S. Y. Ong, Y. A. Chin, H. Than et al., "Rivaroxaban for heparin-induced thrombocytopenia: adding to the evidence," *Annals of Hematology*, vol. 96, no. 3, pp. 525–527, 2017.

[11] H. J. Ng, H. Than, and E. C. Y. Teo, "First experiences with the use of rivaroxaban in the treatment of heparin-induced thrombocytopenia," *Thrombosis Research*, vol. 135, no. 1, pp. 205–207, 2015.

[12] M. Sharifi, C. Bay, Z. Vajo, W. Freeman, M. Sharifi, and F. Schwartz, "New oral anticoagulants in the treatment of heparin- induced thrombocytopenia," *Thrombosis Research*, vol. 135, no. 4, pp. 607–609, 2015.

[13] K. A. Davis and D. O. Davis, "Direct acting oral anticoagulants for the treatment of suspected heparin-induced thrombocytopenia," *European Journal of Haematology*, vol. 99, no. 4, pp. 332–335, 2017.

[14] P. R. Kunk, J. Brown, M. McShane, S. Palkimas, and B. Gail Macik, "Direct oral anticoagulants in hypercoagulable states," *Journal of Thrombosis and Thrombolysis*, vol. 43, no. 1, pp. 79–85, 2017.

[15] I. Kopolovic and T. E. Warkentin, "Progressive thrombocytopenia after cardiac surgery in a 67-year-old man," *Canadian Medical Association Journal*, vol. 186, no. 12, pp. 929–933, 2014.

[16] P. Hantson, C. Lambert, and C. Hermans, "Rivaroxaban for arterial thrombosis related to heparin-induced thrombocytopenia," *Blood Coagulation & Fibrinolysis*, vol. 26, no. 2, pp. 205-206, 2015.

[17] L. Abouchakra, Z. Khabbaz, S. Abouassi, and G. Badaoui, "Rivaroxaban for treatment of heparin-induced thrombocytopenia after cardiac surgery: a case report," *The Journal of Thoracic and Cardiovascular Surgery*, vol. 150, no. 2, pp. e19–20, 2015.

[18] B. Tardy-Poncet, M. Piot, A. Montmartin, A. Burdier, E. Chalayer, and B. Tardy, "Delayed-onset heparin-induced thrombocytopenia without thrombosis in a patient receiving

postoperative thromboprophylaxis with rivaroxaban," *Thrombosis and Haemostasis*, vol. 114, no. 3, pp. 652–654, 2015.

[19] M. Samoš, T. Bolek, J. Ivanková et al., "Heparin-induced thrombocytopenia presenting with deep venous thrombosis and pulmonary embolism successfully treated with rivaroxaban: clinical case report and review of current experiences," *Journal of Cardiovascular Pharmacology*, vol. 68, no. 5, pp. 391–394, 2016.

[20] J. M. Casan, G. Grigoriadis, N. Chan, and S. Chunilal, "Rivaroxaban in treatment refractory heparin-induced thrombocytopenia," *BMJ Case Reports*, vol. 2016, 2016.

[21] M. Sartori, E. Favaretto, M. Cini, C. Legnani, and B. Cosmi, "Rivaroxaban in the treatment of heparin-induced thrombocytopenia," *Journal of Thrombosis and Thrombolysis*, vol. 40, no. 3, pp. 392–394, 2015.

[22] M. Vavlukis, I. Kotlar, H. Taravari, L. Poposka, and S. Kedev, "Can rivaroxaban be a drug of choice for treating heparin-induced thrombocytopenia in a patient with pulmonary thromboembolism?" *The Anatolian Journal of Cardiology*, vol. 18, no. 1, pp. 77–79, 2017.

[23] A. Tvito, T. Bakchoul, J. M. Rowe, A. Greinacher, and C. Ganzel, "Severe and persistent heparin-induced thrombocytopenia despite fondaparinux treatment," *American Journal of Hematology*, vol. 90, no. 7, pp. 675–678, 2015.

[24] O. G. Rivera, S. O. Corsi, J. A. Pavlovic, S. A. Aizman, and A. P. Varas, "Rivaroxaban para el tratamiento de la trombocitopenia inducida por heparina. Caso clínico," *Revista Médica de Chile*, vol. 145, no. 9, pp. 1213–1217, 2017.

[25] A. Barlow, B. Barlow, T. Reinaker, and J. Harris, "Potential role of direct oral anticoagulants in the management of heparin-induced thrombocytopenia," *Pharmacotherapy: The Journal of Human Pharmacology and Drug Therapy*, vol. 39, no. 8, pp. 837–853, 2019.

[26] H. Huang, Y. Lin, R. X. Yao, M. Q. He, and X. J. Lin, "Successful treatment of severe heparin-induced thrombocytopenia with intravenous immunoglobulin, platelet transfusion and rivaroxaban: a case report," *Chinese Medical Sciences Journal*, vol. 34, no. 1, pp. 60–64, 2019.

[27] M. J. Bienz, P. Obrocki, J. Russell, R. Jena, and I. A. Mendichovszky, "Heparin-induced thrombocytopaenia presenting as acute aortic mural thrombosis," *BJR Case Reports*, vol. 5, no. 1, 2018.

[28] F. Manji, T. E. Warkentin, J.-A. I. Sheppard, and A. Lee, "Fondaparinux cross-reactivity in heparin-induced thrombocytopenia successfully treated with high-dose intravenous immunoglobulin and rivaroxaban," *Platelets*, vol. 31, no. 1, pp. 124–127, 2020.

[29] T. Bakchoul, O. Borst, R. Riessen et al., "Autoimmune heparin-induced thrombocytopenia after transcatheter aortic valve implantation: successful treatment with adjunct high-dose intravenous immunoglobulin," *TH Open*, vol. 3, no. 2, pp. e200–e202, 2019.

An Unusual Cause of Secondary ITP in a 34-Year-Old Hispanic Male

Ayrton Bangolo ,[1] Mohamed Ahmed,[1] Ali Atoot,[2] Ashraf Mahmoud,[3] Chibuzo Agbakwuru-Onyike,[1] Maria Karina Larni Y. Palad,[4] Michael Sciarra,[5] and Adam Atoot[1]

[1] *Department of Internal Medicine, Hackensack Meridian Health Palisades Medical Center, North Bergen, NJ, USA*
[2] *Department of Anesthesia, Hackensack University Medical Center, Hackensack, NJ, USA*
[3] *Department of Family Medicine, Hackensack Meridian Health Palisades Medical Center, North Bergen, NJ, USA*
[4] *University of the East Ramon Magsaysay, Quezon, Philippines*
[5] *Department of Gastroenterology, Hackensack Meridian Health Palisades Medical Center, North Bergen, NJ, USA*

Correspondence should be addressed to Ayrton Bangolo; ayrtonbangolo@yahoo.com

Academic Editor: Tomas Jose Gonzalez-Lopez

Secondary immune thrombocytopenic purpura (ITP) associated with *Helicobacter pylori* (*H. pylori*) infection has been described in the literature. It appears to have a geographic distribution; mostly encountered in countries with a higher prevalence for *H. pylori* such as Italy or Japan. *H. pylori* eradication has been recommended in the management of ITP with studies showing improvement in the platelet count in some patients. Substantial platelet count increases in patients with severe thrombocytopenia (platelet counts $<30\times10^3$ microliter), however, are uncommon with *H. pylori* treatment alone. Here, we present a 34-year-old Hispanic male with worsening chronic thrombocytopenia that resolved following eradication of his *H. pylori* infection. Herein, we highlight a rare and reversible cause of secondary ITP. With this case report, we hope to encourage physicians to include *H. pylori* testing in the evaluation of thrombocytopenia.

1. Introduction

Immune thrombocytopenic purpura (ITP) is an acquired disorder in which there is immune-mediated destruction of platelets with possible inhibition of platelet release from the megakaryocytes [1]. In adults, it is a more chronic disease; however, some will experience spontaneous remission which will usually occur within months of the initial diagnosis. ITP is considered secondary if it is associated with an underlying disorder [1]. Several studies have recently shown improvement in platelet counts after eradicating *Helicobacter pylori* (*H. pylori*) infection which suggests an association between the two conditions [2]. It appears that response rates are higher in countries where *H. pylori* infection is endemic and in patients with milder degrees of thrombocytopenia [3, 4]. Herein, we present a 34-year-old male with ITP and worsening platelet levels who was found to have *H. pylori* infection. Following treatment of his infection, the patient had significant improvement and normalization of his platelet count. With this case report, we aim to encourage clinicians to include *H. pylori* in the differential diagnosis of ITP.

2. Case Presentation

This is a 34-year-old Hispanic male with no significant past medical history who presented to the clinic for evaluation of a gnawing, moderate, intermittent epigastric pain that started 3-4 months prior to the visit. The pain improves with meals and is associated with reflux and early satiety. Notably, the patient was told he had "low platelets" on his annual physical the year prior to our encounter. He denied

Table 1: Laboratory values.

	Laboratory values
White blood cells	5.5 × 10*3 (3.4–10.8 × 10*3) microliter (uL)
Red blood cells	5.0 × 10*6 (4.14–5.80 × 10*6) uL
Platelet count on admission	50 × 10*3 (150–450 × 10*3) uL
Platelet count a year ago	91 × 10*3 (150–450 × 10*3) uL
Platelet count 1 week into therapy	105 × 10*3 (150–450 × 10*3) uL
Platelet count 5 weeks after triple therapy	178 × 10*3 (150–450 × 10*3) uL
Erythrocyte sedimentation rate	3 (0–15) millimeter per hour (mm/hr)
C-reactive protein	<1 (0–10) milligram per liter (mg/L)
Hepatitis B surface antigen	Negative
Hepatitis B surface antibody, quantitative	>10,000 (immunity >9.9) milli-international units per milliliter (mIU/mL)
Aspartate aminotransferase	19 (0–40) international units per liter (IU/L)
Alanine transaminase	25 (0–44) IU/L
Human immunodeficiency virus antigen/antibody 4th generation	Nonreactive
Hepatitis C antibody	<0.1 (0.0–0.9) signal-to-cutoff ratio (s/co ro)
Antinuclear antibody	Negative
Serotonin release assay	Negative

any diarrhea, nausea, vomiting, spontaneous bruising, epistaxis, or gingival bleeding. He also denied any intravenous drug use or any dangerous sexual behaviors. He has never been hospitalized and did not undergo any surgical procedures in the past. The family history was noncontributory.

Physical examination was significant for epigastric tenderness on palpation but was otherwise unremarkable. Laboratory results revealed a positive urea breath test as well as worsening thrombocytopenia with a platelet count of 50×10^3 microliter (uL) ($150–450 \times 10^3$) from a platelet count of 91×10^3 uL the year prior as shown in Table 1. The remainder of the laboratory evaluation, including a complete blood count, lipid profile, and urinalysis was unremarkable. The abdominal ultrasound was unremarkable except for a trace effusion between the liver and diaphragm. Further evaluation with a noncontrast computed tomography (CT) of the abdomen/pelvis showed no abdominal pathology.

The patient was started on a 10-day regimen triple therapy (amoxicillin, clarithromycin, and lansoprazole) for eradication of *Helicobacter pylori* (*H. pylori*). One week after initiation of therapy, repeat laboratory results revealed significantly improved platelet levels, 105×10^3 uL. Additional workup for thrombocytopenia was ordered including a hepatitis panel, human immunodeficiency virus testing, heparin-induced thrombocytopenia antibodies, and a serotonin release assay which were all within normal limits.

The patient was reevaluated 5 weeks after completion of the triple therapy. He reported complete resolution of his abdominal pain. The urea breath test was negative as well as the stool antigen for *H. pylori*. The laboratory results revealed continuous improvement and normalization of the platelet levels, 178×10^3 uL.

3. Discussion

Immune thrombocytopenia (ITP, also called idiopathic thrombocytopenic purpura or immune thrombocytopenic purpura) is an acquired thrombocytopenia caused by autoantibodies against platelet antigens. It is one of the more common causes of thrombocytopenia in otherwise asymptomatic adults [1]. ITP is termed secondary if it is associated with an underlying disorder; autoimmune disorders, particularly systemic lupus erythematosus (SLE), and infections, such as human immunodeficiency virus (HIV) infections and hepatitis C, are also common causes. The association of ITP with *Helicobacter pylori* (*H. pylori*) infection is unclear [1]. Some studies show that eradication of *H. pylori* with antibiotics result in marked platelet count increases in patients with ITP [3]. Patients with acute *H. pylori* are often asymptomatic or develop mild self-limited dyspeptic symptoms and may not seek medical attention and thus are not immediately investigated [5]. Our patient had a one-year history of acquired unexplained thrombocytopenia and developed dyspeptic symptoms overtime. He was not initially worked up for *H. pylori* a year prior to our encounter, given the lack of dyspeptic symptoms at the time. He did not endorse any signs or symptoms related to thrombocytopenia. The patient also denied any personal or family history of bleeding disorders or autoimmune conditions.

ITP is a diagnosis of exclusion which is made in patients with isolated thrombocytopenia. The diagnosis of ITP requires that other potential causes of thrombocytopenia, such as recent infections, medications, rheumatologic disorders, or liver disease, be excluded [6]. Several guidelines recommend obtaining a peripheral blood smear to confirm that thrombocytopenia is not artifactual due to platelet clumping and HIV and hepatitis C testing [6–8]. Testing for *H. pylori* is appropriate in patients with gastrointestinal symptoms suggestive of infection because of a reported association between ITP and *H. pylori* infection. Routine screening for *H. pylori* may be reasonable in asymptomatic individuals as well [4]. Antiplatelet antibody testing has low sensitivity and is not recommended [9]. Our patient was not taking any medications including any herbal supplementation to explain his findings. He had no history of rheumatologic disorders, and the liver function test was unremarkable. A year prior to our encounter, the patient had unexplained thrombocytopenia but did not have any gastrointestinal symptoms. It was his dyspepsia and early satiety a year later that prompted evaluation for *H. pylori* infection. However, even despite the lack of dyspeptic symptoms, the patient should have been evaluated for *H. pylori* as part of the workup of unexplained thrombocytopenia.

The treatment of ITP uses drugs that decrease reticuloendothelial uptake of the antibody-bound platelet, decrease antibody production, and/or increase platelet production. Patients with platelet counts $>30 \times 10^3\,\mu L$ appear not to have increased mortality related to the thrombocytopenia and usually do not require treatment with intravenous immune globulin (IVIG) or corticosteroids [1]. IVIG or corticosteroids are usually reserved for bleeding, elective surgery, or severe thrombocytopenia ($<30 \times 10^3$ microliter) without bleeding [10]. A systematic review of the English literature concluded that, in secondary ITP, there is improvement of thrombocytopenia with *H. pylori* eradication [4]. Our patient had a platelet level above 30×10^3 uL, was not bleeding, and was not scheduled for any surgeries. Thus, he was not treated with corticosteroids or IVIG. He was found to have a positive urea breath test and was initiated on triple therapy for *H. pylori* eradication. Following *H. pylori* eradication, the platelet levels normalized, an outcome that is consistent with findings in the literature.

4. Conclusion

Immune thrombocytopenic purpura (ITP) is an acquired disorder that can be associated with *Helicobacter pylori* (*H. pylori*) as previously reported in the literature. *H. pylori* eradication has been associated with improvement and normalization of the platelet levels, especially in patients with nonsevere thrombocytopenia. With this case report, we hope to contribute to the growing literature of *H. pylori* associated with ITP. This case report has the objective to encourage clinicians to include *H. pylori* in the workup of unexplained thrombocytopenia, even without gastrointestinal symptoms.

Consent

Written informed consent was obtained from the patient for publication of this case report and any accompanying images.

Disclosure

Adam Atoot and Michael Sciarra are the article's guarantors.

Authors' Contributions

Ayrton Bangolo and Mohamed Ahmed searched the literature and wrote and revised the manuscript. Ali Atoot, Ashraf Mahmoud, Chibuzo Agbakwuru-Onyike, and Maria Karina Larni Y. Palad revised and edited the manuscript. Adam Atoot and Michael Sciarra revised and approved the final version. All authors certify that they contributed sufficiently to the intellectual content and data analysis. Each author has reviewed the final version of the manuscript and approved it for publication.

References

[1] B. A. Konkle, "Disorders of platelets and vessel wall," in *Harrison's Principles of Internal Medicine*, J. L. Jameson, A. S. Fauci, D. L. Kasper, S. L. Hauser, D. L. Longo, and J. Loscalzo, Eds., McGraw-Hill Education, New York, NY, USA, 2018.

[2] N. Rostami, M. Keshtkar-Jahromi, M. Rahnavardi, M. Keshtkar-Jahromi, and F. Soghra Esfahani, "Effect of eradication of *Helicobacter pylori* on platelet recovery in patients with chronic idiopathic thrombocytopenic purpura: a controlled trial," *American Journal of Hematology*, vol. 83, no. 5, pp. 376–381, 2008.

[3] K. Kaushansky, "Thrombocytopenia," in *Williams Hematology*, K. Kaushansky, J. T. Prchal, L. J. Burns, M. A. Lichtman, M. Levi, and D. C. Linch, Eds., McGraw-Hill Education, New York, NY, USA, 2021.

[4] R. Stasi, A. Sarpatwari, J. B. Segal et al., "Effects of eradication of *Helicobacter pylori* infection in patients with immune thrombocytopenic purpura: a systematic review," *Blood*, vol. 113, no. 6, pp. 1231–1240, 2009.

[5] G. A. Rocha, D. M. Queiroz, E. N. Mendes, A. J. Barbosa, G. F. Lima Júnior, and C. A. Oliveira, "*Helicobacter pylori* acute gastritis: histological, endoscopical, clinical, and therapeutic features," *American Journal of Gastroenterology*, vol. 86, no. 11, pp. 1592–1595, 1991.

[6] British Committee for Standards in Haematology General Haematology Task Force, "Guidelines for the investigation and management of idiopathic thrombocytopenic purpura in adults, children and in pregnancy," *British Journal of Haematology*, vol. 120, no. 4, pp. 574–596, 2003.

[7] D. B. Cines and V. S. Blanchette, "Immune thrombocytopenic purpura," *New England Journal of Medicine*, vol. 346, no. 13, pp. 995–1008, 2002.

[8] F. Rodeghiero, R. Stasi, T. Gernsheimer et al., "Standardization of terminology, definitions and outcome criteria in immune thrombocytopenic purpura of adults and children: report from an international working group," *Blood*, vol. 113, no. 11, pp. 2386–2393, 2009.

[9] J. George, S. Woolf, G. Raskob et al., "Idiopathic thrombocytopenic purpura: a practice guideline developed by explicit methods for the American Society of Hematology," *Blood*, vol. 88, no. 1, pp. 3–40, 1996.

[10] B. Godeau, S. Chevret, B. Varet et al., "Intravenous immunoglobulin or high-dose methylprednisolone, with or without oral prednisone, for adults with untreated severe autoimmune thrombocytopenic purpura: a randomised, multicentre trial," *The Lancet*, vol. 359, no. 9300, pp. 23–29, 2002.

40

Clinical Presentation of Acute Pulmonary Embolism in Patients with Coronavirus Disease 2019 (COVID-19)

Nonso Osakwe [1] **and Douglas Hart** [2]

[1]*Department of Infectious Disease, New York Presbyterian Hospital, Bronxville, NY, USA*
[2]*Department of Cardiology, New York Presbyterian Hospital, Bronxville, NY, USA*

Correspondence should be addressed to Nonso Osakwe; noo2002@nyp.org

Academic Editor: Tatsuharu Ohno

The clinical management of severely ill patients with COVID-19-related acute respiratory distress syndrome (ARDS) presents significant challenges. Many COVID-19 patients with ARDS also present with laboratory findings significant for derangement in coagulation function. In this report, we describe acute pulmonary embolism in three patients with COVID-19. We assessed the role of D-dimer assay and anticoagulation treatment in these patients. The aim of this case report is to increase awareness about the use of D-dimer in addition to patient's clinical status for making treatment decision in COVID-19 patients.

1. Background

The novel coronavirus that causes COVID-19 disease is the severe acute respiratory syndrome coronavirus 2 (SARS-CoV-2) first identified in late 2019 in Wuhan, China [1]. Many severely ill patients present with acute respiratory distress syndrome (ARDS) with laboratory findings significant for derangement in coagulation function including elevated D-dimer [1, 2]. Previous studies have suggested increased risk of thromboembolism in patients with COVID-19 infection, yet very few case studies exist on this topic [3–5]. We present three patients with COVID-19 disease who were admitted with respiratory failure from pneumonia and were found to have thromboembolism.

2. Case 1

A 26-year-old female without significant medical history and no recent birth control pill use was admitted for shortness of breath, cough, fever, hemoptysis, and pleuritic chest pain after testing positive for the COVID-19 about a week earlier. On admission, the patient had a temperature of 101.5 F, tachycardia of 111 beats/minute, tachypnea with respiratory rate ranging from 19 to 31 breaths per minute, and an oxygen saturation of 95% on room air. She progressively got short of breath and required nasal cannular oxygen at 2-3 liters per minute. Initial electrocardiogram showed sinus tachycardia with ST and T-wave abnormalities. Initial laboratory finding included a white cell count of 16 K/UL (4.5–11.0), negative troponin, negative procalcitonin, and D-dimer elevated at 437 NG/MLDDU (0–243). Chest X-ray revealed multifocal opacities in the lungs bilaterally. The patient was placed on investigational treatment with hydroxychloroquine and azithromycin. Computed tomography (CT) angiogram of the chest was performed due to worsening symptoms; the results showed an acute pulmonary embolism bronchus intermedius with straightening of the interventricular septum suggesting right heart strain (Figure 1). Ultrasound of the lower extremities was negative for deep vein thrombosis. The patient was then placed on anticoagulation with enoxaparin with progressive improvement of symptoms.

3. Case 2

A 65-year-old male without significant medical history was admitted for shortness of breath, cough, and fever. He also tested positive for COVID-19. On admission, he was

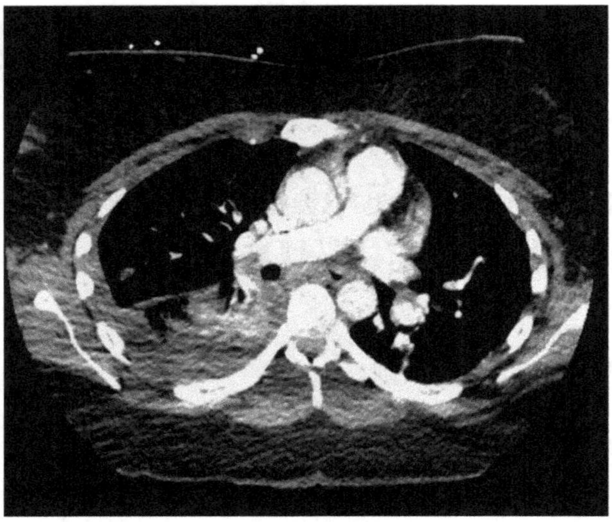

Figure 1: Pulmonary embolism at the level of the bronchus intermedius.

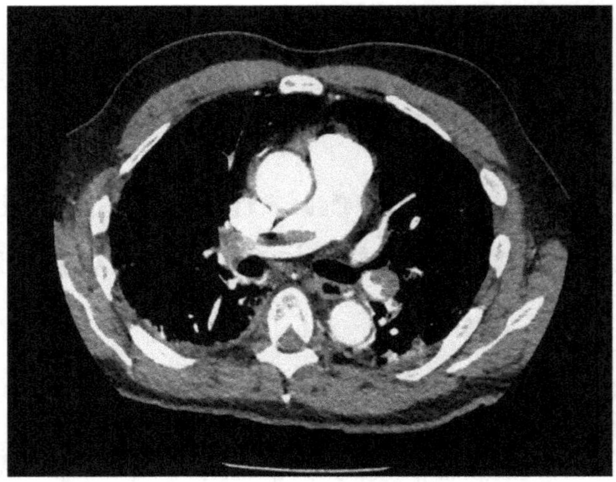

Figure 2: CT angiogram with saddle embolus.

hypoxic and was started on 4 liters of oxygen via nasal cannula. He was febrile with a temperature of 102 F, respiratory rate in the 20 s, and electrocardiogram with nonspecific T-wave abnormalities. Initial laboratory findings included a white cell count of 5.8 K/UL (4.5–11.0), negative initial troponin, negative procalcitonin, and D-dimer >11000 NG/MLDDU (0–243). Chest X-ray showed patchy mid-to-lower lung predominant airspace opacities concerning for multifocal pneumonia. The patient received investigational hydroxychloroquine and azithromycin; however, respiratory status progressively deteriorated and required nonrebreather oxygen at 15 liters/min. Troponins increased to 1.810 NG/ML (<0.120). Computed tomography (CT) angiogram of the chest was performed (Figure 2) that showed saddle embolus with extension of embolus into the right and left interlobar arteries, the right upper lobe artery, the right middle lobe artery, the left upper lobe artery and segmental arteries of the right upper lobe, the right lower lobe, the left upper lobe, the lingula, and the left lower lobe. The patient was started on heparin drip and subsequently transitioned to apixaban with progressive improvement in symptoms.

4. Case 3

A 66-year-old male with medical history of type 2 diabetes mellitus, hypertension, and hyperlipidemia was admitted for worsening cough, fever, and chills. The patient tested positive for COVID-19. On admission, the temperature was 101.7 F and he was hypoxic requiring a venturi mask FiO2 of 40% to maintain oxygen saturation at 93% and tachypneic with a respiratory rate of 25 breaths per minute. Initial electrocardiogram revealed minimal voltage criteria for left ventricular hypertrophy. Initial laboratory findings included a white cell count of 5.4 K/UL and D-dimer of 152 NG/MLDDU (0–243). The chest radiograph revealed patchy airspace opacities bilateral mid-to-lower lung zones. The patient received investigational treatment with hydroxychloroquine and azithromycin. Respiratory status worsened requiring a nonrebreather mask to maintain oxygen saturation at 90–93%. A repeat D-dimer was 6425 NG/MLDDU (0–243). Computer tomography angiogram due to worsening symptoms and elevated D-dimer revealed pulmonary emboli in the distal right and left pulmonary arteries and segmental and subsegmental bilateral upper lobe pulmonary arteries (Figure 3). The patient was placed on subcutaneous enoxaparin with progressive improvement in symptoms. He was transitioned to apixaban and discharge home.

5. Discussion

Wang et al. reported that 71.4% of COVID-19 deaths meet International Society of Thrombosis and Hemostasis (ISTH) criteria for DIC predominantly prothrombotic DIC [2]. Given that D-dimer is a nonspecific marker of inflammation, it is not surprising that the levels increase in COVID-19 cases. Most recently, Chen et al. suggested that patients with COVID-19 pneumonia are at high risk for acute pulmonary embolism when D-dimer remarkably increases [5]; another study suggested that D-dimer values were significantly different between mild and severe disease [1]. In this report, index Case 1 compared to Case 2 had a mildly elevated D-dimer, yet both patients exhibited progressively worsening symptoms. We propose more use of D-dimer elevation as part of treatment decision criteria for acute pulmonary embolism in patients with COVID-19-related ARDS and also encourage a low threshold for further evaluation including CT angiogram especially in patients with worsening or poorly improving clinical status. Closer monitoring of D-dimer in the course of disease may also highlight progression. The clinical question worth exploring is whether higher dose of prophylactic or therapeutic anticoagulation should be administered in patients with COVID-19-related ARDS.

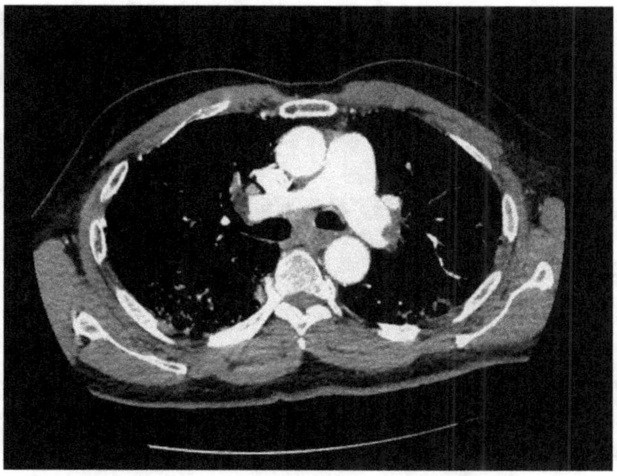

FIGURE 3: CT angiogram showing pulmonary emboli in the distal right and left pulmonary arteries.

Consent

No written consent has been obtained from the patients as there are no patient identifiable data included in this case report.

References

[1] H. Han, L. Yang, R. Liu et al., "Prominent changes in blood coagulation of patients with SARS-CoV-2 infection," *Clinical Chemistry and Laboratory Medicine (CCLM)*, vol. 58, no. 7, p. 1116, 2020.

[2] J. Wang, N. Hajizadeh, E. E. Moore et al., "Tissue plasminogen activator (tPA) treatment for COVID-19 associated acute respiratory distress syndrome (ARDS): a case series," *Journal of Thrombosis and Haemostasis*, vol. 18, no. 7, p. 1752, 2020.

[3] E. Driggin, M. V. Madhavan, B. Bikdeli et al., "Cardiovascular considerations for patients, health care workers, and health systems during the COVID-19 pandemic," *Journal of the American College of Cardiology*, vol. 75, no. 18, pp. 2352–2371, 2020.

[4] G. B. Danzi, M. Loffi, G. Galeazzi, and E. Gherbesi, "Acute pulmonary embolism and COVID-19 pneumonia: a random association?" *European Heart Journal*, vol. 41, no. 19, 2020.

[5] J. Chen, X. Wang, S. Zhang et al., "Findings of acute pulmonary embolism in COVID-19 patients (3/1/2020)," *Social Science Research Network*, vol. 51, 2020.

41

Diagnostic and Treatment Challenges of Paroxysmal Nocturnal Hemoglobinuria in Uganda

Boniface Amanee Elias Lumori and Daniel Muyanja

Department of Internal Medicine, Mbarara University of Science and Technology (MUST), Mbarara, Uganda

Correspondence should be addressed to Boniface Amanee Elias Lumori; bonifacelumori@gmail.com

Academic Editor: Marie-Christine Kyrtsonis

Introduction. Paroxysmal nocturnal hemoglobinuria (PNH) is a very rare disorder of the hematopoietic stem cells which is often underdiagnosed. Its incidence is about 5 cases per million inhabitants in a year, and currently, there are only 1610 patients in the International PNH Registry. In this report, we describe a case of PNH in southwestern Uganda. *Case Presentation.* A 34-year-old man, subsistence farmer, with a history of multiple prior presentations with anemia, jaundice, and dark-colored urine requiring blood transfusions presented to us again in July 2018 with a week's history of palpitations, dizziness, and dark-colored urine. Investigations done suggested a direct antiglobulin test- (DAT-) negative hemolytic anemia, and subsequently, flow cytometry showed a large clone of PNH. He received many blood transfusions and hematinics on several occasions during the course of his admissions. *Conclusions.* Our report showed diagnostic and treatment challenges of PNH in health resource-limited setting.

1. Introduction

Direct antiglobulin test-negative hemolytic anemia is a broad class of diseases characterized by hemolysis and a negative DAT. Paroxysmal nocturnal hemoglobinuria is one of the very rare causes of direct antiglobulin test-negative hemolytic anemia which is often underdiagnosed. It is an acquired hematopoietic stem cells disorder characterized by a variety of clinical features ranging from episodes of hemolysis and its associated symptoms, abdominal pain, erectile dysfunction, and thrombotic events to the renal insufficiency and pulmonary hypertension [1]. The reported incidence of PNH was only about 5 cases per million inhabitants per year [2]; however, it is associated with high morbidity and mortality [1]. Currently, there are only 1,610 patients with confirmed PNH in the International PNH Registry in which variable features of the disease are being studied [3]. To the best of our knowledge, there is no reported case of PNH confirmed by flow cytometry in Uganda. Therefore, in this report, we present a case of a 34-year-old man diagnosed with PNH by flow cytometry after 12 years a diagnostic dilemma.

2. Case Presentation

A 34-year-old man, a subsistence farmer, from southwestern Uganda with a history of multiple prior presentations with anemia, jaundice, and dark-colored urine requiring blood transfusions presented to us again in July 2018 with a week history of palpitations, dizziness, and dark-colored urine.

His condition started in 2006 with an episode of palpitations, yellowing of eyes, and dark-colored urine where he was initially seen in different health facilities close to his home village and later admitted to Mbarara Regional Referral Hospital (MRRH). He recalled being transfused with >4 units of blood during that initial admission and was discharged when all his symptoms subsided.

After discharge, he stayed fairly well for about 3 months before he developed another episode with similar symptoms. These symptoms continued to recur at an interval of 2–4 months, and each episode would require admission and blood transfusion.

In 2012, he was referred to Mulago National Referral Hospital for diagnostics and management. Many investigations were done (Table 1), and he was ultimately given

Table 1: Investigations.

	Blood tests		
Year	Test name	Results	Lab reference range
	CBC		
	(1) WBC	2.2×10^9/L	$3.5–10.5 \times 10^9$/L
	(2) Hb	3.4 g/dl	13.5–17.5 g/dl
	(3) MCV	116 fl	80–96 fl
	(4) PLT	123×10^9/L	$150–450 \times 10^9$/L
	Reticulocyte	10.6%	0.5–2.5%
	Peripheral smear	Pancytopenia, dimorphic, normocytic, and normochromic anemia	
2012	Serum B12 levels	123.2 pmol/L	141–698 pmol/L
	Serum folate levels	45.4 nmol/L	10.4–59 nmol/L
	AST	2.35 ukat/L	0.167–0.667 ukat/L
	Bilirubin total	26 μmol/L	1.7–20.5 μmol/L
	Bilirubin direct	7 μmol/L	5.1 μmol/L
	Antiglobulin test (both direct and indirect)	Negative	
	RDT for malaria	Negative	
	Urine chemistry	Hemoglobin pigments	
	Sickling test	Negative	
	CBC		
	(1) WBC	2.6×10^9/L	$3.5–10.5 \times 10^9$/L
	(2) Hb	5 g/dl	13.5–17.5 g/dl
	(3) MCV	101 fl	80–96 fl
	(4) PLT	130×10^9/L	$150–450 \times 10^9$/L
2013	Serum B12 levels	991.6 pmol/L	141–698 pmol/L
	AST	1.2 ukat/L	0.167–0.667 ukat/L
	Peripheral smear	Macrocytosis	
	Bone marrow aspirate and biopsy report	Erythropiosis: hyperplasia with megaloblastic maturation. No granulopoiesis: hyperplastic, left shift with giant metalocytes, and myeloblast <5%	
	AST	2.29 ukat/L	0.167–0.667 ukat/L
	Bilirubin total	43.2 μmol/L	1.7–20.5 μmol/L
	Bilirubin direct	5.8 μmol/L	5.1 μmol/L
	LDH	45.38 ukat/L	2.67–7.5 ukat/L
2014	Antiglobulin test (both direct and indirect)	Negative	
	HBsAg	Nonreactive	
	Hepatitis C antibodies	Nonreactive	
	HIV rapid test	Nonreactive	
	Urine chemistry	Hemoglobin pigments	
2015	Serum homocysteine levels	21 μmol/L	5–16 μmol/L
	Urine methylmalonic acid	0.0 mmol/mol crt	0.0–3.6 mmol/mol crt
2016	Serum B12 levels	1475.6 pmol/L	141–698 pmol/L
	CBC		
	(1) WBC	3.4×10^9/L	$3.5–10.5 \times 10^9$/L
	(2) Hb	3.5 g/dl	13.5–17.5 g/dl
	(3) MCV	111 fl	80–96 fl
2018	(4) PLT	120×10^9/L	$150–450 \times 10^9$/L
	Abdominal ultrasound scan	Normal	
	Echocardiography	Dilated chambers of the heart with moderate tricuspid and mitral insufficiency. No features of pulmonary arterial hypertension	

CBC, complete blood count; WBC, white blood count; Hb, hemoglobin; MCV, mean corpuscular volume; PLT, platelets; RDT, rapid diagnostic test; HBsAg, hepatitis B surface antigen; AST, leukocyte aspartate aminotransferase; LDH, lactate dehydrogenase.

a diagnosis of vitamin B12 deficiency. He was then treated for 1 year with vitamin B12 injections (no records of the doses available). Despite this treatment, he continued to have episodes of yellowing of eyes, palpitations, and dark-colored urine at approximately similar intervals (2–4 months).

In 2013, investigations were repeated, and in addition, bone marrow aspiration was done. The serum B12 level was found to be high, and the vitamin B12 injections were stopped. However, similar symptoms continued to recur at similar intervals over the following 2 years.

In 2015, he was restarted on B12 injections when found to have high serum levels of homocysteine despite a negative urine methylmalonic acid. The injections were stopped again a year later when found to have a very high serum B12 levels. Symptoms continued to recur at similar intervals till his recent admission in July 2018. Apart from B12 injections, the patient was given oral prednisolone on two occasions in the past but without significant improvement.

On this admission, he presented with predominant symptoms of palpitations, dizziness, generalized body weakness, yellow eyes, and dark-colored urine for about 7 days. This time, he also reported a 5-month history of erectile dysfunction and intermittent mild to moderate abdominal pain without associated vomiting, diarrhea, or dark/bloody stools. Reviews of the other systems were uneventful. He has no other chronic diseases or history of allergies. He has not been on any chronic medications in the past, apart from the tablets of folic acid and ferrous sulfate and vitamin B12 injections. He reported no history of a similar condition in any of his family members or a history of hereditary anemias or hematological malignancies. He reported no history of radiation or toxin exposure and further denied any history of taking traditional remedies.

His physical examination in the latest admission revealed severe pallor and jaundice of the mucous membranes. He had a displaced point of maximum cardiac impulse (6th left intercostal space and anterior axillary line) and grade-3 mitral and tricuspid murmurs of mitral and tricuspid regurgitation, respectively. He has no skin rashes, and the rest of his systemic examination was unremarkable. Many tests done during the course of his illness are displayed in Table 1.

Due to the recurrence of the symptoms, DAT-negative hemolytic anemia, and new onset of erectile dysfunction, we did a flow cytometry including fluorescent aerolysin (FLAER) in which a large PNH clone was found. The details of the flow cytometry test are displayed in Table 2.

In this admission, we transfused him with 4 units of blood and later discharged when his symptoms subsided.

3. Discussion

It took 12 years for our patient to be diagnosed with PNH, which is a little bit longer compared to the cases reported from Asia [1]. This is probably due to the lack of awareness of the disease and diagnostic capabilities in our setting and sub-Saharan Africa in general.

Our patient presents with a recurrence of hemolysis with a negative DAT, features which are suggestive of non-autoimmune hemolytic anemia. Causes of nonautoimmune hemolytic anemias include drugs, malaria, microangiopathic anemias, red blood cells enzymatic defects, and hereditary red blood cell membranes defects as well as paroxysmal cold hemoglobinuria and PNH. Unlike PNH, the hereditary anemias such as sickle cell anemias, thalassemia, hereditary spherocytosis, glucose-6-phosphate dehydrogenase (G6PD) deficiency, and pyruvate kinase have characteristic morphologies in the peripheral smear and positive family history [2]. In addition, these anemias do not have a glycosylphosphatidylinositol- (GPI-) anchored protein deficiency. Drugs/toxins exposure can also cause hemolysis but often stops when the insult is removed. Drugs/toxins exposure can typically manifest with recurrence if the patient is reexposed [3]; however, from our patient's history, there was no any exposure to drugs/toxins before the onset of his symptoms.

Malaria is common in Uganda, and it can cause anemia/hemolysis. Severe anemia is a frequent finding in complicated malaria caused by falciparum malaria. It is difficult to completely rule out malaria in our case, despite negative rapid malaria diagnostic test on some occasions of his admissions. Uganda is an endemic area for malaria; hence, it is unlikely to cause severe disease in adults due to the acquired partial immunity [4]. Blackwater fever is another manifestation of severe malaria characterized by hemolysis, hemoglobinuria, and renal failure [5]. These features are similar to those in our case; however, the recurrence pattern of his condition may rule out blackwater fever.

Disseminated intravascular coagulation, hemolytic uremic syndrome, and thrombotic thrombocytic purpura can similarly manifest with DAT-negative hemolysis; however, the absence of schistocytes on the peripheral smear in addition to the deficiency of GPI-anchored proteins in the flow cytometry ruled out these disorders. Few instances of autoimmune hemolytic anemias present with negative DAT similar to PNH and other DAT-negative hemolytic anemias. Most of the hemolysis in autoimmune hemolytic disorders are extravascular, and therefore, hemoglobinemia and hemoglobinuria are less evident [6].

The absence of any specific trigger for hemolysis in our patient may rule out paroxysmal cold hemoglobinuria which can be triggered by infections and cold temperature. Paroxysmal cold hemoglobinuria is also characterized by the presence of Donath–Landsteiner type antibodies but a negative flow cytometry [6].

Unsurprisingly, on several occasions, our patient was found with pancytopenia (Table 1) which is one of the common features reported in the International PNH Registry. These can be explained by the bone marrow suppression associated with this condition and/or lysis of all the blood cells lineage [7].

Erectile dysfunction and abdominal pain in our patient are likely from the smooth muscle dystonia caused by depletion of nitric oxide by the free circulating hemoglobin. In the PNH Registry, abdominal pain and erectile dysfunction were as common as 44% and 38%, respectively [7]. Our patient had intermittent abdominal pain; unfortunately, the abdominal vascular scan was not done to confirm the presence or absence of abdominal veins thrombosis, which is a serious complication in PNH patients. The normal abdominal scan may exclude the presence of biliary cholecystitis.

Our patient has dilated cardiomegaly which was similarly found in one of the cases of PNH in India [1]. The cardiomegaly in PNH can be attributed to recurrent anemia as well as iron deficiency caused by hemoglobinuria [8, 9].

Similar to the case found in India, our patient has features of megaloblastic anemia in peripheral smear and

TABLE 2: Flow cytometry report.

Blood cells type	GPI-linked antigen type	% blood cells GPI-linked antigen(s) deficiency
Red blood cells	CD59	33.9% (32.4% are type III cells and 1.5% are type II cells)
Neutrophils	FLAER CD24 CD55 CD59	99.6%
Monocytes	CD14 FLAER	99%

CD, cluster of differentiation; GPI, glycosylphosphatidylinositol; FLAER, fluorescent aerolysin. Flow cytometry test was done in South Africa through Lancet Laboratories, Uganda.

bone marrow aspirate in addition to the slightly low serum B12 levels. This might suggest the presence of low B12 status or B12 deficiency. Three years later, a negative urine methylmalonic acid but a high serum homocysteine level was found in our patient which seemed to suggest folate deficiency, despite the fact that both serum B12 and folate levels were not done at that time. Folate and B12 deficiencies are common findings in PNH mainly due to increased compensatory hematopoiesis secondary to chronic hemolysis [10].

Paroxysmal nocturnal hemoglobinuria is mostly a disease of adults, although childhood cases have been reported [11]. The median age of onset is in the thirties [12]. In Africa, we only found two published cases of PNH from South Africa about 6 decades ago [13]. Dr. Paul Strubing in 1882 described a young man who presented with fatigue, abdominal pain, and severe nocturnal paroxysms of hemoglobinuria [14]. In 1937, Ham reported that PNH erythrocytes were broken when incubated with normal, acidified serum [15], and this discovery resulted in the first diagnostic test for PNH, the acidified serum (Ham) test. In 1954, the alternative pathway of complement activation was formally proven to cause the hemolysis of PNH red cells. Later in the 1980s, it was discovered that PNH cells display a global deficiency in a group of proteins affixed to the cell surface by a GPI anchor and two of the missing GPI-anchored proteins (CD55 and CD59) regulate complement.

In PNH, hemolysis is complement mediated due to the PNH cells acquiring deficiency of GPI which are complement regulatory factors. The hematopoietic stem cells with severe deficiency of GPI on their surface progressively expand. The extent of this expansion determines the onset of the disease and its severity. The absence of GPI anchor in all PNH cases is caused by the somatic mutation in phosphatidylinositol glycan class A (PIGA), which is an x-linked gene required for the early step in GPI proteins synthesis. This leads to the deficiency of complement inhibitory proteins (CD55 and CD59) that result in chronic complement-mediated lysis of the GPI-deficient blood cells [7].

The International PNH Registry summarizes the clinical features of patients with PNH, and about 93% of 1610 patients in the registry are symptomatic with fatigue (80%), dyspnea (64%), and hemoglobinuria (62%) representing the most frequent features, then followed by abdominal pain (44%), bone marrow suppression (44%), and erectile dysfunction (38%). In addition, chest pain (33%), thrombosis (16%), and renal dysfunction (14%) are rarely reported [12]. Anemia in PNH is often caused by multiple factors with hemolysis and bone marrow failure as the major causes. Thrombosis in PNH occurs commonly in the intra-abdominal (hepatic, portal, mesenteric, splenic, etc) and cerebral (sagittal and cavernous sinus) veins.

The initial evaluation of a suspected patient includes CBC, reticulocyte count, peripheral smear, haptoglobin, LDH, direct and indirect bilirubin in addition to DAT, urine hemoglobin or hemosiderin, and bone marrow aspirate/biopsy. Usually, these tests show features of hemolysis and the bone marrow aspirate, and biopsy may show hypo-, normo-, or hypercellularity. In suspected patients with thrombosis, a Doppler scan is recommended. The current gold standard test for the confirmation or exclusion of PNH is a two lineage flow cytometry. The diagnosis is made when a positive flow cytometry is found in the context of clinical features that are suggestive of the condition. The clone size is best estimated based on the larger the white cells clones (monocytes and granulocytes), and in our case, it was greater than 99% on analysis of neutrophils and monocytes. This is also important in prognostication of these patients as those with small clones have good prognosis [16]. The International PNH Interest Group classifies PNH into three main classes: the classical PNH (consists of hemolytic and thrombotic patients); subclinical PNH (small PNH clones without clinical or laboratory evidence of hemolysis or thrombosis); and PNH secondary to other bone marrow disorders (e.g., aplastic anemia or myelodysplastic syndrome) [7].

Management approach to patients with PNH includes treatment of anemia, pain from smooth muscle dystonia, and thrombosis. Anticomplement therapy constitutes an important drug for treating symptoms of PNH. Eculizumab (Soliris), a humanized monoclonal antibody, inhibits the complement-mediated lysis of the blood cells. It reduces the destruction of red blood cells, needs for blood transfusion, and improves the quality of life especially in patients with classical PNH [17]. Eculizumab prevents the breakdown of C5 to C5a and C5b by binding to the complement component of C5. Complement 5a and C5b are required for the formation of the membrane attack complex (MAC). In patients with PNH, RBCs lack CD59 which normally prevent the formation of MAC and the resulting hemolysis. It is indicated in patients with symptoms of disabling fatiguability, patients requiring multiple blood transfusions, pains from smooth muscle spasms, or end-organ dysfunctions [18]. In our case, the PNH is severe and our patient wholly depends on blood transfusions for survival; hence, eculizumab is the therapy of choice. However, its availability issues in addition to the high cost (estimated about 400,000 US dollars per year) limits it uses in Uganda and other developing countries. Due to this fact, we are stuck and currently supporting him with blood transfusions whenever he develops an attack. It should be remembered that the anticomplement therapy is associated with a high risk of Neisseria meningitidis infections, and therefore, immunization and/or prophylactic antibiotic therapy are required [16].

Albeit allogenic hematopoietic stem cell transplantation is considered as a curative therapy for PNH, and it is associated with a number of toxic effects including transplant-related mortality and graft versus host disease [19]. Therefore, it is not commonly used nowadays.

4. Conclusion

Our case showed diagnostic and treatment challenges of PNH in a health resource-limited setting.

Consent

Written informed consent was given by the patient.

Acknowledgments

The authors acknowledge the patient and all the clinicians who took part in the management of this patient.

References

[1] R. K. Maj, S. D. L. Col, and H. K. Maj, "Diagnostic dilemmas in paroxysmal nocturnal hemoglobinuria," *Medical Journal Armed Forces India*, vol. 50, no. 1, pp. 27–30, 1994.

[2] J. D. Zimbelman, "Hemolytic anemia," in *Berman's Pediatric Decision Making*, pp. 595–597, Elsevier, New York, NY, USA, 5th edition, 2011.

[3] S. L. Schrier, *Hemolytic Anemia Due to Drugs and Toxins*, UpToDate, Waltham, MA, USA, 2015.

[4] G. Winter and M. Wahlgren, "Severe anemia in malaria: defense gone wrong?," *Blood*, vol. 106, no. 10, pp. 3337-3338, 2005.

[5] F. Brunee, B. Gachot, M. Wolff et al., "Resurgence of blackwater fever in long-term European expatriates in Africa: report of 21 cases and review," *Clinical Infectious Diseases*, vol. 32, no. 8, pp. 1133–1140, 2001.

[6] S. Berentsen and T. Sundic, "Red blood cell destruction in autoimmune hemolytic anemia: role of complement and potential new targets for therapy," *BioMed Research International*, vol. 2015, Article ID 363278, 11 pages, 2015.

[7] R. A. Brodsky, "Paroxysmal nocturnal hemoglobinuria," *Blood*, vol. 124, no. 18, pp. 2804–2811, 2014.

[8] K. Schroecksnadel, B. Wirleitner, and D. Fuchs, "Anemia and congestive heart failure," *Circulation*, vol. 108, no. 6, pp. e41–e42, 2003.

[9] N. Hegde, M. W. Rich, and C. Gayomali, "The cardiomyopathy of iron deficiency," *Texas Heart Institute Journal*, vol. 33, no. 3, pp. 340–344, 2006.

[10] H. B. Castellanos-Sinco, C. O. Ramos-Peñafiel, A. Santoyo-Sánchez et al., "Megaloblastic anaemia: folic acid and vitamin B12 metabolism," *Revista Médica Del Hospital General De México*, vol. 78, no. 3, pp. 135–143, 2015.

[11] R. Naithani, M. Mahapatra, P. Dutta, R. Kumar, H. P. Pati, and V. P. Choudhry, "Paroxysmal nocturnal hemoglobinuria in childhood and adolescence-a retrospective analysis of 18 cases," *Indian Journal of Pediatrics*, vol. 75, no. 6, pp. 575–578, 2008.

[12] H. Schrezenmeier, P. Muus, G. Socie et al., "Baseline characteristics and disease burden in patients in the international paroxysmal nocturnal hemoglobinuria registry," *Haematologica*, vol. 99, no. 5, pp. 922–929, 2014.

[13] M. A. Manuel, "Paroxysmal nocturnal haemoglobinuria in two South African Bantu patients," *South African Medical Journal*, vol. 43, no. 13, pp. 351–354, 1969.

[14] J. J. Pu and R. A. Brodsky, "Paroxysmal nocturnal hemoglobinuria from bench to bedside," *Clinical and Translational Science*, vol. 4, no. 3, pp. 219–224, 2011.

[15] T. H. Ham, "Chronic hemolytic anemia with paroxysmal nocturnal hemoglobinuria," *New England Journal of Medicine*, vol. 217, no. 23, pp. 915–917, 1937.

[16] C. Parker, M. Omine, S. Richards et al., "Diagnosis and management of paroxysmal nocturnal hemoglobinuria," *Blood*, vol. 106, no. 12, pp. 3699–3709, 2005.

[17] P. Hillmen, N. S. Young, J. Schubert et al., "The complement inhibitor eculizumab in paroxysmal nocturnal hemoglobinuria," *New England Journal of Medicine*, vol. 355, no. 12, pp. 1233–1243, 2006.

[18] C. Parker, "Eculizumab for paroxysmal nocturnal haemoglobinuria," *The Lancet*, vol. 373, no. 9665, pp. 759–767, 2009.

[19] R. P. de Latour, H. Schrezenmeier, A. Bacigalupo et al., "Allogeneic stem cell transplantation in paroxysmal nocturnal hemoglobinuria," *Haematologica*, vol. 97, no. 11, pp. 1666–1673, 2012.

42

Hemophagocytic Lymphohistiocytosis Associated with Respiratory Syncytial Virus Infection in an Immunocompetent Elderly Patient

Ralph Kamel, Rubal Sharma, Divya Asti, Arshpal Gill, and Yevgeniy Skaradinskiy

Staten Island University Hospital, Northwell Health, 475 Seaview Avenue, Staten Island, New York 10305, NY, USA

Correspondence should be addressed to Ralph Kamel; rkamel@northwell.edu

Academic Editor: Gergely Feher

Hemophagocytic lymphohistiocytosis is a serious and potentially fatal disorder characterized by excessive immune system activation. The disorder is diagnosed mainly based on laboratory, clinical, and pathologic criteria. The spectrum comprises hereditary or "primary" HLH that comprises genetically heterogeneous conditions, occurring during childhood. The secondary form presents later in life and is associated with several conditions mainly malignancy, autoimmune diseases, viral or bacterial infections, and hematological diseases. We present the case of an 80-year-old female patient who initially presented with an acute viral syndrome secondary to respiratory syncytial virus. The hospital course was complicated by disseminated intravascular coagulation and shock with multiorgan failure. Extensive workup revealed that several of the criteria for hemophagocytic lymphohistiocytosis were met. A review of literature fails to identify cases of hemophagocytic lymphohistiocytosis associated with respiratory syncytial virus in immunocompetent adults. This case report provides further insight on RSV as a possible etiologic agent associated with HLH and the importance of early recognition of this fatal disorder in RSV-positive patients who show unpredictable clinical decompensation.

1. Introduction

Hemophagocytic lymphohistiocytosis is a life-threatening disorder characterized by excessive activation of T lymphocytes, natural killer cells (NK cells), and macrophages resulting in a state of hypercytokinemia and subsequent organ damage [1]. The condition was first described in 1939 by Scott and Robb-Smith after analyzing a group of patients presenting with similar clinical features that included fever, lymphadenopathy, and hepatosplenomegaly that later progressed into cytopenias and eventually death [2]. HLH can be classified into 2 main groups, depending on the etiology. "Primary" or "familial" HLH is caused by mutations in genes that govern lymphocyte cytotoxicity, and "secondary" HLH is due to infections, neoplasms, and autoimmune diseases [3]. The true incidence of the disease has been difficult to calculate in adults due to diagnostic challenges, although consecutive cohort studies conducted between 1996 and 2011 and published by Parikh et al. estimated the incidence to be 1/2000 for adult critical care admissions, with the majority of patients being male, and cancer being the most common reported cause. The median age was 49 years, and the median overall survival was 2.1 months [4]. Diagnosis still represents a challenge and frequently occurs late in the disease course. The current consensus adopts the HLH-2004 criteria, and patients are diagnosed with the disease if they meet 5 out of 8 criteria that include fever, cytopenia, splenomegaly, hypertriglyceridemia, hypofibrinogenemia, hyperferritinemia, low or absent NK cell activity, elevated IL-2 receptor levels, and biopsy-proven hemophagocytosis [5]. HLH is often triggered by viral infections, and among those the most commonly reported are human immunodeficiency virus (HIV) and Epstein–Barr virus (EBV) infections [6]. Respiratory syncytial virus infection has seldom been reported in the literature as a trigger of HLH in elderly immunocompetent patients. We present the unusual case of an 80-year-old female patient diagnosed with RSV infection with subsequent dramatic clinical deterioration, who subsequently met the required number of criteria for diagnosis of HLH.

2. Case Presentation

We report the case of an 80-year-old female patient with a past medical history of atrial fibrillation, hypertension, hyperlipidemia, nonischemic cardiomyopathy, and chronic obstructive pulmonary disease who presented to the emergency department with 1 week of upper respiratory symptoms that progressed to chest pain, dyspnea, and nonbloody nonbilious vomiting the day prior to presentation.

On admission, she had a low-grade fever with a temperature of 100.3, and she was tachycardic and normotensive and had a normal oxygen saturation with mild tachypnea. A chest X-ray was performed and showed no consolidation, effusion, or pneumothorax.

Her complete blood count revealed leukocytosis of 19,960 (the differential count was not performed). Her basic metabolic panel was consistent with hyperkalemia, high anion gap metabolic acidosis, acute kidney injury, and elevated lactate level. Her transaminase and bilirubin levels were normal.

The rapid respiratory viral panel showed a positive respiratory syncytial virus (RSV) PCR and a negative influenza A and influenza B PCR.

The patient was started on vancomycin, azithromycin, and cefepime as well as a 5-day course of prednisone 40 mg.

The next day, her complete blood count showed worsening leukocytosis with a neutrophilic predominance along with thrombocytopenia. She was also found to have evidence of myocardial injury with elevated troponin T level. The patient was started on maintenance IV fluid. A CT scan of the abdomen and pelvis showed no evidence of abdominal or pelvic pathology.

Overnight, the patient became hypotensive with worsening tachycardia and increased oxygen requirements. She was started on pressor support. Her laboratory studies revealed worsening thrombocytopenia (Figure 1), hyponatremia, and acute kidney injury. She was also found to have evidence of shock liver. She was started on argatroban infusion for suspicion of heparin-induced thrombocytopenia as well as N-acetylcysteine infusion in light of a diagnosis of subfulminant liver failure.

The acute viral hepatitis panel, chronic liver disease workup, and vasculitis panel were negative. An echocardiogram revealed a decreased ejection fraction of 22%.

Hematology opinion was sought given worsening thrombocytopenia as well as the mottled cyanotic appearance of the extremities, and the differential diagnoses included disseminated intravascular coagulation (DIC), thrombotic thrombocytopenic purpura (TTP), and heparin-induced thrombocytopenia (HIT). A peripheral smear revealed the burr cells but the absence of schistocytes and blasts. Her 4T score indicated an intermediate probability of HIT with negative heparin/platelet factor IV antibody. Consequently, the argatroban infusion was stopped. The patient's coagulation panel revealed evidence of DIC, and her ferritin level was elevated at 12,760 ng/mL.

A venous and arterial dopplers of the lower and upper extremities showed no deep venous thrombosis and normal arterial flow, respectively.

Given the presence of elevated ferritin levels, the presence of pyrexia and the decreased fibrinogen level, concern about hemophagocytic lymphohistiocytosis (HLH) was raised. The patient had no splenomegaly, her triglyceride level was normal at 96 mg/dL, her IL-2 receptor level was also normal (less than 31.2 pg/mL), and her natural killer cell absolute number and percentage were within normal limits, 29 cells/μL and 5% of total lymphocytes, respectively. A bone marrow biopsy was performed to rule out the presence of hemophagocytes. Her soluble CD25 level was elevated at 3990 pg/mL.

A flow cytometry performed on the bone marrow specimen revealed no increase in myeloid immaturity and normal myeloid antigen maturation pattern and normal lymphocyte immunophenotypic findings. Given the lack of improvement of mental status and worsening respiratory distress, a goals-of-care discussion was performed with the family, who decided to pursue comfort measures only and limit all medical interventions. The patient expired soon after. After her death, the hemopathology report of the bone marrow aspirate showed cellular bone marrow (20 to 40%) with trilineage maturing hematopoiesis with the presence of hemophagocytosis and decreased iron stores (Figures 2 and 3). 5 out of 8 criteria for the diagnosis of HLH have therefore been met.

3. Discussion

As presented in this case, diagnosis of HLH poses a clinical challenge and occurs late during the course of the disease.

The first definition of HLH was outlined by the Histiocyte Society in 1994 and was later revised in 2004 for the HLH-2004 trial. The revised diagnostic criteria comprise the presence of gene mutations consistent with HLH or the fulfillment of 5 of the following criteria: fever equal to or higher than 38.5°C, splenomegaly, cytopenia affecting at least 2 of the 3 lineages (hemoglobin level < 9 g/dL, platelet count < 100,000/mL, or neutrophil count < 1000/mL), hypertriglyceridemia (fasting level > 265) or hypofibrinogenemia (<150 mg/dL), presence of hemophagocytes in the reticulo-endothelial system, low or absent NK cell activity, elevated ferritin level >500 ng/mL, and elevated CD25 [7]. In this case, one of the earliest clinical manifestations was end-organ damage that presented as acute kidney injury, hypotension, myocardial injury, and fulminant hepatic failure which created additional confusion with regard to diagnosis, as septic shock and cardiogenic shock were primarily suspected early on. HLH was low on the differential diagnosis due, in part, to RSV being the infectious agent in question. As mentioned, HLH can be triggered by multiple factors and infection remains an important etiology. Meta-analyses performed previously have identified EBV, CMV, and HIV as the most common triggering viral infections [8]. Cases of HLH induced by

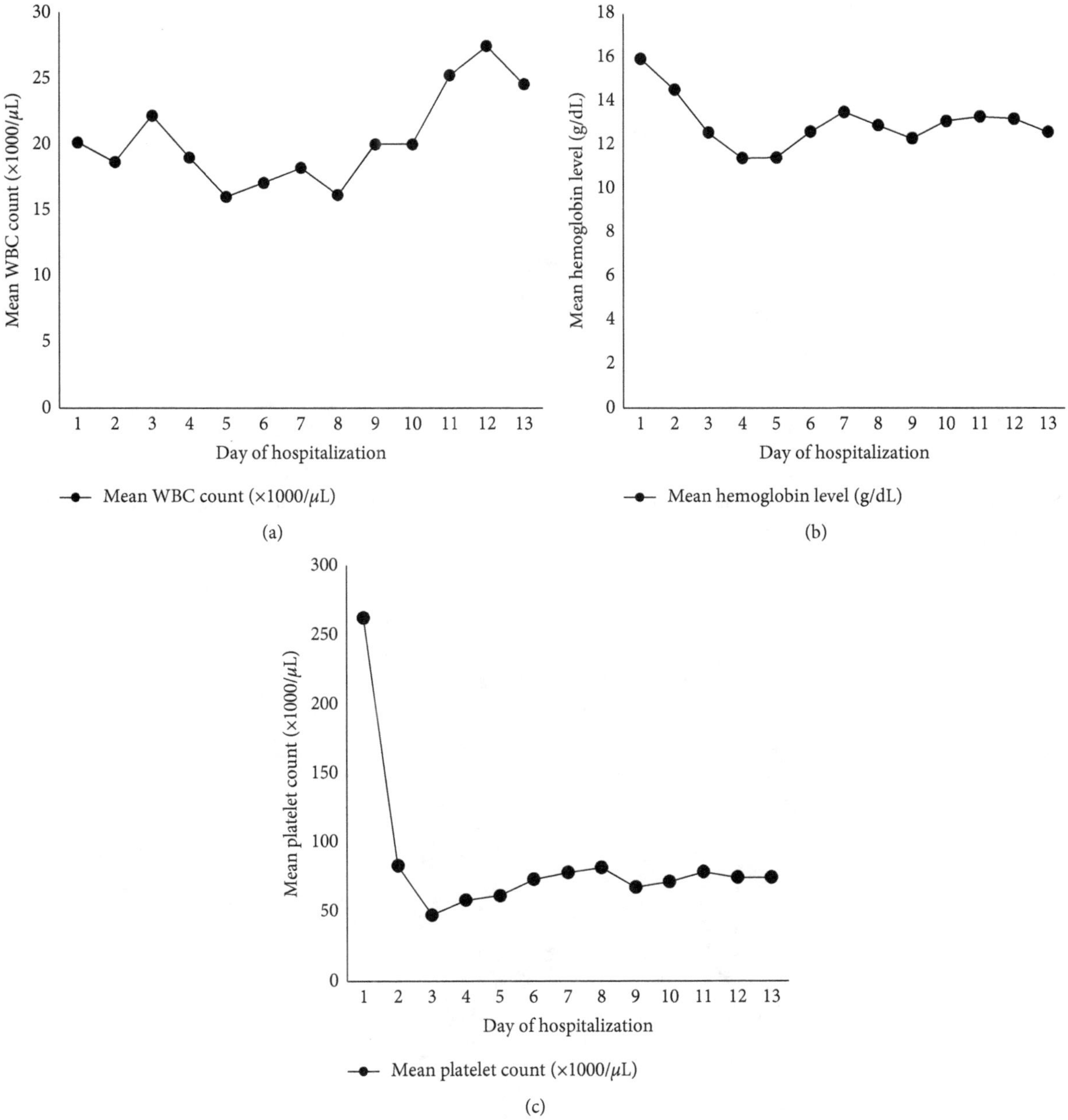

FIGURE 1: Graphs showing the variation of the mean count of each bone marrow lineage as a function of time. (a) Mean white blood cell count (×1000 cells/μL) over time. Leukocytosis was noted since admission with no significant drop in white blood cell count observed during hospitalization. (b) Variation of mean hemoglobin level (g/dL) over time with acute drop in hemoglobin level observed within 3 days of admission. (c) Variation of mean platelet count (×1000 platelets/μL) over time showing a significant decrease of platelet count within 3 days of admission.

RSV infection in adult and elderly immune-competent patients are seldom described in the literature.

Early diagnosis is critical as some therapeutic options may increase the overall survival. The first therapeutic study launched in 1994 by the Histiocyte Society used dexamethasone taper and etoposide as initial therapy followed by hematopoietic stem cell transplant or a continuation therapy combining dexamethasone, etoposide, and cyclosporine A in patients with severe, relapsed, or refractory disease awaiting bone marrow transplant. In 2004, a newer protocol that deviated from the HLH-94 protocol, called HLH-2004, added cyclosporine as part of the initial combination therapy. The newer HLH-2004 protocol was associated with nonstatistically significant reduction in pre-HSCT mortality; however, time to HSCT was significantly reduced [9]. The most recent study, an open-label, single-group study published in 2020, analyzed the efficacy of emapalumab, a human anti-interferon g, in addition with dexamethasone in children with primary HLH and showed promising results [10]. It is important to

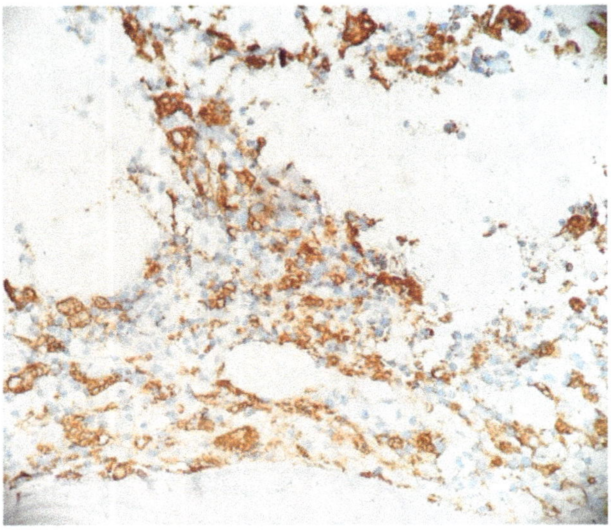

FIGURE 2: Bone marrow biopsy specimen. Immunopathology reveals positive staining for CD163, indicating moderately increased number of macrophages, some of them with hemophagocytosis.

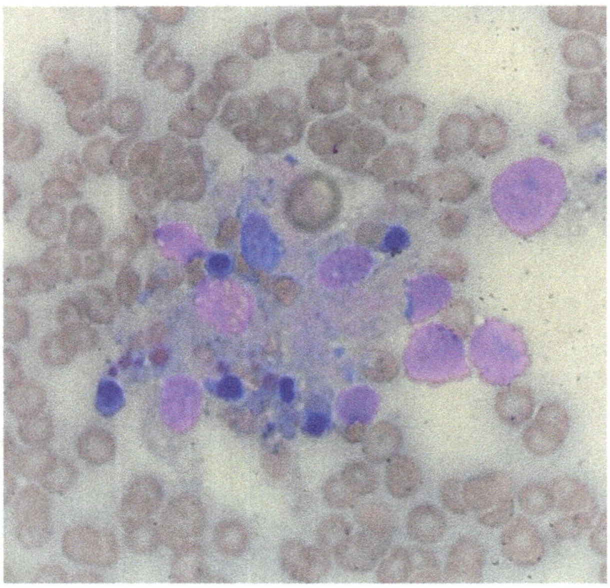

FIGURE 3: Microscopic analysis of a peripheral smear specimen with hematoxylin and eosin staining revealing the presence of macrophages with hemophagocytosis.

mention that most studies found in the literature have mainly focused on the pediatric population. More studies including adult patients are needed before a protocol with proven efficacy is adopted.

In our specific case, no targeted treatment was instituted for 2 main reasons: severe clinical decompensation despite supportive therapy, and final diagnosis made postmortem as only at that time had the 5 criteria been met.

4. Conclusion

In conclusion, our case is unique in that RSV infection in an immunocompetent elderly patient has never been described in the literature as a triggering factor for the development of HLH. This case should aware the clinicians about a possible association between RSV infection and HLH, and the importance of considering HLH as a part of the differential diagnosis in RSV patients that show dramatic clinical decompensation. It should also be mentioned that HLH is a poorly understood disease, with insidious and nonspecific presentation, and that relying on presumed associated conditions for its consideration as a differential diagnosis could potentially prove misleading.

Disclosure

The abstract of this manuscript has been submitted to the 2020 Academic Competition and Research Symposium of the Donald and Barbara Zucker School of Medicine Academic Works. All authors are current employees of Northwell Health, Staten Island University Hospital.

References

[1] H. Al-Samkari and N. Berliner, "Hemophagocytic lymphohistiocytosis," *Annual Review of Pathology: Mechanisms of Disease*, vol. 13, no. 1, pp. 27–49, 2018.

[2] Y. M. Esteban, J. L. O. de Jong, and M. S. Tesher, "An overview of hemophagocytic lymphohistiocytosis," *Pediatric Annals*, vol. 46, no. 8, pp. e309–e313, 2017.

[3] M. B. Jordan, C. E. Allen, J. Greenberg et al., "Challenges in the diagnosis of hemophagocytic lymphohistiocytosis: recommendations from the North American Consortium for Histiocytosis (NACHO)," *Pediatric Blood & Cancer*, vol. 66, no. 11, 2019.

[4] S. A. Parikh, P. Kapoor, L. Letendre, S. Kumar, and A. P. Wolanskyj, "Prognostic factors and outcomes of adults with hemophagocytic lymphohistiocytosis," *Mayo Clinic Proceedings*, vol. 89, no. 4, pp. 484–492, 2014.

[5] S. Konkol and M. Rai, *Lymphohistiocytosis (Hemophagocytic Lymphohistiocytosis)*, StatPearls Publishing, Treasure Island, FL, USA, 2020, http://www.ncbi.nlm.nih.gov/pubmed/32491708.

[6] Z. K. Otrock and C. S. Eby, "Clinical characteristics, prognostic factors, and outcomes of adult patients with hemophagocytic lymphohistiocytosis," *American Journal of Hematology*, vol. 90, no. 3, pp. 220–224, 2015.

[7] M. B. Jordan, C. E. Allen, S. Weitzman, A. H. Filipovich, and K. L. McClain, "How I treat hemophagocytic lymphohistiocytosis," *Blood*, vol. 118, no. 15, pp. 4041–4052, 2011.

[8] C. E. Allen and K. L. McClain, "Pathophysiology and epidemiology of hemophagocytic lymphohistiocytosis," *Hematology*, vol. 2015, no. 1, pp. 177–182, 2015.

[9] E. Bergsten, A. Horne, M. Aricó et al., "Confirmed efficacy of etoposide and dexamethasone in HLH treatment: long-term results of the cooperative HLH2004 study," *Blood*, vol. 130, no. 25, pp. 2728–2738, 2017.

[10] F. Locatelli, M. B. Jordan, C. Allen et al., "Emapalumab in children with primary hemophagocytic lymphohistiocytosis," *New England Journal of Medicine*, vol. 382, no. 19, pp. 1811–1822, 2020.

43

A Case of Secondary Hemophagocytic Lymphohistiocytosis Presenting with Severe Dyserythropoeisis in a Patient with Autoimmune Hemolysis

Kai J. Rogers and Sharathkumar Bhagavathi

Department of Pathology, University of Iowa Hospitals and Clinics, Iowa, IA, USA

Correspondence should be addressed to Kai J. Rogers; kai-rogers@uiowa.edu

Academic Editor: Pier Paolo Piccaluga

The diagnosis of hemophagocytic lymphohistiocytosis (HLH) requires that several clinical criteria are met, and often relies on the identification of rare hemophagocytic cells in the bone marrow. Given the challenge in making the diagnosis, additional signs of immune dysregulation in the bone marrow would have practical clinical use in cases where overt hemophagocytosis is not seen. We present here a case of secondary HLH in a patient with autoimmune hemolysis ultimately diagnosed as Evans syndrome that initially presented with profound dyserythropoeisis in both the peripheral blood and bone marrow. We also explore an association between dyserythropoeisis and HLH in a series of cases previously seen at our institution.

1. Introduction

Hemophagocytic lymphohistiocytosis (HLH) is a hyperinflammatory syndrome caused by a dysregulated immune response. In all cases, HLH is triggered by an inciting event, often viral illness, and in a subset of cases patients are genetically predisposed to such responses due to deficiencies in cytolytic activity of leukocytes (primary HLH) thereby disrupting the ability to maintain immune homeostasis [1]. Additionally, there exists a subset of secondary HLH called macrophage activation syndrome (MAS or MAS-HLH) which occurs secondary to various autoimmune processes, and which can be clinically indistinguishable from HLH when the inciting event is ambiguous. Given the rarity and nonspecific clinical presentation, HLH is often challenging to diagnose resulting in delayed treatment and increased morbidity and mortality. Here we report a case of secondary HLH that presented with severe dyserythropoeisis in the bone marrow and peripheral blood smear of a patient with Evans syndrome. This case builds on a prior case-series correlating cellular dysplasia with HLH [2] and provides further evidence for this association.

2. Case Presentation

The patient is a 52 year-old Asian female with a reported history of hepatitis C and nonalcoholic steatohepatitis who presented with 4 days of weakness, back pain, nausea, and vomiting. Upon admission, she was found to be profoundly anemic (Hgb 2.1 g/dl) with a positive direct antiglobulin test (DAT), elevated lactate dehydrogenase, (1,995 U/L) and decreased haptoglobin (<10 mg/dl), initially concerning for acute autoimmune hemolytic anemia. In addition, she had general signs of severe inflammation with ferritin elevated to 75,415 μg/L and elevated c-reactive protein at 15.9 mg/dl, and organ dysfunction with creatinine 1.5 mg/dl, ALT 243 U/L, AST 539 U/L, and total bilirubin 16.5 mg/dl. Shortly after admission, the patient suffered cardiopulmonary arrest, at which point she was stabilized, intubated, and admitted to the medical intensive care unit for further evaluation. After receiving 5 units of packed RBCs, 1 unit of fresh frozen plasma, and 2 units of platelets, a complete blood count was obtained which revealed the following: hemoglobin 7.2 g/dl (normal 11.9–15.5), white blood cell count $11.3\times10^3/\mu$l (normal 3.7–10.5), a platelet count of

$36 \times 10^3/\mu l$ (normal 150–400), and 10 nucleated RBCs/100WBCs (normal 0). Given the overall clinical picture, including multiorgan dysfunction and concern for hemolysis, a bone marrow biopsy was performed. Review of the peripheral blood smear revealed numerous nucleated RBCs, a large subset of which exhibited signs of dysplasia, with abnormal nuclear contours, nuclear budding, and karyorrhexis (Figure 1(a)). The bone marrow aspirates showed a markedly decreased myeloid: erythroid ratio (0.3) and red cell precursors demonstrated profound dysplasia (>50% of cells) including multinucleate forms, nuclear budding, dysmaturation, and karyorrhexis (Figure 1(b)). Granulocyte and megakaryocyte morphology were normal. Given the profound dyserythropoeisis, the initial impression was that this was consistent with a myelodysplastic syndrome, however, on further review of the smears, numerous hemophagocytic histiocytes were identified raising concern for hemophagocytic lymphohistiocytosis (HLH) (Figure 1(c)). As the cytogenetics performed on the bone marrow specimen were normal and no mutations were identified by molecular analysis, MDS was considered less likely, and the bone marrow was ultimately signed out as concerning for HLH based on the presence of hemophagocytic cells. It should be noted that hemophagocytosis has been observed in the setting of recent transfusion and/or hemolysis [3] and thus we recommended this finding be considered in the context of the patient's constellation of symptoms. After review of the biopsy, the patient was found to meet 5/8 criteria for HLH according to the HLH-2004 criteria [4] (Table 1), sufficient for diagnosis, and she improved rapidly on high-dose corticosteroids and intravenous immunoglobulin (IVIG). Given that secondary HLH is a reactive process, a significant workup was performed in the search for an inciting event. From an infectious disease perspective, the patient had no evidence of infection with CMV, EBV, HIV, HAV, HBV, HCV (reported as having a history but PCR negative), or HHV-8. She was, however, found to be PCR positive in a peripheral blood sample for parvovirus B19, and at the time this was presumed to be the underlying cause of her HLH leading to the diagnosis of secondary HLH over MAS-HLH. Of note, the patient was readmitted ~1 year later with a similar presentation of autoimmune hemolytic anemia and immune-mediated thrombocytopenia. While repeat bone marrow biopsy was not performed, ferritin at the time was elevated to 1,964 $\mu g/L$ and flow cytometry of the peripheral blood showed increased numbers of CD38+/HLA-DR + CD4+ and CD8+ T-lymphocyte populations which have been shown to be consistent with HLH [5], arguing in favor of the diagnosis, although a definitive workup was not pursued. In addition, given the prior assumption that her HLH was secondary to parvovirus B19 infection, PCR was sent, and she was found to be negative. During her second admission, she was ultimately diagnosed with Evans syndrome, an autoimmune disorder presenting with bicytopenias (commonly autoimmune hemolytic anemia and immune thrombocytopenia) that subsequently triggered the dysregulated immune response manifesting as secondary HLH vs. MAS-HLH. She was treated with high-dose solumedrol and IVIG and later transitioned to eltrombopag with recovery of her RBC and platelet counts. She was discharged and has done well on a combination of eltrombopag and rituximab with no further episodes to date.

3. Discussion

As HLH is a clinical syndrome that occurs secondary to dysregulated inflammation, it can be quite difficult to definitively diagnose. Furthermore, as primary HLH is frequently noted during childhood, it is worth noting that the criteria for diagnosis of HLH are often not validated in adult populations which can lead to misdiagnosis in patients with ambiguous presentations [6]. Patients who raise clinical concern for HLH are often critically ill and fall just short of meeting the diagnostic criteria, leading the clinical team to order a bone marrow biopsy and request pathologists to evaluate for the presence of hemophagocytic cells. Such cells are often challenging to find and clear evidence of hemophagocytosis is uncommon, leading to inconclusive results that can delay treatment while awaiting the results of send-out tests with a slow turnaround time of several days such as NK cell activity and soluble IL-2 receptor levels. As such, additional signs and symptoms that consistently predict HLH are of high clinical interest. In this endeavor, a 2000 study by Imashuku et al. was the first to suggest a connection between HLH and reactive dysplasia [7], followed shortly by a 2001 case-series focusing specifically on dyserythropoeisis [2]. This correlation was subsequently observed in the context of Kikuchi disease [8], and we report our experience here in order to strengthen this connection.

To briefly evaluate the possible association between dyserythropoeisis and HLH, we retrospectively reviewed prior cases of HLH at our institution and found dyserythropoeisis in 9/22 cases of secondary HLH that received a bone marrow biopsy (40.1%). In contrast to the case we present here, the dyserythropoeisis was typically less severe, and in no case were dysplastic cells observed in the peripheral blood, a striking and unique feature of our case. Interestingly, in 5/9 cases meeting criteria for HLH with dyserythropoeisis, no hemophagocytic cells were identified, leaving dysplasia as the only morphologic evidence of disease. This is an important point as obvious dysplasia is easily identified and may serve as a marker of profound bone marrow stress providing evidence supporting the diagnosis and prompting a more thorough review when obvious hemophagocytic cells are not initially identified. It is also worth noting that other groups have identified myeloid neoplasms which may also present with dyserythropoeisis such as MDS, AML, and MPNs as triggers for HLH [9, 10] making their exclusion an important part of the diagnostic workup.

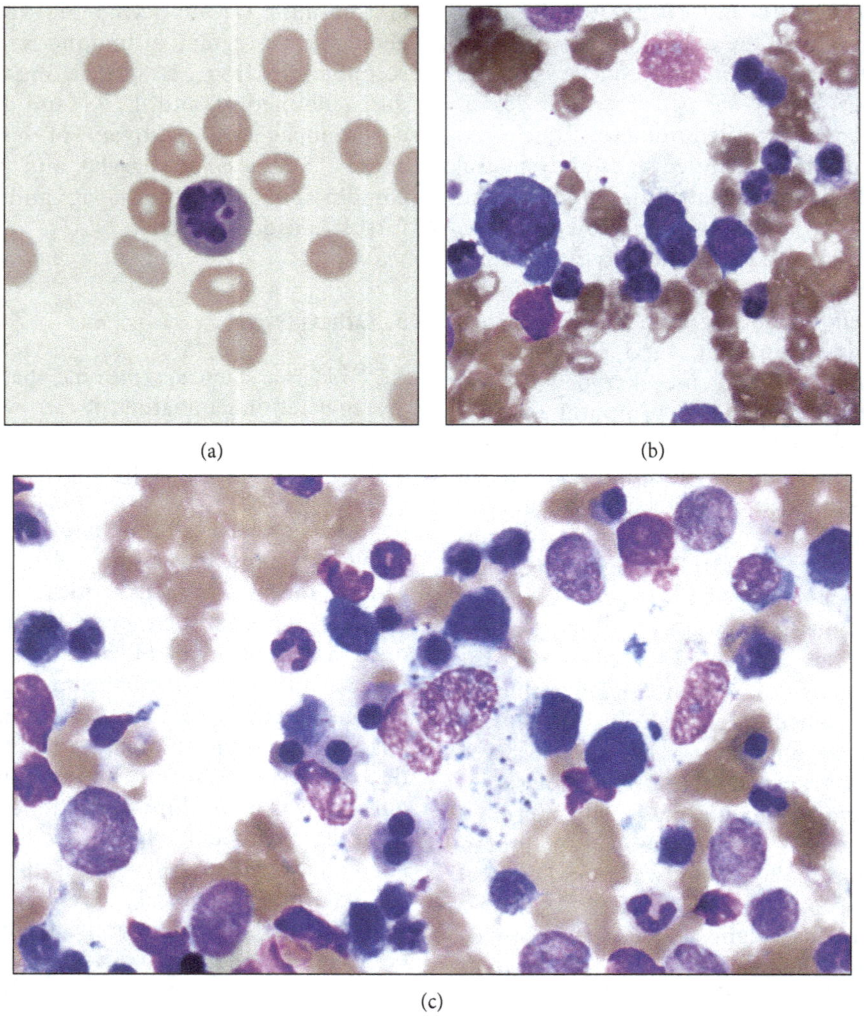

FIGURE 1: (a) The peripheral blood showed increased nucleated red blood cells with signs of dysplasia (100× objective), (b) the aspirate smears showed profound dyserythropoeisis (50× objective), (c) aspirate smears also revealed readily identifiable hemophagocytic cells, consistent with hernophagocytic lymphohistiocytosis (50× objective).

TABLE 1: Diagnostic criteria for HLH in our patient.

Diagnostic criteria	Patient value	Criterion met?
Fever ≥38.5°C for >7 days	Patient was afebrile, Tmax = 37.4°C	No
Splenomegaly	12.3 cm craniocaudal length by ultrasound	No
Cytopenia of 2+ cell lines	Bicytopenia (Hgb nadir of 5.8 g/dL, platelet nadir of 18,000 cells/μL)	Yes
Hypertriglyceridemia (fasting triglycerides >265 mg/dL)	437 mg/dL	Yes
Hemophagocytosis in bone marrow, spleen, lymph node, or liver	Extensive hemophagocytosis in bone marrow	Yes
Low or absent NK activity	Non-detectable	Yes
Serum ferritin concentration ≥500 μg/L	Patient value ranged from 2,759 to 75,415 μg/L	Yes
Soluble CD25 (IL-2 receptor) ≥2400 U/mL	1,035 U/mL, reference range 137–838 U/mL	No

4. Conclusion

This case describes a rarely reported association between dyserythropoeisis and secondary HLH that has been observed in ~40% of cases at our institution. Given the small number of reports to date, the mechanistic link between HLH and cellular dysplasia remains unexplored, although future work in this area may prove insightful. While evidence of hemophagocytic cells remains the key diagnostic feature of HLH from the pathologist's perspective, it is important to note that any abnormality not directly attributable to another disease process should prompt consideration of HLH in the appropriate clinical context.

References

[1] S. Gupta and S. Weitzman, "Primary and secondary hemophagocytic lymphohistiocytosis: clinical features, pathogenesis and therapy," *Expert Review of Clinical Immunology*, vol. 6, no. 1, pp. 137–154, 2010.

[2] M. Macheta, A. M. Will, J. B. Houghton, and R. F. Wynn, "Prominent dyserythropoiesis in four cases of haemophagocytic lymphohistiocytosis," *Journal of Clinical Pathology*, vol. 54, no. 12, pp. 961–963, 2001.

[3] E. McGinnis, N. Medvedev, M. J. Richards, L. Y. C. Chen, and M. P. Wong, "Post-transfusion hemophagocytosis without hemophagocytic lymphohistiocytosis," *Mayo Clinic Proceedings: Innovations, Quality & Outcomes*, vol. 3, no. 4, pp. 517–522, 2019.

[4] J. I. Henter, A. Horne, M. Arico et al., "HLH-2004: diagnostic and therapeutic guidelines for hemophagocytic lymphohistiocytosis. *Pediatr Blood Cancer*," *Pediatric Blood and Cancer*, vol. 48, no. 2, pp. 124–131, 2007.

[5] V. Chaturvedi, R. A. Marsh, A. Zoref-Lorenz et al., "T-cell activation profiles distinguish hemophagocytic lymphohistiocytosis and early sepsis," *Blood*, vol. 137, no. 17, pp. 2337–2346, 2021.

[6] P. La Rosee, A. Horne, M. Hines et al., "Recommendations for the management of hemophagocytic lymphohistiocytosis in adults," *Blood*, vol. 133, no. 23, pp. 2465–2477, 2019.

[7] S. Imashuku, K. Kitazawa, M. Ishii et al., "Bone marrow changes mimicking myelodysplasia in patients with hemophagocytic lymphohistiocytosis," *International Journal of Hematology*, vol. 72, no. 3, pp. 353–357, 2000.

[8] Z. Xu and R. Van der Jagt, "Dyserythropoiesis due to reactive hemophagocytic lymphohistiocytosis," *Blood*, vol. 128, no. 17, p. 2190, 2016.

[9] Y. Sun, C. Blieden, B. Y. Merritt, R. Sosa, and G. Rivero, "Hemophagocytic lymphohistiocytosis and myelodysplastic syndrome: a case report and review of the literature," *Journal of Medical Case Reports*, vol. 15, no. 1, p. 98, 2021.

[10] A. Setiadi, A. Zoref-Lorenz, C. Y. Lee, M. B. Jordan, and L. Y. C. Chen, "Malignancy-associated haemophagocytic lymphohistiocytosis," *The Lancet Haematology*, vol. 9, no. 3, pp. e217–e227, 2022.

44

The Diagnosis is in the Smear: A Case and Review of Spur Cell Anemia in Cirrhosis

Gabriella A. Raffa,[1] Diana M. Byrnes,[2] and John J. Byrnes[3]

[1]*Internal Medicine Residency Program, Jackson Memorial Hospital, Miami, FL, USA*
[2]*Hematology/Oncology Fellowship Program, Jackson Memorial Hospital, Miami, FL, USA*
[3]*Department of Medicine, Division of Hematology, University of Miami, Miami, FL, USA*

Correspondence should be addressed to Gabriella A. Raffa; gabriella.raffa@jhsmiami.org

Academic Editor: Kostas Konstantopoulos

The etiology of anemia in liver cirrhosis is multifactorial; one less recognized cause is hemolytic anemia due to spur cells, known as spur cell anemia. We present the case of a 57-year-old woman with alcoholic cirrhosis who presented with symptomatic macrocytic anemia with a hemoglobin level of 7.4 g/dL and signs of decompensated liver disease. Notably, she had no signs of overt bleeding. Further workup was consistent with hemolysis, with peripheral smear demonstrating spur cells. The patient was treated with both steroids and IVIG, although she eventually expired. The characteristic morphology of spur cells is due to alteration of the lipid composition of the erythrocyte membrane, changing its shape and leading to splenic sequestration and destruction. Characteristic of this disorder is an increased ratio of cholesterol to phospholipid on the membrane, as well as low levels of apolipoproteins and low- and high-density lipoproteins. The presence of spur cells is an indicator of poor prognosis and high risk of mortality. Currently, the only definitive cure is liver transplantation. There is a paucity of literature on the prevalence of this phenomenon and even less about treatment. This case highlights the importance of recognition of spur cell anemia as a cause of anemia in cirrhosis as well as the importance of the peripheral smear in the diagnostic workup. Early recognition can lead to avoidance of unnecessary procedures. Further research is needed to elucidate the true prevalence of spur cell anemia and examine further treatment options.

1. Introduction

The systemic sequelae of liver cirrhosis are vast and consist of hematological abnormalities, including anemia. The etiology of anemia in cirrhotic patients is multifactorial and can be secondary to red blood cell destruction by splenic sequestration and hypersplenism, bone marrow suppression, vitamin deficiencies, and occult or chronic bleeding from varices or gastropathy [1]. Less commonly generated in the differential, although unmistakable on peripheral smear, is that of spur cell anemia (SCA) which induces a hemolytic anemia in patients with liver disease. SCA is associated with high mortality and treatment options are limited. Here, we report a case of SCA in the setting of alcoholic liver cirrhosis.

2. Case Report

We present the case of a 57-year-old Hispanic woman with a past medical history of alcoholic cirrhosis (MELD-Na 30 on admission, Child-Pugh Class C) complicated by Grade I esophageal varices and portal hypertensive gastropathy, as well as recently diagnosed stage I colorectal adenocarcinoma (treatment naïve), who presented to the hospital with a one-week history of fatigue, dyspnea, and dizziness. On admission, the patient was noted to be hypotensive with a blood pressure of 89/48, afebrile with a temperature of 98.4 °F, and tachycardic with a heart rate of 100 beats per minute. Physical exam was notable for appearance of weakness, although the patient was awake, alert, and oriented, with scleral icterus, jaundice, splenomegaly, ascites, and mild abdominal distension. Laboratory exams in the initial days of presentation are noted in Table 1 and are significant for macrocytic anemia with a hemoglobin of 7.4 g/dL and a mean corpuscular volume of 109.4 fL. Studies were consistent with hemolysis, with an elevated LDH of 263 U/L, indirect hyperbilirubinemia of 9.2 mg/dL, undetectable haptoglobin (<10 mg/dL), and elevated reticulocyte count of 16.1% (Table 1). Her macrocytosis was most likely secondary to reticulocytosis due to hemolysis, although workup of vitamin deficiencies was initiated, demonstrating normal folate levels and elevated vitamin B12 levels, likely in the setting of severe liver disease [2, 3]. Peripheral smear demonstrated mostly acanthocytes (spur cells), spherocytes, rare schistocytes, target cells, and few burr cells (Figure 1). The patient was resuscitated with packed red blood cells and fluids and briefly placed on vasopressors. Notably, the patient had no clinical evidence of upper or lower gastrointestinal bleeding. For this reason, the patient did not undergo endoscopy or colonoscopy during her admission.

On further workup of her hemolytic anemia, the patient was tested for paroxysmal nocturnal hemoglobinuria with FLAER, which was negative, as was direct Coombs testing. Of note, three months prior to this presentation, during a previous admission, the patient had a direct Coombs test that was positive for IgG antibody; elution testing revealed a warm autoantibody. It was speculated that perhaps the patient had a low level of antibodies, not detectable during this admission, and that she perhaps had warm autoimmune hemolytic anemia (WAIHA). However, during her previous admission, when she tested positive, she had also received a blood transfusion at that time which could have contributed to a false positive. Additional workup included CT of the abdomen and pelvis to assess for lymphadenopathy given the association of lymphoproliferative disorders and WAIHA, which was negative for lymphadenopathy although remarkable for splenomegaly of 14.4 cm. She was initially treated for WAIHA with steroids at 1 mg/kg for three days, increased to 1.5 mg/kg for five days with no clinical response in terms of her hemolysis panel; therefore, a steroid taper was started. Due to the refractory nature, she was treated with IVIG 1 mg/kg for two days. The new leading diagnosis was SCA because of findings on peripheral smear and lack of response to steroid therapy. Lipid levels, including apolipoprotein levels, were obtained, given the association with SCA and defects in lipid metabolism, and were notable for decreased total cholesterol, LDL, and apolipoproteins AI and B (Table 2). After receiving IVIG, her hemolysis panel was unchanged, except for the indirect bilirubin which continued to worsen (Table 3). Unfortunately, several days later, the patient continued to decompensate and expired from acute respiratory distress syndrome secondary to pneumonia.

Table 1: Laboratory data from admission.

Complete blood count	
WBC (4.0–10.5 $10^3/\mu L$)	9.4
Hgb (11.1–14.6 g/dL)	7.4
Hct (33.2–43.4%)	22.1
MCV (80–100 fL)	109.4
Plt (140–400 $10^3/\mu L$)	51
Serum chemistries	
Sodium (135–146 mmol/L)	131
Potassium (3.5–5.5 mmol/L)	5.0
Chloride (98–110 mmol/L)	101
Bicarbonate (19–34 mmol/L)	20
BUN (6–20 mg/dL)	16
Creatinine (0.4–1.1 mg/dL)	0.58
Total bilirubin (0–1.2 mg/dL)	15.4
Direct bilirubin (0.0–0.3 mg/dL)	6.2
Total protein (6.1–8.1 g/dL)	4.5
Albumin (3.5–5.2 g/dL)	2.3
AST (10–40 U/L)	48
ALT (0–33 U/L)	33
Alkaline phosphatase (35–130 U/L)	118
Anemia workup	
Vitamin B12 (232–1,245 pg/mL)	1,925
Folate (>7.3 ng/mL)	11.1
Iron (37–145 mcg/dL)	148
TIBC (200–400 mcg/dL)	220
Ferritin (13–150 mg/mL)	203
%transferrin sat. (14–50%)	67.3
Reticulocyte%	16.1
LDH (135–214 U/L)	263
Indirect bilirubin (calculated)	9.2
Haptoglobin (30–200 mg/dL)	<10
PNH with FLAER (GPI-linked CD59) negative	
Direct Coombs	Negative
Coagulation studies	
PTT (23.4–36.0 sec)	46.1
PT (12.0–14.5 sec)	28.5
INR (0.88–1.12)	2.7
Fibrinogen (164–498 mg/dL)	206

Note that iron studies were obtained after transfusion.

3. Discussion

Acanthocytes, or spur cells, consist of characteristic spicules seen on peripheral smear. The mechanism is thought to be alteration of lipid metabolism on the erythrocyte membrane, leading to the characteristic morphology that has a propensity for hemolysis. As delineated previously, the etiologies of anemia in liver disease are vast. Portal hypertension can lead to enlargement of the spleen (as seen in this patient), causing sequestration and destruction of red and white blood cells as well as platelets. Another important consideration is disseminated intravascular coagulation (DIC), which has a number of causes, including cirrhosis and malignancy, and should be on the differential in any patient with elevation of coagulation tests and thrombocytopenia. Although this patient's normal fibrinogen, rare schistocytes on smear, and chronically elevated coagulation studies do not wholly support acute DIC, the chronic form is an important concern and could exacerbate an occult bleed from varices or gastropathy, leading to anemia. Specifically, the differential of hemolytic anemia in alcoholics with liver disease, in addition to SCA, includes a pathology known as Zieve syndrome, a condition characterized by hemolytic anemia, jaundice, and transient hyperlipidemia. The pathophysiology is attributed to alcohol toxicity to the erythrocyte membranes, leading to hemolysis and release of lipid into the circulation [4]; spur cells are usually not seen on peripheral smear [5]. Zieve syndrome is seen in milder liver disease, and the prognosis is markedly different: cessation of alcohol use usually resolves the anemia and other sequelae.

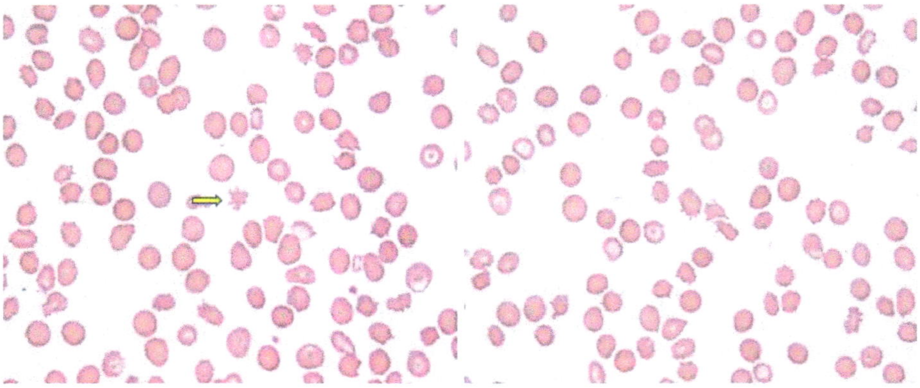

FIGURE 1: Peripheral smear using 100x objective lens demonstrating numerous acanthocytes (spur cells), spherocytes, target cells, and occasional burr cells. An example of a spur cell is identified with a yellow arrow.

TABLE 2: Comparison of lipid panel before admission and during hospitalization.

Lipid Panel	5 months prior	Current
Cholesterol (<240 mg/dL)	257	132
Triglycerides (<150 mg/dL)	76	74
HDL (>49 mg/dL)	46	59
LDL (<130 mg/dL)	193	59
Apolipoprotein A1 (>125 mg/dL)	71	
Apolipoprotein B (<90 mg/dL)	40	

TABLE 3: Hemolysis panel during hospitalization.

	Day 2	Pre-steroids (Day 6)	Pre-IVIG* (Day 13)	Post-IVIG (Day 15)
Hgb	7.4	9.0	7.4	7.0
Haptoglobin	<10	<10	<10	<10
Indirect bili	9.2	8	11.4	17.3
LDH	263	393	285	292

*Patient was initiated on steroids on Day 6 at 1 mg/kg for three days, increased to 1.5 mg/kg for five days (day 8 through 13) with no clinical response, and was subsequently placed on a taper which was continued until her death.

The liver plays a key role in the metabolism and homeostasis of lipids, and thus, liver dysfunction has modification of lipid homeostasis as a known side effect. In alcoholic cirrhosis, fat accumulation in the liver contributes to this dysfunction [6]. It has been observed that in liver disease, the erythrocyte membrane has an increased ratio of cholesterol to phospholipid [7, 8]. This is in part due to the fact that in the setting of liver disease, the activity of serum lecithin cholesterol acyltransferase, an enzyme which converts free cholesterol into cholesterol ester, is decreased, and consequently, the free cholesterol is elevated. This cholesterol accumulation increases erythrocyte surface area, altering its shape [7, 9], leading to splenic sequestration and subsequent destruction [10].

Other lipid profile abnormalities have been observed in liver disease. For example, Duhamel et al. noted that significantly low levels of apolipoprotein A (apoA)-II, high-density lipoprotein (HDL) III, and low-density lipoprotein (LDL) appeared characteristic of alcoholic cirrhotics with spur cells, with a trend toward lower apolipoprotein B (apoB) levels [11]. Although we do not have a baseline apoB for our patient, her level was on the low end of normal (40 mg/dL) when measured during admission. Cicognani et al. demonstrated an inverse relationship between levels of LDL, HDL, and total serum cholesterol level with severity of liver disease [12]. Notably, decreased levels of Apo-AI, as seen in our patient, seem to be a marker of fibrosis in alcoholic patients, potentially secondary to binding to fibronectin [6]. Indeed, studies have demonstrated a worsening lipid profile with increasing severity of liver disease [13, 14]. It is worth noting tht five months prior to presentation, the patient had a MELD-Na of 25 and was Child-Pugh Class B (compared to MELD-Na 30 with Child-Pugh Class C on presentation) with the lipid panel as seen in Table 2, with a trend toward decreasing total cholesterol and LDL (albeit with an increase in HDL). The presence of spur cell anemia has been associated with poor prognosis in cirrhotic patients; one study reported a median survival of 1.9 months in patients with >5% spur cells [15]. Similarly, a study by Vassiliadis et al. observed that presence of >5% spur cells correlated with lower 3-month survival rates [5].

Other sequelae of SCA include a prolonged INR. This elevation is in part secondary to the diminished synthesis of coagulation factors seen in liver disease and often concomitant vitamin K deficiency that is seen with malnutrition and alcoholism, although in the setting of SCA, it is also postulated to be due to the alteration of the phospholipid components of thromboplastin reagents [5, 16]. In addition, it has been reported that platelets also have alteration of membrane lipids, warping the meshwork used in clot formation [16]. However, the additional cholesterol on platelet membranes appears to induce platelet aggregation [17]. Sundaram et al. hypothesized that this hypercoagulable state may offset the bleeding diathesis that would otherwise be expected in the setting of a pronounced coagulopathy. Both the Child-Pugh and MELD scores, used as an estimation of cirrhosis severity and for liver transplant allocation, respectively, utilize the INR in their calculation. Given the association of SCA with severe liver disease, the effect of the pathologic mechanisms of SCA on the already present coagulopathy may be serendipitous, as this would increase the MELD score and the likelihood for a transplant.

There is a paucity of literature on the true prevalence of spur cell anemia, and even less so on treatment modalities. The only definitive cure for spur cell anemia is liver transplant, and complete reversal of anemia has been reported after transplantation [18]. Unfortunately, our patient was not a candidate for liver transplant given her active workup for colorectal adenocarcinoma. Plasmapheresis has historically been attempted. One study comparing lipid profiles before and after plasmapheresis demonstrated an increase in concentrations of total cholesterol, phospholipids, and apo-AI after treatment, although low levels of lipoprotein (a), LDL, and apo-AII persisted. Reticulocyte counts and hemoglobin levels were also noted to improve, although other markers of hemolysis were constant [19]. A case of spur cell anemia has been reported with successful improvement of hemolysis panel, decrease in number of spur cells, and decrease in the amount of free cholesterol in the blood with combination therapy of flunarizine, pentoxifylline, and cholestyramine, with remission achieved for almost a year with cholestyramine alone [20].

This case serves as a review of spur cell anemia as a cause of hemolytic anemia in advanced cirrhosis and highlights the importance of the peripheral smear in its diagnosis. Clinician awareness of the differential of hemolytic anemia in alcoholic liver disease should prompt ordering of a lipid profile, which is otherwise not normally ordered in an anemic cirrhotic patient. Early recognition could not only lead to early treatment but also prevent unnecessary procedures, namely, an elaborate endoscopic search for a gastrointestinal bleed. In addition, this report details the lack of efficacy of steroids and IVIG in treating this form of hemolytic anemia. Further research is needed to define treatment options and more accurately delineate the true prevalence of this etiology of anemia.

References

[1] A. A. Qamar and N. D. Grace, "Abnormal hematological indices in cirrhosis," *Canadian Journal of Gastroenterology*, vol. 23, no. 6, pp. 441–445, 2009.

[2] T. Sugihara, M. Koda, T. Okamoto et al., "Falsely elevated serum vitamin B12 levels were associated with the severity and prognosis of chronic viral liver disease," *Yonago Acta Medica*, vol. 60, no. 1, pp. 31–39, 2017.

[3] J. Dou, W. Xu, B. Ye, Y. Zhang, and W. Mao, "Serum vitamin B12 levels as indicators of disease severity and mortality of patients with acute-on-chronic liver failure," *Clinica Chimica Acta*, vol. 20, no. 23-24, pp. 1809–1812, 2012.

[4] A. Gremida, S. Paleti, E. T. Perez, and D. McCarthy, "Hemolysis in alcoholic liver disease: Zieve's syndrome," *Digestive Diseases and Sciences*, vol. 63, no. 3, pp. 601–604, 2018.

[5] T. Vassiliadis, A. Mpoumponaris, S. Vakalopoulou et al., "Spur cells and spur cell anemia in hospitalized patients with advanced liver disease: incidence and correlation with disease severity and survival," *Hepatology Research*, vol. 40, no. 2, pp. 161–170, 2010.

[6] G. Privitera, L. Spadaro, S. Marchisello, G. Fede, and F. Purrello, "Abnormalities of lipoprotein levels in liver cirrhosis: clinical relevance," *International Surgery*, vol. 87, no. 4, pp. 201–204, 2002.

[7] R. A. Cooper, "Anemia with spur cells: a red cell defect acquired in serum and modified in the circulation," *Journal of Clinical Investigation*, vol. 48, no. 10, pp. 1820–1831, 1969.

[8] G. Privitera and G. Meli, "An unusual cause of anemia in cirrhosis: spur cell anemia, a case report with review of the literature," *Gastroenterol Hepatol Bed Bench*, vol. 9, no. 4, pp. 335–339, 2016.

[9] S. M. Sabesin, H. L. Hawkins, L. Kuiken, and J. B. Ragland, "Abnormal plasma lipoproteins and lecithin-cholesterol acyltransferase deficiency in alcoholic liver disease," *Gastroenterology*, vol. 72, no. 3, pp. 510–518, 1977.

[10] R. A. Cooper, "Hemolytic syndromes and red cell membrane abnormalities in liver disease," *Seminars in Hematology*, vol. 17, no. 2, pp. 103–112, 1980.

[11] G. Duhamel, P. Forgez, B. Nalpas, P. Berthelot, and M. J. Chapman, "Spur cells in patients with alcoholic liver cirrhosis are associated with reduced plasma levels of apoA-II, HDL3, and LDL," *Journal of Lipid Research*, vol. 24, no. 12, pp. 1612–1625, 1983.

[12] C. Cicognani, M. Malavolti, A. M. Morselli-Labate, L. Zamboni, C. Sama, and L. Barbara, "Serum lipid and lipoprotein patterns in patients with liver cirrhosis and chronic active hepatitis," *Archives of Internal Medicine*, vol. 157, no. 7, pp. 792–796, 1997.

[13] M. R. Ghadir, A. A. Riahin, A. Havaspour, M. Nooranipour, and A. A. Habibinejad, "The relationship between lipid profile and severity of liver damage in cirrhotic patients," *Hepatitis Monthly*, vol. 10, no. 4, pp. 285–288, 2010.

[14] A. Abbasi, A. R. Bhutto, N. Butt, K. Lal, and S. M. Munir, "Serum cholesterol: could it be a sixth parameter of child-pugh scoring system in cirrhotics due to viral hepatitis?" *Journal of the College of Physicians and Surgeons Pakistan*, vol. 22, no. 8, pp. 484–487, 2012.

[15] A. Alexopoulou, L. Vasilieva, T. Kanellopoulou, S. Pouriki, A. Soultati, and S. P. Dourakis, "Presence of spur cells as a highly predictive factor of mortality in patients with cirrhosis," *Journal of Gastroenterology and Hepatology*, vol. 29, no. 4, pp. 830–834, 2014.

[16] V. Sundaram, A. M. S. Al-Osaimi, J. J. Lewis, T. Lisman, and S. H. Caldwell, "Severe prolongation of the INR in spur cell anemia of cirrhosis: true-true and related?" *Digestive Diseases and Sciences*, vol. 51, no. 7, pp. 1203–1205, 2006.

[17] M. Watanabe, K. Shiraishi, M. Itakura, and S. Matsuzaki, "Relationship between platelet membrane lipid compositions and platelet aggregability in alcoholic liver disease," *Alco-*

holism: Clinical and Experimental Research, vol. 22, no. S3, pp. 97S–102S, 1998.

[18] P. Malik, D. Bogetti, P. Sileri et al., "Spur cell anemia in alcoholic cirrhosis: cure by orthotopic liver transplantation and recurrence after liver graft failure," *International Journal of Hematology*, vol. 73, no. 3, pp. 351–355, 2001.

[19] K. Miki, T. Maruki, and S. Imashuku, "Plasmapheresis for spur cell anemia in a patient with alcoholic liver cirrhosis," *Case Reports in Hematology*, vol. 2018, Article ID 9513946, 4 pages, 2018.

[20] K. Aihara, H. Azuma, Y. Ikeda et al., "Successful combination therapy-flunarizine, pentoxifylline, and cholestyramine- for spur cell anemia," *International Journal of Hematology*, vol. 73, no. 3, pp. 351–355, 2001.

45

Chronic Atrophic Gastritis with Negative Intrinsic Factor and Parietal Cell Antibody Presenting as a Severe Hemolytic Anemia

G. F. Cittolin-Santos, S. Khalil, J. K. Bakos, and K. Baker

Medical University of South Carolina, Department of Internal Medicine, Charleston, SC, USA

Correspondence should be addressed to G. F. Cittolin-Santos; cittolin@musc.edu

Academic Editor: Tom S. J. Gonz lez L pez

A 28-year-old Caucasian male with Hashimoto's disease and vitiligo presented with two weeks of dizziness on exertion following pharyngitis which was treated with prednisone 40 mg by mouth once a day for five days. Initial workup revealed anemia, elevated lactate dehydrogenase (LDH), and low haptoglobin. He underwent workup for causes of hemolytic anemia which was remarkable for a peripheral blood smear with hypersegmented neutrophils and low vitamin B12 levels concerning for pernicious anemia. Parietal cell and intrinsic factor antibodies were negative, and he then underwent an esophagogastroduodenoscopy with biopsy. The biopsy was negative for *Helicobacter pylori*, and the immunohistochemical stains were suggestive of chronic atrophic gastritis. He was started on vitamin B12 1,000 mcg intramuscular injections daily. His hemoglobin, LDH, and haptoglobin normalized. Given the absence of the parietal cell antibody and intrinsic factor antibody, this is a rare case of seronegative pernicious anemia.

1. Introduction

Pernicious anemia is often associated with other autoimmune diseases such as Hashimoto's disease and vitiligo [1]. Severe cases of vitamin B12 deficiency can cause ineffective erythropoiesis and a hemolytic anemia [2–5]. The differential and workup for a hemolytic anemia is broad and can be clouded by concomitant infections and other autoimmune conditions. Historically, the Schilling test was used to diagnose pernicious anemia; however, advances in testing have led to the measurement of intrinsic factor level, anti-parietal cell antibody, anti-intrinsic factor antibody, and histologic analysis [6, 7]. Here, we report a case of hemolytic anemia and ineffective erythropoiesis associated with atrophic gastritis due to seronegative atrophic gastritis causing pernicious anemia.

2. Case Presentation

A 28-year-old male with a past medical history of Hashimoto's disease and vitiligo presented with two weeks of exertional dizziness, fatigue, nausea, pallor, and an intermittent generalized maculopapular rash. He denied fevers, chills, joint pain, easy bruising, recent travel, or sick contacts. He had also been recently treated for pharyngitis by his primary care physician with prednisone 40 mg by mouth once a day for five days due to the severe throat pain with improvement of symptoms. He denied any prior personal or family history of blood disorders. He denied any new medications other than prednisone use for his pharyngitis. His only medication was levothyroxine 150 mcg by mouth once a day. On admission, his temperature was 37.2°C, pulse 102 bpm, blood pressure 119/81 mmHg, respiratory rate 16, and oxygen saturation 100% while breathing ambient air. He had pale conjunctiva and skin without bruising, petechiae, or rashes. He had splenomegaly, but the remainder of the physical examination was normal. Initial workup was remarkable for macrocytic anemia, elevated LDH, low haptoglobin, and undetectable vitamin B12 levels (Table 1). An infectious workup and serologic workup for autoimmune anemia and pernicious anemia were also performed (Table 2). Patient had normal hemoglobin electrophoresis. Initially, flow cytometry testing for paroxysmal nocturnal hemoglobinuria (PNH) was not performed, while the DAT

Table 1: Laboratory data.

Variable	Reference range	Day 1	Day 2*	Day 3**	Day 4*	Day 5	Day 6	Day 7	Day 8	Day 15	Day 22
Hematocrit (%)	41–53	16.2	14.2	15.9	18	17.5	20.9	21.9	24	32.6	38.2
HB (g/dL)	12–18	6.1	5.2	6.5	6.2	7.1	7.1	7	7.5	10.7	12.5
Retic index		0.29				0.15	0.21	3.61	5.28	2.26	
Platelets (K/μL)	140–440	94	90	65	73	62	70	82	66	383	252
MCV (fL)	77–106	109									
WBC (K/CUMM)	4.8–10.8	5.6	5.35	4.47	4.48	5.67	6.51	5.04	4.24	6.7	5.6
LDH (U/L)	100–240	6941					6170	4048	3487		
AST (U/)	10–36	270	191	189			172	109	71		
ALT (U/L)	12–78	163	127	128			170	169	71		
Fibrinogen (mg/dL)	231–486	264									
Total bilirubin (mg/dL)	0.2–1.3	1.4	1.4	2.3			1.2	0.9	1		
Haptoglobin (mg/dL)	14–258	<8					<8				23
Serum iron (mg/dL)	50–175	163									
Ferritin (mg/mL)	21.8–322	662									
TIBC (mcg/dL)	245–425	182									
G6PD (U/g Hb)	9.9–16.6	14.2									
Folate (ng/ml)	7–31.4	12.9									
Vit B12 (pg/mL)	211–911	<146				>1700					991
Erythropoietin (mIU/mL)	2.6–18.5	114									
TSH (mIU/mL)	0.35–4.94	4.56									

G6PD = glucose-6-phosphate dehydrogenase; TSH = thyroid-stimulating hormone; *one unit of packet RBC (pRBC) was transfused that day; **daily B12 injections were started that day.

Table 2: Infectious and autoimmune workup.

CMV PCR	Negative
EBV PCR	Negative
HIV PCR	Negative
Hepatitis C antibody	Negative
Coombs test	Negative
Parietal cell antibody	Negative
Intrinsic factor antibody	Negative
Cryoglobulin	Trace after 24 h
Direct antiglobulin test*	Negative

*Direct antiglobulin test (DAT) includes DAT polyspecific, immunoglobulin G (IgG), complement 3/complement 3d antibodies, 4C low ionic strength saline (LISS) wash antibodies, polyethylene glycol antibodies, IgG and IgA gel antibodies, and acid eluate.

results were pending, although PNH was a diagnosis on the differential. Peripheral smear was notable for hypersegmented neutrophils, macrocytic normochromic anemia, thrombocytopenia, and lacked schistocytes (Figure 1). Abdominal ultrasound was significant for splenomegaly.

The hypersegmented neutrophils in the peripheral smear without schistocytes, the laboratory findings of hemolytic anemia, and the undetectable B12 levels were all consistent with the diagnosis of pernicious anemia. The patient was started on intramuscular vitamin B12 1,000 mcg on day three of admission. On the second and fourth day of hospitalization, the patient's hemoglobin was 5.2 and 6.2 g/dL, so the patient was transfused one unit of packed red blood cells (pRBCs) each day with a hemoglobin response to 6.5 and 7.1 g/dL, respectively. On hospital day eight, his hemoglobin improved without transfusion to 7.5 g/dL, so he was deemed stable for discharge with close follow-up. The patient underwent regular B12 replacement—weekly for a month and then monthly thereafter. He then underwent an outpatient esophagogastroduodenoscopy (EGD), which demonstrated widespread atrophy of the stomach. Biopsies were taken of the mucosa that suggested chronic atrophic gastritis with histologic and immunohistochemical findings consistent with pernicious anemia without evidence of *Helicobacter pylori* (Figure 2). The patient was continued on B12 replacement and presented for outpatient follow-up on day 15, 25, and 60 after his initial hospital presentation with hemoglobin level 10.7, 12.5, and 14.5, respectively. He had no further evidence of hemolysis and did not require any further intervention other than the B12 injections. This is an unusual case of hemolytic anemia from ineffective erythropoiesis secondary to seronegative pernicious anemia and B12 deficiency.

3. Discussion

Identifying the culprit for an acute episode of anemia can be challenging. There are multiple etiologies of acute anemia including hemolysis, and the cause of hemolysis can vary greatly [8, 9]. Anemia due to B12 deficiency is not usually associated with hemolysis, and it is not classified as a hemolytic anemia [10, 11]. Despite that, it is important to consider B12 deficiency as the cause of hemolysis when faced with an increase in LDH levels higher than 5–10 times the upper normal limit, especially with accompanying cytopenia. Although uncommon, B12 deficiency causes one of the highest peaks in LDH due to the ineffective erythropoiesis and premature RBC death. Paroxysmal nocturnal hemoglobinuria also causes a marked LDH peak and sometimes is associated with cytopenias and should be considered in this setting as well [9]. There are well-known algorithms for the workup of anemia; however, standard algorithms do not always apply and can be obscured by confounding diseases. As previously described (Barcellini and Fattizzo, 2015), the

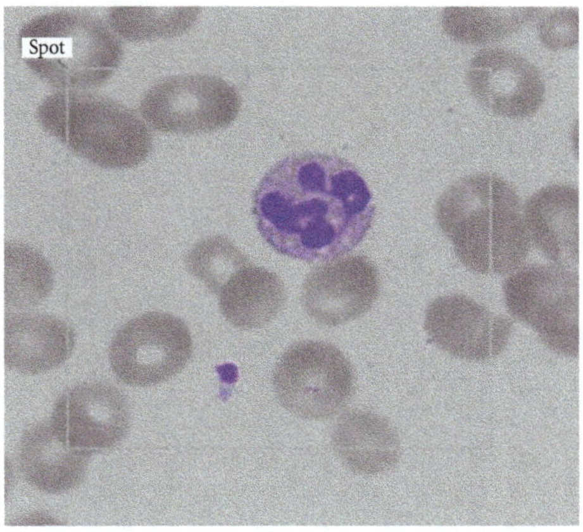

FIGURE 1: Peripheral smear with hypersegmented neutrophils.

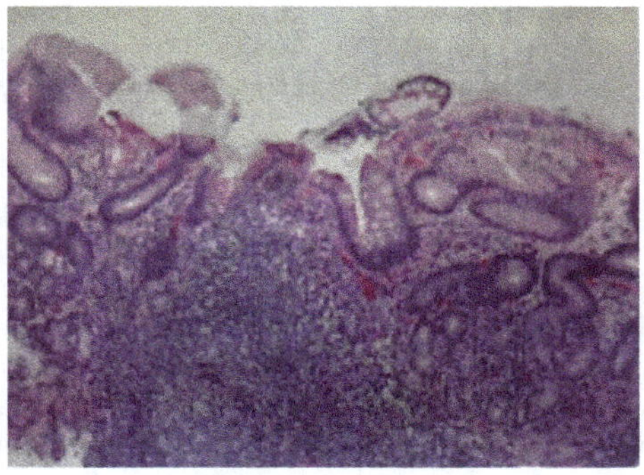

FIGURE 2: Gastric biopsy showing lymphoplasmacytic cells in the lamina propria of gastric tissue. No neutrophilic activity is identified. Atrophy was noted without dysplastic alterations.

utilization of clinical and hemolytic markers is helpful in diagnosing hemolytic anemias [9]. Reaching the correct diagnosis is important because each condition requires specific treatment and follow-up.

We faced a case of acute hemolytic anemia in a patient with known autoimmune disease. It is known that patients with autoimmune conditions are especially prone to develop autoimmune hemolytic anemia [5]. However, a majority of patients with pernicious anemia present with subacute to chronic symptoms [12], and the case above is an atypical presentation. Although B12 deficiency has been previously associated with intramedullary hemolysis and ineffective erythropoiesis, hemolysis due to B12 deficiency is rare. We also considered PNH as a possible cause due to the markedly elevated LDH levels. However, the patient had improvement with B12 treatment when the final DAT testing resulted, so we did not order a flow cytometry testing for PNH due to the low likelihood of this diagnosis at that time. Furthermore, the sensitivity of antiparietal antibodies is high, and it is uncommon for both antiparietal and anti-intrinsic factor antibodies to be negative. It has been shown that these antibodies are present in ninety percent of patients with pernicious anemia. Seronegativity may be explained by complete antibody-to-antigen binding so that no free antigen is circulating by antibody production failure or by the disappearance of the antibody due to antigen disappearance. In our case, the recent course of prednisone may have altered the antibody response. Type-I auto-antibodies that block the binding of the intrinsic factor and vitamin B12 were only demonstrated in approximately seventy percent of patients with pernicious anemia. Type-II auto-antibodies that bind to another site separate from the vitamin B12-binding site are also only present in approximately thirty-five to forty percent of these patients [13]. This explains how patients with pernicious anemia may have seronegative findings.

Hypersegmented neutrophils on the peripheral smear were compatible with B12 deficiency (Figure 1). The paucity of schistocytes in the peripheral smear leads us to believe that the hemolytic process was intramedullary, a phenomenon which has been previously described in cases of extreme B12 deficiency. Also, marked intravascular hemolysis is usually associated with dark "brownish" urine discoloration due to the presence of hemosiderin bound to iron in the urine, which was not present in this case [9, 14]. We observed a response in reticulocyte count and Hgb levels around seven days after starting intramuscular vitamin B12 1,000 mcg daily injections. Besides a two-time pRBC transfusion and daily vitamin B12 injections, the patient did not require any other interventions, and his symptoms resolved shortly thereafter. The patient underwent an outpatient EGD with gastric biopsy following discharge that confirmed the presumptive diagnosis by demonstrating atrophy with lymphoplasmacytic cells in the lamina propria of gastric tissue similar to atrophy and diffuse lymphoplasmacytic cells seen in a typical case of pernicious anemia (Figure 2).

This case is an atypical presentation of B12 deficiency due to the acute onset of severe symptomatic anemia and the negative serologic workup for pernicious anemia. However, the patient's resolution in anemia and hemolysis following vitamin B12 injections along with the biopsy result of chronic atrophic gastritis confirmed the diagnosis of seronegative pernicious anemia. Anemia due to B12 deficiency is often successfully treated with supplementation without even evaluating serology, but having a confirmatory test diagnosing pernicious anemia is important due to possible complications if the condition is left untreated. Patients with untreated pernicious anemia may develop neurological symptoms that range from paresthesia to ataxia, generating a clinical scenario of combined sclerosis of the spinal cord that may lead to irreversible sequelae. Also, the autoimmune gastritis of pernicious anemia is associated with susceptibility of gastric tumors—carcinoid, carcinomas, and non-Hodgkin's malignant lymphoma. Thus, surveillance of gastric tumors is warranted, and the patients should be referred to a gastroenterologist [15]. This case illustrates why one should keep pernicious anemia in the differential diagnosis for hemolytic anemias, especially when LDH levels are exceedingly high and associated with cytopenias, despite negative antiparietal cell or intrinsic factor antibodies.

References

[1] A. A. Zulfiqar and E. Andres, "Association pernicious anemia and autoimmune polyendocrinopathy: a retrospective study,"

Journal of Medicine and Life, vol. 10, no. 4, pp. 250–253, 2017.

[2] R. Khalil, S. Naqvi, and V. Chastain, "Vitamin B12 deficiency as a cause of hemolytic anemia," *Journal of Hospital Medicine*, vol. 7, 2012.

[3] E. Andres, S. Affenberger, J. Zimmer et al., "Current hematological findings in cobalamin deficiency. A study of 201 consecutive patients with documented cobalamin deficiency," *Clinical and Laboratory Haematology*, vol. 28, no. 1, pp. 50–56, 2006.

[4] U. Acharya, J.-T. Gau, W. Horvath, P. Ventura, C.-T. Hsueh, and W. Carlsen, "Hemolysis and hyperhomocysteinemia caused by cobalamin deficiency: three case reports and review of the literature," *Journal of Hematology & Oncology*, vol. 1, no. 1, p. 26, 2008.

[5] G. F. Bass, E. T. Tuscano, and J. M. Tuscano, "Diagnosis and classification of autoimmune hemolytic anemia," *Autoimmunity Reviews*, vol. 13, no. 4-5, pp. 560–564, 2014.

[6] D. Cattan, "Pernicious anemia: what are the actual diagnosis criteria?" *World Journal of Gastroenterology*, vol. 17, no. 4, pp. 543-544, 2011.

[7] E. Lahner and B. Annibale, "Pernicious anemia: new insights from a gastroenterological point of view," *World Journal of Gastroenterology*, vol. 15, no. 41, pp. 5121–5128, 2009.

[8] G. Dhaliwal, P. A. Cornett, and L. M. Tierney Jr., "Hemolytic anemia," *American Family Physician*, vol. 69, no. 11, pp. 2599–2606, 2004.

[9] W. Barcellini and B. Fattizzo, "Clinical applications of hemolytic markers in the differential diagnosis and management of hemolytic anemia," *Disease Markers*, vol. 2015, Article ID 635670, 7 pages, 2015.

[10] V. Hoffbrand and D. Provan, "ABC of clinical haematology: macrocytic anaemias," *BMJ*, vol. 314, no. 7078, p. 430, 1997.

[11] Q. A. Hill, A. Hill, and S. Berentsen, "Defining autoimmune hemolytic anemia: a systematic review of the terminology used for diagnosis and treatment," *Blood Advances*, vol. 3, no. 12, pp. 1897–1906, 2019.

[12] S. P. Stabler, "Vitamin B12 deficiency," *New England Journal of Medicine*, vol. 368, no. 2, pp. 149–160, 2013.

[13] B.-H. Toh, I. R. van Driel, and P. A. Gleeson, "Pernicious anemia," *New England Journal of Medicine*, vol. 337, no. 20, pp. 1441–1448, 1997.

[14] A. Cheema, J. Bramson, R. Bajwa, M. A. Hossain, and A. Asif, "Hemolytic anemia an unusual presentation of Vitamin B12 deficiency," *Journal of Hematology & Thromboembolic Diseases*, vol. 6, no. 1, p. 1, 2018.

[15] E. Andres and K. Serraj, "Optimal management of pernicious anemia," *Journal of Blood Medicine*, vol. 3, pp. 97–103, 2012.

46

Transient Complete Recovery of Chronic Refractory Idiopathic Thrombocytopenic Purpura after Treatment with Monoclonal Antibody Targeting SARS-CoV-2 Spike Protein

Pooja Gogia and Yiqing Xu

Department of Medicine, Division of Hematology/Oncology, Maimonides Medical Center, Brooklyn, NY, USA

Correspondence should be addressed to Yiqing Xu; yxu@maimonidesmed.org

Academic Editor: Håkon Reikvam

Idiopathic thrombocytopenic purpura (ITP), also known as immune thrombocytopenic purpura, is an immune-mediated acquired disease characterized by transient or persistent decrease of the platelet count due to autoimmune-related destruction of platelets. Therapy for ITP relies on competing and inhibiting the autoantibody binding and destruction (intravenous immunoglobulin and anti-D immunoglobulin and spleen tyrosine kinase (Syk) inhibitor fostamatinib), augmenting platelet production (thrombopoietin receptor agonists), immunosuppression to reduce the autoantibody production, as well as splenectomy. Studies on autoantigens on the platelets suggested epitopes to be located predominantly on the GP IIb/IIIa receptor or integrin $\alpha IIb\beta 3$, though the trigger for the development of ITP is unclear. We report a case here of a 37-year-old gentleman who has chronic ITP managed on eltrombopag, who after receiving monoclonal antibody against SARS-CoV-2 (mAb) i.e. casirivimab and imdevimab for his COVID-19 infection, demonstrated complete recovery of his platelet count for a short period of time. We discuss a few potential mechanisms of action and propose further studies to elucidate the therapeutic effect of COVID-19 mAb in ITP.

1. Introduction

Idiopathic thrombocytopenic purpura (ITP) is an acquired autoimmune disorder characterized by transient and persistent decrease in the platelet counts (less than 100×10^9/L) caused by increased platelet destruction and impaired platelet production in the absence of secondary causes [1]. The initiation of the treatment of ITP usually starts when the platelet count is below $20–30 \times 10^9$/L or when the patient starts to have bleeding events. A number of treatment strategies have been developed, including glucocorticoids, immunoglobulin (IVIG), anti-D immunoglobulin, thrombopoietin receptor agonists (TPO-RAs), rituximab, spleen tyrosine kinase (Syk) inhibitor, other immunosuppressive agents, and combination therapy [2]. Splenectomy has demonstrated the greatest chance of achieving sustained remission [3].

Glucocorticoids have been reported to result in long-term remissions in only approximately 20% of cases [4]; while rituximab may be associated with a 40–60% long-term remission rate [5, 6]. The response rate of eltrombopag reaches 79%, but prolonged maintenance is required, and rebound thrombocytopenia would occur when the treatment is discontinued [7, 8]. The ITP-specific antigens have not been clearly elucidated; IVIG or anti-D immune globulin, working by interfering the Fc receptor-mediated macrophage clearance of autoantibody bound platelets, has demonstrated a response rate of 67%, which is usually temporary [9, 10].

In this report, we present a case description of a young man with a diagnosis of chronic relapsing ITP for the last 8 and half years who has been maintained on eltrombopag with improved platelet count, and showed a temporary but complete resolution of thrombocytopenia after receiving treatment with monoclonal antibodies to SARS-CoV-2 and casirivimab i.e. imdevimab, after contracting COVID-19 infection.

2. Case Presentation

A 37-year-old man presented in July 2021 to the emergency room (ER) with chief complaints of cough, fever, and malaise of 3 days duration and was diagnosed with SARS-CoV-2 viral infection. Eight years ago, he was first diagnosed with ITP after he had a minor nose bleed. His platelet count was 27×10^9/L (normal platelet count 150–400 $\times 10^9$/L). He has no family history of blood disorders. His other medical history was hypothyroidism and took levothyroxine 100 micrograms a day. He denied the use of tobacco, alcohol, recreational drugs, or herbal supplements. Initial laboratory workup revealed normal coagulation parameters. ANA screen and lupus anticoagulation syndrome workup and viral infection work up including HIV antigen, hepatitis panel, *H. pylori*, hepatitis C, and Epstein-Barr IgM were all negative.

He was initially treated with pulse dose of steroids with dexamethasone 40 mg daily for 4 days and had an immediate, but short response. He was then treated with prednisone 40 mg daily with response; but his thrombocytopenia recurred with a platelet count of 18×10^9/L when prednisone was tapered down to 20 mg daily. He responded to IVIG and was further treated with anti-D immunoglobulin every 2-3 months for 7 years. During that period, the peak platelet count was 122×10^9/L, and the nadir was 14×10^9/L. He was initiated on eltrombopag 25 mg a day, 9 months prior to the presentation in the ER. The dose was increased to 50 mg daily 3 months later, and the platelet count stabilized to 40–60 $\times 10^9$/L. The dose was further increased to 75 mg three months later. Fifteen days prior to the presentation, his platelet count was 62×10^9/L.

On presentation to the ER, he was found to be positive by the PCR test for SARS-CoV-2 from a nasopharyngeal swab. He did not receive prior vaccination against COVID-19. He was diagnosed with COVID-19 infection of moderate severity. On physical examination, he was febrile with a temperature of 39°C, respiration rate of 18 breaths/min, heart rate 92 beats/min, and oxygen saturation 96–98% on room air. Physical exam was unremarkable except a BMI of 42. He was treated with monoclonal antibody (mAb) against SARS-CoV-2, i.e., casirivimab 600 mg and imdevimab 600 mg.

Laboratory studies on the day of ER visit prior to the mAb treatment showed platelet count of 82×10^9/L and lymphopenia of 1.1×10^9/L. Patient's symptoms subsided over the next 1-2 weeks. On his subsequent outpatient follow-up, 14 days after the mAb infusion, his platelet count was 292×10^9/L, so eltrombopag was held. On the 17th day after mAb infusion, the platelet count was 199×10^9/L. On the 24th day after mAb treatment, his platelet count declined to 45×10^9/L, and eltrombopag was reinitiated at 50 mg daily. On the 74th day after ER visit, his platelet count was 34×10^9/L, and his dose of eltrombopag was increased to 75 mg daily. On the 90th day after mAb treatment, his platelet count was 73×10^9/L.

The trend of his platelet counts in relationship to his treatments is shown in Figure 1.

3. Discussion

ITP has long been considered an autoimmune disease and autoantibody-associated platelet destruction is the mechanism of thrombocytopenia [11]. It may be associated with viral infections and a number of chronic disorders such as systemic lupus erythematosus and chronic lymphocytic leukemia [11]. Studies on uncovering the epitopes on the platelets for autoantibody production has revealed GP IIb/IIIa receptor or integrin αIIbβ3 to be the predominant target. Other potential sources are GP Ib/IX, IV, and Ia/IIa; however, GP IV or Ia/IIa are never the sole targets [12, 13]. Regardless, a reliable gold standard test has not been established, and the diagnosis of ITP remains a diagnosis of exclusion [14].

The therapeutic application and success of IVIG or anti-D immune globulin corroborates the autoimmune mechanism of thrombocytopenia in ITP. IVIG interferes with the uptake of autoantibody-coated platelets by the macrophages; while anti-D immunoglobulin aims to saturate the macrophage Fc receptors with anti-D-coated red blood cells (RBCs) and therefore works to inhibit the destruction and clearance of the platelets [10]. Although a rapid therapeutic response is usually expected, its efficacy is inevitably short acting, averaging about 3-4 weeks [10].

Casirivimab and imdevimab are monoclonal antibodies that bind to different sites on the receptor-binding domain of the spike protein of SARS-CoV-2 and, thereby, block its attachment to the human ACE2 receptor and subsequent entry to the human cells [15]. The combination use has been shown to effectively decrease the progression of COVID-19 infection and to decrease the rate of hospitalization in high-risk patients [16]. It has been approved by US Food and Drug Agency (FDA) for Emergency Use Authorization to patients who have mild COVID-19 infection who do not exhibit hypoxia and who do not need hospitalization and, subsequently, also for postexposure prophylaxis for high-risk patients [16].

The observation of the improvement of platelet count in this ITP patient after contracting COVID-19 infection and receiving casirivimab and imdevimab treatment is both intriguing and fascinating. The patient had a platelet count of 80×10^9/L prior to mAb treatment, and this level of platelet count was the expected response to eltrombopag. However, with a complete recovery of count to 292×10^9/L after the COVID-19 monoclonal antibody treatment, it is compelling to hypothesize that the improvement in the platelet count was the result of the treatment effect from casirivimab and imdevimab, instead of the effect of eltrombopag.

Several mechanisms of action may be proposed. First, mAb might have exerted an effect with a similar mechanism as IVIG or anti-D immunoglobulin, as nonspecific competition with platelets coated with autoantibodies for the Fc receptors for macrophage-mediated destruction. We noted that the dose of immunoglobulin in the monoclonal antibody treatment (1200 mg total) was significantly lower than that in the therapeutic IVIG dose (1000 mg/kg x 2 days), and

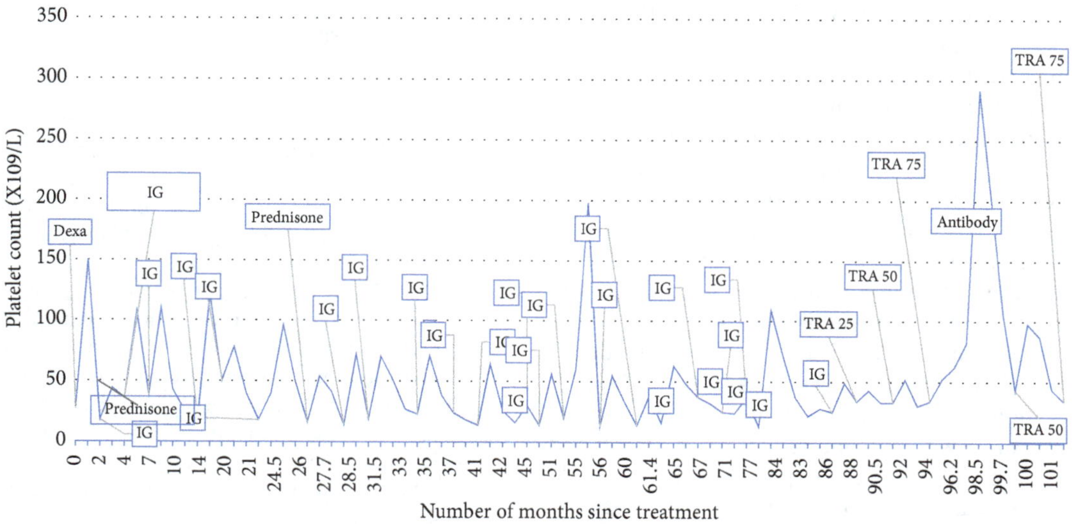

FIGURE 1: Depicting trend in platelet counts with various treatments dexa: dexamethsone (pulse dose of steroids). Prednisone: prednisone 1 mg/kg. IG: anti-D immunoglobulin. TRA (thrombopoietin receptor agonist) 25: eltrombopag 25 mg. TRA 50: eltrombopag 50 mg. TRA 75: eltrombopag 75 mg antibody: monoclonal antibody (mAb) against SARS-COV2.

this low dose may not function effectively as a nonspecific competition mechanism.

A second possibility is specific binding and competition of the platelet-specific autoantigen by the therapeutic antibodies. In that speculation, we hypothesize that there might be shared epitopes between the autoantigens in ITP and the SARS-CoV-2 spike protein. In fact, a molecular mimicry between the spike or other proteins from the virus and the platelet specific antigens has been proposed as a mechanism of increased platelet destruction leading to thrombocytopenia in COVID-19 infection [17]. One would ask why would therapeutic antibody casirivimab and imdevimab, similarly binding to shared platelet antigens, lead to platelet stabilization, while binding from the self-produced antibody to the viral spike protein lead to platelet destruction? One may raise a hypothesis that the unique feature of the Fc fragment of those monoclonal antibodies may fail to elicit strong Fc receptor binding and clearance, different from the polyclonal Fc fragments from self-produced antibodies. In that regard, it is known that depending on the properties in the Fc region of the IgG molecule, interaction of IgG with Fc receptor can be activating or inhibitory; and a large body of preclinical studies have investigated possible alteration of effector function by modulating the amino acid sequence and glycosylation pattern in IgG Fc [18].

Third, viral particles or viral fragments coated with casirivimab or imdevimab could compete with autoantibodies for Fc receptors, thus decreasing platelet destruction.

Presumably, a simple laboratory test can be done to test the above hypothesis. Serum from patients with ITP may be added to the viral spike proteins-coated microtiter plates to test for binding. The caveats for this experiment could be low titer or low affinity of the autoantibodies to the spike protein. If this proof-of-concept experiment shows supportive result, further studies should be performed in ITP patients to test the therapeutic effect in rapid raise in platelet count with casirivimab and imdevimab.

The association of COVID-19 infection and thrombocytopenia has been well studied and is typically mild [19, 20]. Severe thrombocytopenia can be seen in COVID-19-infected patients who have preexisting ITP [21]. Multiple mechanisms of thrombocytopenia associated with COVID-19 infection have been postulated, in addition to the above-discussed molecular mimicry theory. Decreased production by infected bone marrow cells resulting in abnormal hematopoiesis and consumption by damaged lung tissues and pulmonary endothelial cells is one of them [17]. Particularly, as most of the patients show increase in the D-dimer level in the initial phase of COVID-19 infection, a consumptive process may be a more important mechanism, especially in the early stage of the COVID-19 infection, when autoantibodies have not been fully produced.

On the other hand, the vaccination with ChAdOx1 nCoV-19 vaccine may rarely elicit a different type of antibody, which targets platelet factor 4 (PF4) and causes the development of immune thrombotic thrombocytopenia, which results in thrombosis and clinically mimics autoimmune heparin-induced thrombocytopenia and thrombosis (HITT) [22, 23]. Our case scenario does not suggest an autoimmune process with that mechanism.

Eltrombopag is a thrombopoietin receptor agonist that acts on the axis of increasing the production of platelets [24]. The efficacy appears to be dose dependent, and few cases of patients going into remission without the need for unremitting treatment have been reported [7]. In a retrospective analysis of 260 patients, 201 achieved complete remission, and out of which in 62 patients, eltrombopag was discontinued without need of continuous treatment [7]. In this case, the patient responded to the increased dose of eltrombopag well with higher platelet count, and his response was as predicted. Nonetheless, he required resumption of eltrombopag treatment about 3-4 weeks after mAb treatment, which was consistent with the wearing-off of the therapeutic effect from the monoclonal antibody, rather than the remission-induction effect from eltrombopag. In addition, the time course of his decline of platelet to his baseline of 45×10^9/L on day 24 from mAb treatment is consistent with the time course of the effect seen after IVIG treatment.

In conclusion, we report an interesting case of the possible therapeutic effect on ITP from monoclonal antibody developed for COVID-19 treatment, i.e., casirivimab and imdevimab. This report may be the first case report in this aspect. The impressive result prompted us to hypothesize various possible mechanisms, including nonspecific competition of mAbs with platelet-specific autoantibodies for Fc receptor binding and macrophage clearance; specific competitive binding of molecularly similar platelet autoantigen leading to platelet stabilization and competition of viral particles coated with therapeutic mAb with autoantibodies for Fc receptors-mediated clearance. This notion requires further careful preclinical and clinical studies, and a prospective study to examine the therapeutic effects of mAb in thrombocytopenia associated ITP may be considered.

Consent

Written informed consent of the patient was obtained for this study.

References

[1] F. Rodeghiero, R. Stasi, and T. Gernsheimer, "Standardization of terminology, definitions and outcome criteria in immune thrombocytopenic purpura of adults and children: report from an international working group," *Blood*, vol. 113, p. 2386, 2009.

[2] C. Neunert, D. R. Terrell, and D. M. Arnold, "American Society of Hematology 2019 guidelines for immune thrombocytopenia," *Blood*, vol. 3, pp. 3829–3866, 2019.

[3] K. Kojouri, S. K. Vesely, and D. R. Terrell, "Splenectomy for adult patients with idiopathic thrombocytopenic purpura: a systematic review to assess long-term platelet count responses, prediction of response, and surgical complications," *Blood*, vol. 104, p. 2623, 2004.

[4] S. Mithoowani, K. Gregory-Miller, and J. Goy, "High-dose dexamethasone compared with prednisone for previously untreated primary immune thrombocytopenia: a systematic review and meta-analysis," *The Lancet. Haematology*, vol. 3, p. e489, 2016.

[5] S. Chugh, S. Darvish-Kazem, and W. Lim, "Rituximab plus standard of care for treatment of primary immune thrombocytopenia: a systematic review and meta-analysis," *The Lancet. Haematology*, vol. 2, p. e75, 2015.

[6] W. Ghanima, A. Khelif, and A. Waage, "Rituximab as second-line treatment for adult immune thrombocytopenia (the RITP trial): a multicentre, randomised, double-blind, placebo-controlled trial," *The Lancet. Haematology*, vol. 385, p. 1653, 2015.

[7] T. J. González-López, C. Pascual, M. T. Álvarez-Román et al., "Successful discontinuation of eltrombopag after complete remission in patients with primary immune thrombocytopenia," *American Journal of Hematology*, vol. 90, no. 3, pp. E40–E43, 2015.

[8] B. Ghadaki, I. Nazi, J. G. Kelton, and D. M. Arnold, "Sustained remissions of immune thrombocytopenia associated with the use of thrombopoietin receptor agonists," *Transfusion*, vol. 53, no. 11, pp. 2807–2812, 2013.

[9] B. Godeau, M. T. Caulier, L. Decuypere, C. Rose, A. Schaeffer, and P. Bierling, "Intravenous immunoglobulin for adults with autoimmune thrombocytopenic purpura: results of a randomized trial comparing 0.5 and 1 g/kg b.w," *British Journal of Haematology*, vol. 107, no. 4, pp. 716–719, 1999.

[10] A. H. Lazarus and A. R. Crow, "Mechanism of action of IVIG and anti-D in ITP," *Transfusion and Apheresis Science*, vol. 28, no. 3, pp. 249–255, 2003 Jun.

[11] G. Moulis, J. Germain, T. Comont et al., "Newly diagnosed immune thrombocytopenia adults: clinical epidemiology, exposure to treatments, and evolution. Results of the CARMEN multicenter prospective cohort," *American Journal of Hematology*, vol. 92, no. 6, pp. 493–500, 2017.

[12] R. He, D. M. Reid, C. E. Jones, and N. R. Shulman, "Spectrum of Ig classes, specificities, and titers of serum antiglycoproteins in chronic idiopathic thrombocytopenic purpura," *Blood*, vol. 83, no. 4, pp. 1024–1032, 1994.

[13] K. Fujisawa, T. E. O'Toole, P. Tani et al., "Autoantibodies to the presumptive cytoplasmic domain of platelet glycoprotein IIIa in patients with chronic immune thrombocytopenic purpura [published erratum appears in Blood 1991 Dec 1; 78(11):3109]," *Blood*, vol. 77, no. 10, pp. 2207–2213, 1991.

[14] M. Swinkels, M. Rijkers, G. Vidarsson, F. W. G. Leebeek, and A. J. G Jansen, "Emerging concepts in immune thrombocytopenia," *Frontiers in Immunology*, vol. 9, p. 880, 2018.

[15] "An EUA for Casirivimab and Imdevimab for COVID-19," *The Medical letter on drugs and therapeutics*, vol. 62, 2020.

[16] "Fact sheet for health care providers. Emergency Use Authorization (EUA) of casirivimab and imdevimab," 2021, https://bit.ly/36NmbDm.

[17] P. Xu, Q. Zhou, and J. Xu, "Mechanism of thrombocytopenia in COVID-19 patients," *Annals of Hematology*, vol. 99, no. 6, pp. 1205–1208, 2020.

[18] E. A. Fitzpatrick, J. Wang, and S. E. Strome, "Engineering of Fc multimers as a protein therapy for autoimmune disease," *Frontiers in Immunology*, vol. 11, p. 496, 2020.

[19] Y. Liu, W. Sun, Y. Guo et al., "Association between platelet parameters and mortality in coronavirus disease 2019 retrospective cohort study," *Platelets*, vol. 31, no. 4, pp. 490–496, 2020.

[20] S. Bhattacharjee and M. Banerjee, "Immune thrombocytopenia secondary to COVID-19 a systematic review," *Springer Nature Comprehensive Clinical Medicine*, vol. 2, pp. 2048–2058, 2020.

[21] Z. Hu, W. Chen, W. Liang, C. Xu, W. Sun, and Y. Yi, "Severe exacerbation of immune thrombocytopenia and COVID-19: the favorable response to corticosteroid-based therapy-a case report," *Annals of Hematology*, vol. 100, no. 8, pp. 2135–2137, 2020.

[22] N. H. Schultz, I. H. Sørvoll, A. E. Michelsen et al., "Thrombosis and thrombocytopenia after ChAdOx1 nCoV-19 vaccination," *New England Journal of Medicine*, vol. 384, no. 22, pp. 2124–2130, 2021.

[23] D. B. Cines and J. B. Bussel, "SARS-CoV-2 vaccine-induced immune thrombotic thrombocytopenia," *New England Journal of Medicine*, vol. 384, no. 23, pp. 2254–2256, 2021.

[24] J. R. Gonzalez-Porras and J. M. Bastida, "Eltrombopag in immune thrombocytopenia: efficacy review and update on drug safety," *Therapeutic Advances in Drug Safety*, vol. 9, no. 6, pp. 263–285, 2018.

47

Severe Thrombocytopenia Two Weeks Following Immunization with the Janssen Ad26.CoV2.S Vaccine

Bana Antonios, Markie Zimmer, Emma Herrman, and Ramona Berghea

Department of Internal Medicine, William Beaumont Hospital, Royal Oak, MI, USA

Correspondence should be addressed to Bana Antonios; bana.antonios@beaumont.org

Academic Editor: Massimo Breccia

Immune thrombocytopenia (ITP) has been associated with immunizations with various proposed mechanisms, including overactivation of the immune system and production of antibodies against circulating platelets. ITP has also been associated with several viral infections, including HCV, HIV, and most recently, active SARS-CoV-2 infection. Here, we present a case of a 52-year-old male with no past medical history who sought evaluation with his primary care physician for upper and lower extremity ecchymosis of one week duration. Outpatient laboratory studies were notable for severe isolated thrombocytopenia with platelet count of 8×10^9/L. Interestingly, he received the Johnson and Johnson COVID-19 vaccine 16 days prior to his presentation. Clinical work up and laboratory investigations led to the diagnosis of ITP.

1. Introduction

In February 2021, the Janssen COVID-19 immunization by Johnson and Johnson pharmaceutical company was FDA-approved as a single-dose intramuscular immunization for adults over 18 years of age [1]. By April 2021, 7.98 million doses had been administered with high efficacy [2]. However, the vaccine adverse events reporting system reported 13,725 cases of arterial or venous thrombosis along with thrombocytopenia, a new hematological condition initially known as vaccine-induced thrombotic thrombocytopenia (VITT), now known as thrombotic thrombocytopenic syndrome (TTS). A diagnosis is established in the setting of recent immunization (4 to 30 days prior), venous or arterial thrombosis, thrombocytopenia, and positive antibodies directed against platelet factor-4 (PF4) [2, 3].

To our knowledge, isolated ITP without any evidence of arterial or venous thrombosis has been reported with mRNA COVID-19 immunizations, i.e., Pfizer and Moderna. Only one case has been published describing isolated thrombocytopenia following the Johnson and Johnson vaccine.

2. Case Presentation

A 52-year-old male with no past medical history sought evaluation with his primary care physician for upper and lower extremity ecchymosis of one week duration. Outpatient laboratory studies were notable for severe thrombocytopenia with platelet count of 8×10^9/L, and he was ultimately referred to the emergency department for hospital admission. He denied any recent flu-like symptoms, gingival bleeding, epistaxis, headaches, visual changes, abdominal pain, shortness of breath, leg pain, or swelling. He did not take any medication other than occasional nonsteroidal anti-inflammatory drugs for chronic back pain. He also denied any family history of bleeding or autoimmune disorders. Interestingly, the patient mentioned that he recently received the Janssen Ad26.CoV2.S immunization 16 days prior to his hospital admission.

Initial workup in the emergency department revealed a leukocyte count of 6.8 10^9/L (normal range 3.5–10.1 10^9/L), hemoglobin 150 g/L (normal range 130–170 g/L), hematocrit 0.45 (normal range 0.40–0.5), MCV 92 μm^3 (normal range 80–100 μm^3), MCH 31 pg/cell (normal range 28–33 pg/cell), MCHC 31 g/dL (normal range 32–36 g/dL), RDW CV 12%

(normal range 12–15%), and platelet *f* 8 x 10^9/L (normal range 150–400 x 10^9/L). The baseline platelet count was 190 x 10^9/L in years prior. Serum chemistries, including electrolytes, renal function, and hepatic function were all unremarkable. Total bilirubin was 5.13 μmol/L (normal range 5.13–20.5 μmol/L), with direct 1.7 μmol/L (normal range 0.0–6.8 μmol/L). The reticulocyte count was 86 × 10^9/L (normal range 21–100 10^9/L) and immature reticulocyte fraction was 0.07 (normal range 0.01–0.16). The prothrombin time (PT) was 12.0 seconds (normal range 9.2–13.5 seconds), activated partial thromboplastin time (aPTT) was 29.9 seconds (normal range 25–38 seconds), and international normalized ratio (INR) was 1.1. D-dimer was 413 mg FEU/L (normal range 0–499 mg FEU/L) and fibrinogen 4736 μmol/L (normal range 3420–6480 μmol/L). Vitamin B12 and folate levels were within normal limits and iron studies were not available. HIV, HCV, ANA, TSH, and *H. pylori* were all unremarkable. Peripheral smear revealed normal morphology of neutrophils and monocytes, with small and mature lymphocytes; normocytic normochromic red blood cells without significant anisopoikilocytosis; severe thrombocytopenia with normal platelet morphology. ELISA results of IgG antibodies against platelet factor-4 (PF4) were negative with 0.131 OD (optical density normal range <0.400 OD). Abdominal ultrasound revealed patent hepatic vasculature and unremarkable liver and spleen, with spleen measuring 11.4 cm in length.

The differential diagnosis for severe thrombocytopenia is broad, particularly in a patient with no known prior medical history. Serum chemistries were unremarkable, including a disseminated intravascular coagulation (DIC) screen, making DIC unlikely, further supported by lack of hemolysis on peripheral smear. He was not infectious, ruling out sepsis. Viral causes, such as SARS-CoV-2, HIV, and HCV were negative. Nutritional investigations, including vitamin B12 and folate, were within normal limits. He had no history of alcohol use disorder, making toxic marrow suppression unlikely. Abdominal imaging revealed a normal-sized spleen and patent hepatic vasculature, ruling out hepatic vasculopathy or hypersplenism. Additionally, his coagulation studies were within normal limits. ANA was negative, and with his age and no personal or family history of autoimmune conditions or other symptoms, systemic lupus erythematosus was effectively ruled out.

Thus, ITP, thrombotic thrombocytopenic purpura (TTP), heparin-induced thrombocytopenia (HIT), and drug side effects were the highest on the remaining differential diagnosis. PLASMIC score, which predicts ADAMTS13 deficiency in TTP, was 5 at admission, indicating an intermediate risk for TTP. However, ADAMTS13 level was not checked, nor was plasmapheresis initiated. Though he had no exposure to heparin, the pretest scoring system for HIT, so-called 4 T score was 3, corresponding to a low HIT probability and antibodies directed against PF4 were negative. There was concern for TTS in the setting of recent vaccination against COVID-19 with the Janssen Ad26.CoV2.S vaccine. There was negative HPF4 serology and no evidence of thrombosis, effectively ruling out VITT and finalizing a diagnosis of ITP.

Hematology/oncology consultation was obtained from the emergency department. He was transfused with one unit of apheresed platelets with a minimum of 2.9 × 10^{11} platelets and started on dexamethasone 40 mg daily for four days in the setting of high suspicion for ITP. Heparin products were avoided during the investigations.

The patient was discharged from the hospital to complete his last planned dose of dexamethasone 40 mg PO at home that evening. His platelet count across hospitalization is shown in Figure 1.

Based on available outpatient medical records across 48 days since hospital discharge, the patient had close follow-up with his primary care physician and hematology/oncology. Unfortunately, he had relapse of thrombocytopenia and was again started on prednisone with slow taper course, but at the time of this writing, was deemed steroid dependent and Hematology/oncology was planning to initiate a thrombopoietin receptor (TPO) agonist.

3. Discussion

Immune thrombocytopenia (ITP) is a rare disease characterized by immune-mediated destruction of platelets leading to thrombocytopenia and increased bleeding risk. Immunizations are a recognized cause of secondary ITP. The proposed mechanism of this entity is molecular mimicry, where the epitope of the antigen shares properties with a self-peptide. Autoantibodies form and target platelet surface glycoproteins, most commonly GPIIb-IIIa and/or GPIb-IX, causing destruction of platelets and subsequent isolated thrombocytopenia [1, 3, 4].

ITP is usually a diagnosis of exclusion. Initial work up usually aims at excluding potential causes such as viral or bacterial infections, most commonly HIV, hepatitis C, and *Helicobacter pylori*. Low B12 and folate levels could also cause thrombocytopenia but is often associated with anemia or leukopenia. Evaluation for underlying autoimmune disease is also important to rule out, such as systemic lupus erythematosus and antiphospholipid syndrome, where thrombocytopenia is a common finding. Physical exam and abdominal imaging assessing for underlying organomegaly is important to exclude liver disease or hypersplenism.

Multiple case reports have now described ITP in patients diagnosed with SARS-CoV-2 infection as well as following administration of the mRNA immunizations—Moderna and Pfizer-BioNTech BNT16B2b2 [3, 5]. A case series at Cleveland Clinic hospitals noted an incident of 0.34% of COVID-19-induced thrombocytopenia. Reported results concluded response to corticosteroids, as well as the use of thrombopoietin receptor agonists (TPRAs) as second-line treatment [6]. A case series completed only months after Moderna and Pfizer use was widespread amongst the public population described 20 cases of thrombocytopenia within 2 weeks of receiving Moderna or Pfizer vaccines [3].

To our knowledge, ITP has not been reported following the Janssen Ad26.CoV2.S immunization. However, there have been reported cases of thrombosis with thrombocytopenia syndrome following its administration. The term vaccine-induced thrombotic thrombocytopenia (VITT) was

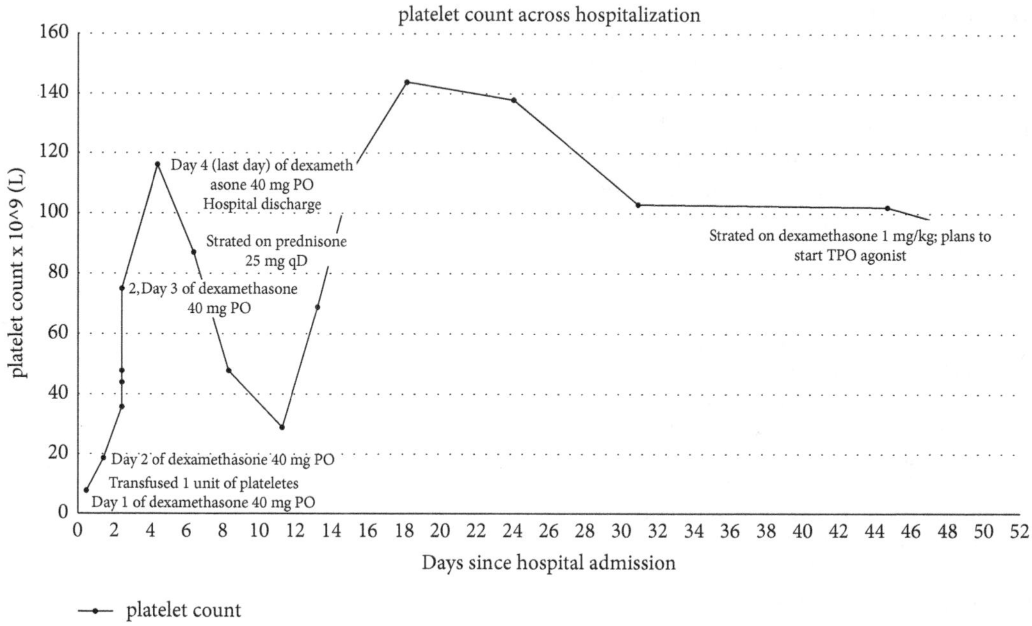

Figure 1: Platelet count across hospitalization.

proposed to describe this novel entity to avoid confusion with HIT [7] but has since been renamed thrombosis with TTS. TTS is rare and characterized by arterial or venous thrombosis in the presence of new-onset thrombocytopenia. In one case series, 12 of the 15 thrombotic events that occurred were a cerebral venous sinus thrombosis (CVST). Administration of the Janssen Ad26.CoV2.S vaccine was initially suspended after 6 patients developed CVST [7]. Interestingly, CVST has been observed following the AstraZeneca immunization approved in Europe as well, but has not been observed following administration of the mRNA immunizations. AstraZeneca and Janssen Ad26.CoV2.S have similar mechanisms, with AstraZeneca being a chimpanzee adenoviral vector, and Janssen Ad26.CoV2.S being a human adenoviral vector. In case reports of those who developed TTS following AstraZeneca administration, it appeared via a similar mechanism as heparin-induced thrombocytopenia, with elevated antibodies directed against PF4 despite lack of recent administration of heparin [8]. Antibodies directed against PF4 were included in our work up despite the fact that our patient did not have a recent heparin use, given the recently raised awareness of thrombotic thrombocytopenic syndrome associated with certain types of the SARS-CoV-2 vaccines.

General guidelines of ITP treatment vary based upon presentation and severity of thrombocytopenia. In cases presenting with critical bleeding, it is important to rapidly raise the platelets count when it is below $10 \times 10\hat{9}/L$ with platelet transfusions. However, for ITP cases presenting with minor bleeding and patients who remain asymptomatic, treatment is reserved for platelet count of below $50 \times 10\hat{9}/L$ and below $20 \times 10\hat{}/L$, respectively. Glucocorticoids are the preferable initial therapy, with either a pulse dose of dexamethasone, usually 40 mg daily for four days or methylprednisolone 1 g daily for three days, or 1 mg/kg of prednisone followed by a slow taper. Intravenous immunoglobulin (IVIG) is another option that can increase platelet count rapidly and is generally reserved for cases refractory to glucocorticoids [3, 4]. Bone marrow aspiration is usually reserved for patients over 60 years old to rule out myelodysplastic syndrome or other potential malignancies such as leukemias and aplastic anemia. However, in ITP patients, it is not a requirement for diagnosing but is considered in steroid-resistant cases [8–10].

Another small case series evaluated ITP cases observed within two weeks after administration of mRNA COVID-19 vaccine. Fifteen cases followed the Pfizer-BioNTech version and thirteen cases followed the Moderna version. Most of the patients were treated with glucocorticoids and IVIG. However, as the majority of them required more than one line of treatment, we note that vaccine-induced ITP appears to be resistant to steroids therapy. Unfortunately, the data about these cases are brief and limited, and two patients suffered lethal consequences [11].

To the best of our knowledge, this is an early case of ITP following the administration of the Janssen Ad26.CoV2.S immunization at the time of presentation. There has only been one reported case of isolated thrombocytopenia without thrombosis since. Certainly, there is no definitive evidence to argue that this was not an initial episode of primary ITP coincidentally surrounding the immunization administration. Strikingly, the timeline of events, as well as the thorough workup to exclude other secondary causes, leads us to believe that the Janssen Ad26.CoV2.S immunization caused secondary ITP in this patient.

Consent

Informed consent was obtained from the patient.

Authors' Contributions

All the authors were involved with manuscript presentation, draft revision, and have revised and approved the manuscript for submission. M.Z and E.H contributed equally as co-authors in reviewing literature on similar cases. B.R has mentored and supervised the manuscript in its entirety.

References

[1] S. E. Oliver, J. W. Gargano, H. Scobie et al., "The advisory committee on immunization practices' interim recommendation for use of janssen COVID-19 vaccine—United States, february 2021," *MMWR Morbidity and Mortality Weekly Report*, vol. 70, no. 9, pp. 329–332, 2021.

[2] D. K. Shay, J. Gee, J. R. Su et al., "Safety monitoring of the janssen (Johnson & Johnson) COVID-19 vaccine—United States, march-april," vol. 70, pp. 680–684, 2021.

[3] E. J. Lee, D. B. Cines, T. Gernsheimer et al., "Thrombocytopenia following pfizer and Moderna SARS-CoV-2 vaccination," *American Journal of Hematology*, vol. 96, no. 5, pp. 534–537, 202119.

[4] C. Perricone, F. Ceccarelli, G. Nesher et al., "Immune thrombocytopenic purpura (ITP) associated with vaccinations: a review of reported cases," *Immunologic Research*, vol. 60, pp. 226–235, 2014.

[5] G. Bomhof, P. G. N. J. Mutsaers, F. W. G. Leebeek et al., "COVID-19-associated immune thrombocytopenia," *British Journal of Haematology*, vol. 190, no. 2, pp. 61–64, 2020.

[6] T. Kewan, T. N. Gunaratne, K. Mushtaq, D. Alayan, H. Daw, and A. Haddad, "Outcomes and management of immune thrombocytopenia secondary to covid- 19: cleveland clinic experience," *Transfusion*, vol. 61, 2021.

[7] A. Greinacher, T. Thiele, T. E. Warkentin, K. Weisser, P. A. Kyrle, and S. Eichinger, "Thrombotic thrombocytopenia after ChAdOx1 nCov-19 vaccination," *New England Journal of Medicine*, vol. 384, no. 22, pp. 2092–2101, 2021.

[8] J. R. MacNeil, J. R. Su, K. R. Broder et al., "Updated recommendations from the advisory committee on immunization practices for use of the janssen (Johnson & Johnson) COVID-19 vaccine after reports of thrombosis with thrombocytopenia syndrome among vaccine recipients—United States, April 2021," *MMWR. Morbidity and Mortality Weekly Report*, vol. 70, no. 17, pp. 651–656, 2021.

[9] D. Kuter, "Immune Thrombocytopenia," *Merck Manuals*, https://www.merckmanuals.com/professional/hematology-and-oncology/thrombocytopenia-and-platelet-dysfunction/immune-thrombocytopenia-itp, 2020.

[10] A. Purohit, M. Aggarwal, P. K. Singh et al., "Re-evaluation of need for bone marrow examination in patients with isolated thrombocytopenia contributors," *Indian Journal of Hematology and Blood Transfusion*, vol. 32, no. 2, pp. 193–196, 2016.

[11] K. J. Welsh, J. Baumblatt, W. Chege, R. Goud, and N. Nair, "Thrombocytopenia including immune thrombocytopenia after receipt of mRNA COVID-19 vaccines reported to the Vaccine Adverse Event Reporting System (VAERS)," *Vaccine*, vol. 39, no. 25, pp. 3329–3332, 2021.

Permissions

All chapters in this book were first published by Hindawi Publishing Corporation; hereby published with permission under the Creative Commons Attribution License or equivalent. Every chapter published in this book has been scrutinized by our experts. Their significance has been extensively debated. The topics covered herein carry significant findings which will fuel the growth of the discipline. They may even be implemented as practical applications or may be referred to as a beginning point for another development.

The contributors of this book come from diverse backgrounds, making this book a truly international effort. This book will bring forth new frontiers with its revolutionizing research information and detailed analysis of the nascent developments around the world.

We would like to thank all the contributing authors for lending their expertise to make the book truly unique. They have played a crucial role in the development of this book. Without their invaluable contributions this book wouldn't have been possible. They have made vital efforts to compile up to date information on the varied aspects of this subject to make this book a valuable addition to the collection of many professionals and students.

This book was conceptualized with the vision of imparting up-to-date information and advanced data in this field. To ensure the same, a matchless editorial board was set up. Every individual on the board went through rigorous rounds of assessment to prove their worth. After which they invested a large part of their time researching and compiling the most relevant data for our readers.

The editorial board has been involved in producing this book since its inception. They have spent rigorous hours researching and exploring the diverse topics which have resulted in the successful publishing of this book. They have passed on their knowledge of decades through this book. To expedite this challenging task, the publisher supported the team at every step. A small team of assistant editors was also appointed to further simplify the editing procedure and attain best results for the readers.

Apart from the editorial board, the designing team has also invested a significant amount of their time in understanding the subject and creating the most relevant covers. They scrutinized every image to scout for the most suitable representation of the subject and create an appropriate cover for the book.

The publishing team has been an ardent support to the editorial, designing and production team. Their endless efforts to recruit the best for this project, has resulted in the accomplishment of this book. They are a veteran in the field of academics and their pool of knowledge is as vast as their experience in printing. Their expertise and guidance has proved useful at every step. Their uncompromising quality standards have made this book an exceptional effort. Their encouragement from time to time has been an inspiration for everyone.

The publisher and the editorial board hope that this book will prove to be a valuable piece of knowledge for researchers, students, practitioners and scholars across the globe.

List of Contributors

Sonal Prasad
Ross University School of Medicine, Bridgetown, Barbados

Roopam Jariwal, Moujidin Adebayo, Sara Jaka, Greti Petersen and Everardo Cobos
Department of Internal Medicine, UCLA at Kern Medical Center, Bakersfield, CA 93306, USA

Natasha Mupeta Kaweme, Sahar Mounir Nagib Butress and Hamakwa Muluti Mantina
University Teaching Hospital, Private Bag RW1X Ridgeway, Nationalist Road, Lusaka 10101, Zambia

Ahmed Arfa, Nivin Omar, Kulsum Bano and Natasha M. Savage
Department of Pathology, Medical College of Georgia at Augusta University, Augusta, Georgia

Le Zhong, Juskaran Chadha and Ali Ameri
Department of Medicine, Zucker School of Medicine at Hofstra/Northwell at Lenox Hill Hospital, 100 E 77th St., New York, NY 10075, USA

Yoshinori Hashimoto, Rina Hosoda, Hiromi Omura and Takayuki Tanaka
Department of Hematology, Tottori Prefectural Central Hospital, Tottori, Japan

Fnu Jaydev, Vinod Kumar, Jaikumar Khatri and Shobha Shahani
Division of Internal Medicine and Geriatrics, Indiana University School of Medicine, Indianapolis, IN, USA

Sead Beganovic
Indiana University Health Central Indiana Cancer Center, Indianapolis, IN, USA

Korin Karabulut and Ana Andronikashvili
Steward Carney Hospital, 2100 Dorchester Avenue, Boston, MA 02124, USA

Ahmet Hakki Kapici
Robert Wood Johnson University Hospital, 1 Robert Wood Johnson Place, New Brunswick, NJ 08901, USA

G. A. C. Gamakaranage, C. Kulathilake, K. H. B. P. Fernandopulle, C. S. Moonesinghe, D. Gunawardena and R. S. Gamage
Department of Pathology, Faculty of Medical Sciences, University of Sri Jayewardenepura, Nugegoda, Sri Lanka

P. G. N. Nadeeshani
Professorial Medical Unit, Colombo South Teaching Hospital, Dehiwala-Mount Lavinia, Sri Lanka

N. Perera and J. Indrakumar
Department of Medicine, Faculty of Medical Sciences, University of Sri Jayewardenepura, Nugegoda, Sri Lanka

Scott Mayer, Nikhilesh Srinivasan, Ryan Spilman and Dmitriy Scherbak
HCA HealthONE, Lone Tree, CO, USA

Jenny Nguyen
Rocky Vista University School of Osteopathic Medicine, Lone Tree, CO, USA

Eigo Ikushima, Manabu Hisahara, Takuya Nishijima, Hikaru Uchiyama, Tatsushi Onzuka, Yoshie Ochiai and Shigehiko Tokunaga
Department of Cardiovascular Surgery, Japan Community Healthcare Organization (JCHO) Kyushu Hospital, 1-8-1, Kishinoura, Yahatanishi-ku, Kitakyushu, Fukuoka 806-8501, Japan

Tsuyoshi Muta
Department of Hematology/Oncology, Japan Community Healthcare Organization (JCHO) Kyushu Hospital, 1-8-1, Kishinoura, Yahatanishi-ku, Kitakyushu, Fukuoka 806-8501, Japan

Binoy Yohannan and Mark Feldman
Department of Internal Medicine, Texas Health Presbyterian Hospital, Dallas, Texas 75231, USA

Dai Chu N. Luu
Department of Internal Medicine, Division of Hematology and Oncology, Texas Health Presbyterian Hospital, Dallas, Texas 75231, USA

Ayrton Bangolo, Mahabuba Akhter, Amer Jarri, Manpreet Kaur, Parul Jandir, Mahmood Ibrahim and Adam Atoot
Hackensack, Meridian Health Palisades Medical Center, Department of Internal Medicine, North Bergen, NJ, USA

Ali Atoot
Hackensack University Medical Center, Department of Anesthesia, Hackensack, NJ, USA

Lochana Manandhar
Hackensack Meridian Health Palisades Medical Center, Department of Nephrology, North Bergen, NJ, USA

Shigeru Koba, Tomoya Yamaguchi, Kenji Miki and Hiroshi Makihara
Department of Internal Medicine, Uji-Tokushukai Medical Center, Uji 611-0041, Japan

Shinsaku Imashuku
Department of Laboratory Medicine, Uji-Tokushukai Medical Center, Uji 611-0041, Japan

Gurchetan Randhawa
Maimonides Medical Center, Department of Medicine, Brooklyn, NY, USA

Chia-Yu Chiu and Thanunthorn Suban Na Ayutthaya
Lincoln Medical Center, Department of Medicine, The Bronx, NY, USA

Kern Y. Chai, Cara J. Quijano and Shingirai Chiruka
Department of Haematology, Dunedin Hospital, 201 Great King Street, Dunedin 9016, New Zealand

Azhar Kareem Razzaq
College of Medicine-University of Basrah, Department of Haematology, Baghdad, Iraq

Ameer Al-Jasim
College of Medicine-University of Baghdad, Baghdad, Iraq

Imran Gani, George Hinnant and Rajan Kapoor
Department of Nephrology, Hypertension and Transplant Medicine, Augusta University Health, Augusta, Georgia

Natasha Savage
Department of Pathology, Augusta University Health, Augusta, Georgia

Alexis Lordi
St. Joseph's University Medical Center, 703 Main St., Paterson, NJ 07503, USA
St. George's University School of Medicine, True Blue, Grenada

Nida Ansari
St. George's University School of Medicine, True Blue, Grenada
Rowan University School of Osteopathic Medicine, Stratford, New Jersey, NJ 08084, USA

Michael Maroules and Anusha Manjegowda
St. Joseph's University Medical Center, 703 Main St., Paterson, NJ 07503, USA
Department of Hematology and Oncology, St. Joseph's University Medical Center, 703 Main St., Paterson, NJ 07503, USA

Carlo Guerrero
Department of Medicine, Houston Methodist Hospital, Houston, TX, USA

Tania Jain
Adult Bone Marrow Transplantation Service, Memorial Sloan Kettering Cancer Center, New York, NY, USA

Katalin Kelemen
Department of Laboratory Medicine and Pathology, Mayo Clinic, Phoenix, AZ, USA

Ethan Burns, Kartik Anand, Gonzalo Acosta, Malcolm Irani and Lawrence Rice
Houston Methodist Hospital, Department of Medicine, 6550 Fannin St, Houston, TX 77030, USA

Betty Chung
Houston Methodist Hospital, Department of Pathology and Genomic Medicine, 6550 Fannin St, Houston, TX 77030, USA

Abhishek Maiti
The University of Texas MD Anderson Cancer Center, Division of Cancer Medicine, 1515 Holcombe Blvd, Houston, Texas 77030, USA

Ibrahim Ibrahim
University of Texas Southwestern, Department of Internal Medicine, Division of Hematology/Oncology, 5323 Harry Hines Blvd, Dallas, TX 75390, USA

Essohana Padaro and Kossi Agbétiafa
Hematology Department, Campus Teaching Hospital, University of Lome, Lome, Togo

Baguilane Douaguibe
Gynecology Department, Campus Teaching Hospital, University of Lome, Lome, Togo

Irénée Kueviakoe and Ahoefa Vovor
Hematology Department, Tokoin Teaching Hospital, University of Lome, Lome, Togo

Ikuo Inoue, Yuichi Ikegami, Daigo Saito and Akira Shimada
Department of Endocrinology and Diabetes, Faculty of Medicine, Saitama Medical University, 38 Morohongo, Moroyama, Iruma, Saitama 350-0495, Japan

Yasuhiro Takenaka
Department of Endocrinology and Diabetes, Faculty of Medicine, Saitama Medical University, 38 Morohongo, Moroyama, Iruma, Saitama 350-0495, Japan
Department of Physiology, Graduate School of Medicine, Nippon Medical School, 1-25-16 Nezu, Bunkyo, Tokyo 113-0031, Japan

Yoshitora Kin
Department of Internal Medicine, Fukaya Red Cross Hospital, 5-8-1 Kamishibatyohnishi, Fukaya, Saitama 366-0052, Japan

Satoshi Yamazaki
Kumagaya-geka Hospital, 3811-1 Sayata, Kumagaya, Saitama 360-0023, Japan

Kenji M. Cunnion
Department of Pediatrics, Eastern Virginia Medical School, 700 West Olney Road, Norfolk, VA 23507, USA
Children's Specialty Group, 811 Redgate Avenue, Norfolk, VA 23507, USA
Children's Hospital of the King's Daughters, 601 Children's Lane, Norfolk, VA 23507, USA
Department of Microbiology and Molecular Cell Biology, Eastern Virginia Medical School, 700 West Olney Road, Norfolk, VA 23507-1696, USA

Lisa M. Feagin
Department of Pharmacy, Children's Hospital of the King's Daughters, 601 Children's Lane, Norfolk, VA 23507, USA

Michael F. Chicella and Jessica Price
Department of Pediatrics, Eastern Virginia Medical School, 700 West Olney Road, Norfolk, VA 23507, USA
Department of Pharmacy, Children's Hospital of the King's Daughters, 601 Children's Lane, Norfolk, VA 23507, USA

Cortney L. Kaszowski and Pamela S. Hair
Department of Pediatrics, Eastern Virginia Medical School, 700 West Olney Road, Norfolk, VA 23507, USA

William C. Owen
Department of Pediatrics, Eastern Virginia Medical School, 700 West Olney Road, Norfolk, VA 23507, USA
Children's Specialty Group, 811 Redgate Avenue, Norfolk, VA 23507, USA
Children's Hospital of the King's Daughters, 601 Children's Lane, Norfolk, VA 23507, USA

H. G. C. S. Karunathilaka, D. P. Chandrasiri, V. Ratnamalala and A. H. N. Fernando
National Hospital of Sri Lanka, Colombo, Sri Lanka

P. Ranasinghe
Department of Pharmacology, Faculty of Medicine, University of Colombo, Colombo, Sri Lanka

Sara Alhaj and James Tran
Texas Tech University Health Sciences Center School of Medicine, Amarillo, TX, USA

Muhammad Nazim and Hassan Ahmed
Department of Surgery, Texas Tech University Health Sciences Center School of Medicine, Amarillo, TX, USA

Praveen Tumula
Texas Oncology, Amarillo, TX, USA

Muhammad Husnain
Division of Hematology/Oncology, Department of Medicine, Miller School of Medicine, University of Miami, Miami, FL, USA

Maikel Valdes
Sylvester Comprehensive Cancer Center, University of Miami, Miami, FL, USA

Trent Wang, James Hoffman and Lazaros Lekakis
Division of Hematology/Oncology, Department of Medicine, Miller School of Medicine, University of Miami, Miami, FL, USA
Sylvester Comprehensive Cancer Center, University of Miami, Miami, FL, USA

Jorge D. Guerra
Department of Internal Medicine, Baylor Scott & White Medical Center, Texas A&M University College of Medicine, Temple, TX, USA

Jasmine Gowarty, Jordan Buess, James Mason and Kathleen Halka
Department of Hematology and Medical Oncology, Baylor Scott & White Medical Center, Texas A&M University College of Medicine, Temple, TX, USA

William Forehand III, Germame Ajebo, Anand Jillella and Paul Dainer
Division of Hematology-Oncology, Medical College of Georgia, Augusta University, Georgia Cancer Center, Augusta, Georgia

Michael Toscano
Department of Pathology and Laboratory Medicine, Augusta University, Augusta, Georgia

Synne Dragesund Rørvik and Øystein Bruserud
Department of Medicine, Haukeland University Hospital, Bergen, Norway

Kristoffer Stange Larsen
Department of Medicine, Haraldsplass Deaconess Hospital, Bergen, Norway

Lars Helgeland
Department of Pathology, Haukeland University Hospital, Bergen, Norway
Department of Clinical Medicine (K1), University of Bergen, Bergen, Norway

Håvard Dale
Department of Clinical Medicine (K1), University of Bergen, Bergen, Norway
Department of Orthopaedic Surgery, Haukeland University Hospital, Bergen, Norway

Birgitta Ivarsen
Department of Plastic Surgery, Haukeland University Hospital, Bergen, Norway

Tor Henrik Anderson Tvedt
Department of Medicine, Haukeland University Hospital, Bergen, Norway
Department of Haematology, Oslo University Hospital, Rikshospitalet, Oslo 0424, Norway

Ahmad El Alayli, Logeswari Neelakandan and Hicham Krayem
Detroit Medical Center Sinai Grace Hospital, Detroit, MI, USA

Tamer Othman, Ayman Abdelkarim and Karen Huynh
Department of Internal Medicine, Harbor-UCLA Medical Center, Torrance, CA, USA

An Uche and Jennifer Lee
Division of Hematology and Medical Oncology, Harbor-UCLA Medical Center, Torrance, CA, USA

Sulagna Das, Charles Abreu, John Shrader and Satish Sarvepalli
Department of Medicine, Kettering Health, Dayton, OH, USA

Micah Harris
Boonshoft School of Medicine, Wright State University, Dayton, OH, USA

Pradeepthi Badugu and Modupe Idowu
Division of Hematology, Department of Internal Medicine, McGovern Medical School, The University of Texas Health Science Center at Houston, 6411 Fannin Street, Houston 77030, USA

Amanda M. Woodford, Rabhea Chaudhry and Gabriella A. Conte
Department of Medicine, Jersey Shore University Medical Center, Hackensack Meridian Health, Neptune Township, NJ, USA

Varsha Gupta and Madhurima Anne
Department of Hematology and Oncology, Jersey Shore University Medical Center, Hackensack Meridian Health, Neptune Township, NJ, USA

I. Ramasamy
Worcester Royal Hospital, Charles Hastings Way, Worcester WR41DD, UK

Jamie Geringer, Joshua Fenderson and Michael Osswald
San Antonio Uniformed Services Health Education Consortium, 3551 Roger Brooke Drive JBSA, Fort Sam Houston, San Antonio, TX 78234, USA

H. Auge, R. Morizot, C. Moulin, P. Feugier, A. Perrot and L. Filliatre-Clement
Hematology Department, University Hospital of Nancy, 5 Rue du Morvan, 54500 Vandoeuvre les Nancy, France

C. Yguel and H. Busby-Venner
Histopathology Department, University Hospital of Nancy, 5 Rue du Morvan, 54500 Vandoeuvre les Nancy, France

E. Schmitt
Neuroradiology Department, University Hospital of Nancy, 29 Avenue du Mar´echal de Lattre de Tassigny, 54035 Nancy, France

B. Frotscher
Hemostasis Department, University Hospital of Nancy, 5 Rue du Morvan, 54500 Vandoeuvre les Nancy, France

Mohamed Aon
Department of Medicine, Jahra Hospital, Ministry of Health (HOM), Jahra city, Kuwait

Department of Medicine, Faculty of Medicine, Cairo University, Giza, Egypt

Omar Al-Shammari
Department of Medicine, Jahra Hospital, Ministry of Health (HOM), Jahra city, Kuwait

Mohamed Ahmed and Chibuzo Agbakwuru-Onyike
Department of Internal Medicine, Hackensack Meridian Health Palisades Medical Center, North Bergen, NJ, USA

Ashraf Mahmoud
Department of Family Medicine, Hackensack Meridian Health Palisades Medical Center, North Bergen, NJ, USA

Maria Karina Larni Y. Palad
University of the East Ramon Magsaysay, Quezon, Philippines

Michael Sciarra
Department of Gastroenterology, Hackensack Meridian Health Palisades Medical Center, North Bergen, NJ, USA

Nonso Osakwe
Department of Infectious Disease, New York Presbyterian Hospital, Bronxville, NY, USA

Douglas Hart
Department of Cardiology, New York Presbyterian Hospital, Bronxville, NY, USA

Boniface Amanee Elias Lumori and Daniel Muyanja
Department of Internal Medicine, Mbarara University of Science and Technology (MUST), Mbarara, Uganda

Ralph Kamel, Rubal Sharma, Divya Asti, Arshpal Gill and Yevgeniy Skaradinskiy
Staten Island University Hospital, Northwell Health, 475 Seaview Avenue, Staten Island, New York 10305, NY, USA

Kai J. Rogers and Sharathkumar Bhagavathi
Department of Pathology, University of Iowa Hospitals and Clinics, Iowa, IA, USA

Gabriella A. Raffa
Internal Medicine Residency Program, Jackson Memorial Hospital, Miami, FL, USA

Diana M. Byrnes
Hematology/Oncology Fellowship Program, Jackson Memorial Hospital, Miami, FL, USA

John J. Byrnes
Department of Medicine, Division of Hematology, University of Miami, Miami, FL, USA

G. F. Cittolin-Santos, S. Khalil, J. K. Bakos and K. Baker
Medical University of South Carolina, Department of Internal Medicine, Charleston, SC, USA

Pooja Gogia and Yiqing Xu
Department of Medicine, Division of Hematology/Oncology, Maimonides Medical Center, Brooklyn, NY, USA

Bana Antonios, Markie Zimmer, Emma Herrman and Ramona Berghea
Department of Internal Medicine, William Beaumont Hospital, Royal Oak, MI, USA

Index